Transsexual and Other Disorders of Gender Identity

A practical guide to management

Edited by

James Barrett

Consultant Psychiatrist,
Charing Cross Gender Identity Clinic,
London

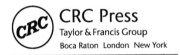

CRC Press
Taylor & Francis Group
Boca Raton   London   New York

CRC Press is an imprint of the
Taylor & Francis Group, an **informa** business

Radcliffe Publishing Ltd
18 Marcham Road
Abingdon
Oxon OX14 1AA
United Kingdom

www.radcliffe-oxford.com
Electronic catalogue and worldwide online ordering facility.

New research and clinical experience can result in changes in treatment and drug therapy. Readers of this book should therefore check the most recent product information on any drug they may prescribe to ensure they are complying with the manufacturer's recommendations concerning dosage, the method and duration of administration, and contraindications. Neither the publisher nor the authors accept liability for any injury or damage arising from this publication.

British Library Cataloguing in Publication Data

A catalogue record for this book is available from the British Library.

ISBN-10: 1 85775 719 X
ISBN-13: 978 1 85775 719 4

Typeset by Aarontype Ltd, Easton, Bristol

Contents

Preface   viii
About the editor   x
List of contributors   xi

1   Disorders of gender identity   1
    James Barrett
2   Second opinions   3
    James Barrett

Part 1   The referral process and screening   7
3   Referrals   9
    James Barrett

4   Diagnosis   11
    James Barrett
        Taking a history   11
        Examination   15

5   Categorisation and differential diagnosis   17
    James Barrett
        Overview   17
        Female transsexuals   18
        Male primary transsexuals   21
        Heterosexual male secondary transsexuals   22
        Homosexual male secondary transsexuals   26

6   Dealing with the differentials   31
    James Barrett
        Transvestites   31
        Autogynaephilia   35
        Dysmorphophobia   37
        'Third sex'   42
        Psychosis   43
        Affective disorders   49
        Chromosomal and hormonal abnormalities   51
        Dementia   52

7   Challenging patient types and circumstances   55
    James Barrett
        Patients in forensic settings   55
        Homosexuals   56

Prostitute patients   59
Sexual deviance   60
Gender reassignment surgery with no role change   62
Bilateral mastectomy without role change   64
Personality disorder   65

Part 2   The real life experience   69
8   The real life experience: introduction   71
    James Barrett

9   Common issues   75
    James Barrett
    Occupational matters   75
    Children's reactions   78
    Family reactions   79
    Parents' reactions   83
    Intimate relationship issues and outcomes   84
    Orchidectomy in a female role   90
    Psychotherapy for gender disorders (*Mark Morris*)   91

10 Challenging patients and circumstances   101
    James Barrett
    Coincidental non-psychotic mental illnesses   101
    Coincidental psychosis   102
    Learning disability (*Daniel Wilson*)   104
    Asperger's syndrome   108
    Physically disabled patients   108
    Forensic patients and the real life experience   113
    Patients in the police or armed services   117
    Hormone treatment without role change   119
    Role change without hormone treatment   123
    Reversion to former gender role during real life experience but   124
        before gender reassignment surgery
    Patients who never quite change gender role   128
    Patients who hesitate at the brink of gender reassignment surgery   131
    Patients who choose not to have gender reassignment surgery   134

Part 3   Non-surgical treatments   137
11 The role of the speech and language therapist   139
    Christella Antoni
    Referral   140
    Initial assessment   141
    Speech and language therapy treatment   143
    Surgical voice modification: the role of the speech and   151
        language therapist
    Length of intervention   152
    Discharge criteria   153
    Summary and conclusions   153

12   The practical management of hormonal treatment in adults with   157
     gender dysphoria
     Leighton J Seal
         Introduction   157
         Disorders that may present with gender confusion   157
         Initiation of hormone therapy   166
         Hormonal regimens in common use   167
         Treatment protocols   167
         Effects of hormone replacement   172
         Safety monitoring   177
         Management of therapy complications   178
         Treatment of capital hair loss   180
         Female-to-male patients   181
         Metabolic derangement   184
         Gynaecological malignancy   184
         Osteoporosis   185
         Obstructive sleep apnoea   185
         Summary   185

13   Feminisation of the larynx and voice   191
     Guri Sandhu
         Introduction   191
         Laryngeal anatomy   191
         The development of the larynx   192
         Voice production   193
         Voice feminisation surgery   194
         Discussion   197

Part 4   Surgical treatments for born males   199
14   Breasts   201
     Dai M Davies and AJ Stephenson
         The breast   201
         Breast augmentation: history   201
         Breast differences   202
         Selection   203
         Implant choices   203
         Placement   203
         Access   204
         Size   204
         Author's preferred technique   204
         Complications   204
         Breast cancer   205

15   Genital surgery   209
     James Bellringer
         History   209
         Current practice   209
         Complications   214

Post-operative care 217
Sexual function 218

16 Advice for patients undergoing vaginoplasty and vulvoplasty 221
James Barrett
Things to do before you come into hospital 221
In hospital 222
Post-operative care at home 224

Part 5 Surgical treatments for born females 225
17 Breasts 227
Dai M Davies and AJ Stephenson
Author's preferred technique 228
Complications 228
Choice of surgeon 228

18 Phalloplasty 229
David Ralph and Nim Christopher
History of modern phalloplasty surgery 229
Surgical stages 230
The ideal phalloplasty 231
Types of phalloplasty 231
Referral criteria 235
Assessment in clinic 235
Preparation for surgery 237
Phalloplasty surgery 238
Associated surgery 241
Post-operative care 243
Dealing with complications 243
Outcome 245

Part 6 Post-operative psychological follow-up 249
19 Relationships 251
James Barrett

20 Reversion to former gender role after gender reassignment surgery 257
James Barrett
Religiously motivated reversion 257
Reversion motivated by a relationship or its breakdown 257
Reversion related to inadequate assessment or diagnosis 258

Part 7 Legal issues 259
21 The Gender Recognition Act 2004 261
Stephen Whittle
How the Gender Recognition Act works 262
Marriage, civil partnership and the family 262
Welfare benefits 263
Pensions 263
Employment law prior to the Gender Recognition Act 264
The impact of gender recognition for employment 264

The 'toilet question'   265
Privacy protection   265
Healthcare providers' obligations regarding privacy for   266
   transsexual people
Conclusion   267

22 Military service   269
   Stephen Whittle
   Transsexualism and homosexuality   269
   Particular issues in relation to military life   271

23 Religious matters   277
   James Barrett
   The Jewish view   277
   The mainstream Church of England View   278
   The Jehovah's Witness view   278
   The Catholic view   278
   The Evangelical Alliance's view   279
   The Buddhist view (*Paramabandhu Groves*)   280
   The Islamic view   282
   The Hindu view (*Chetna Kang*)   282

24 Fertility issues   285
   James Barrett

Recent case law   287

Afterword   289

Index   291

Preface

I conceived and edited this book because when asked for recommended reading on the practicalities of treatment for disorders of gender identity, I had nothing to suggest to others. I was always able to provide lists of books that dealt with the classification of gender identity disorders, and texts rich with competing aetiological theories. There were also fascinating sociopolitical (including post-modern) expositions. The problem always came with recommending practical texts for everyday clinical use. There seemed, particularly in a non-US setting, to be nothing other than the Harry Benjamin *Minimum Standards of Care*.[1] More recently, forthcoming UK intercollegiate guidelines promise to be much more applicable to UK practice. Even so, while both these standards are important, they relate to clinical practice in the same way as the Department of Transport's 'Road Traffic Regulations' does to learning to drive.

This is not a typical academic textbook. It is far too didactic, prescriptive and personal. There has been good research in gender identity disorders, but much of it has centred on surgical outcomes rather than on the clinical process that preceded them. The remainder has tended to be concerned with aetiology rather than outcomes – perhaps because mundane questions are less interesting than profound ones, although no easier to answer.

There is a shortage of accounts of process. While this shortage exists, and people with gender identity disorders need helping, I would modestly proffer this book as a practical help. It is drawn from considerable experience in the Charing Cross Hospital Gender Identity Clinic. As a consequence it is going to be more applicable to UK practice than any other, although the general principles should apply anywhere.

This book contains clinical vignettes. They are the psychiatric equivalent of those photographs of clinical pathology that are so beloved of physicians. As with physicians' books of pathological photographs, I have tried to include material that is subtle as well as spectacularly obvious. The cases are drawn from clinical practice. A very few are based directly on cases where the patient concerned has consented to publication. Most are composites, in that they represent the condensation of many different cases into one fictional case, characteristic of a recognisable type. Chess Denman has described and defended this approach, along with the use of the term 'patient', more eloquently than I could.[2]

Lastly, a word about terminology and the use of English pronouns. In this text 'male' and 'female' are used to mean physical sex assigned at birth. 'Transsexual' appears throughout this book, sometimes as a noun, but mainly as an adjective. 'Transman' and 'transwoman' rarely appear. This reflects use in practice. 'Transsexual' is used throughout the medical world, as a noun and adjective, and would be the key word for literature searches. 'Trans' used as a prefix to 'man', 'woman' or 'person' is isolated to the UK, and is not in common use. When used at all, it would be applied to someone who had already changed gender role and undergone treatment (*see* Chapter 21 on the Gender Recognition Act). Those who use a 'trans' prefix in this context would recognise that a person first arriving at a gender identity clinic might be described as 'transsexual' rather than 'trans' (S Whittle, personal communication).

References

1 *Harry Benjamin International Gender Dysphoria Association's Standards of Care for Gender Identity Disorders* (6e). Minneapolis: Harry Benjamin International Gender Dysphoria Association. www.hbigda.org/soc.htm (accessed 9 November 2006).
2 Denman C. *Sexuality, a Biopsychosocial Approach*. Basingstoke: Palgrave Macmillan 2004.

About the editor

James Barrett is a consultant psychiatrist and lead clinician at the Charing Cross Gender Identity Clinic. This is the oldest and largest gender identity clinic in the world.

He has worked in this field since 1987, and since that time has dealt with approximately two and a half thousand patients.

List of contributors

Ms Christella Antoni
Speech and Language Therapist
Charing Cross Hospital
Fulham Palace Road
London W6 8RF

Mr James Bellringer
Consultant Urologist
Charing Cross Hospital
Fulham Palace Road
London W6 8RF

Mr Nim Christopher
Consultant Uroandrologist
St. Peter's Andrology Centre
Hospital of St John and St Elizabeth
60 Grove End Road
London NW8 9NH

Mr Dai M Davies
Consultant Plastic Surgeon
Plastic Surgery Partners
55 Harley Street
London W1G 8QR

Dr Paramabandhu Groves
Consultant Psychiatrist
Alcohol Advisory Service
309 Grays Inn Road
London WC1X 8QS

Dr Chetna Kang
Specialist Registrar in Psychiatry
Ealing Hospital, West London Mental Health NHS Trust
Uxbridge Road
Southall
Middlesex
UB1 3EU

Dr Mark Morris
Consultant Psychiatrist in Psychotherapy
Tavistock & Portman NHS Trust
120 Belsize Lane
London NW3 5BA

Mr David Ralph
Consultant Uroandrologist
St. Peter's Andrology Centre
Hospital of St John and St Elizabeth
60 Grove End Road
London NW8 9NH

Mr Guri Sandhu
Consultant ENT Surgeon
Charing Cross Hospital
Fulham Palace Road
London W6 8RF

Dr Leighton Seal
Consultant Endocrinologist
Charing Cross Gender Identity Clinic
Claybrook Centre
Claybrook Road
London W6 8LN

Mr AJ Stephenson
Consultant Reconstructive, Plastics and Burns Surgeon
Northern General Hospital
Sheffield S5 7AU

Dr Stephen Whittle
Lecturer in Law
Manchester Metropolitan University
Elizabeth Gaskell Campus
Hathersage Rd
Manchester M13 0JA

Mr Daniel Wilson
Community Learning Disability Nurse
Woodside Road
Abbots Langley
Hertfordshire WD5 0HT

Disorders of gender identity

James Barrett

This is a highly politicised area. It has been subject to the attention of political and sociological theorists, of radical activists and conservatives. It can be viewed in a huge number of different and sometimes sharply opposed ways.

One school of thought holds that people with gender identity disorders have always been with us. Expositions about the two spirit people of North America often follow such statements. This generalises out to the view that such states are part of life's rich tapestry, and ought not to be medicalised. This seems to be anthropology at the expense of anything medical. It has much to commend it, although it is notable that those who propound it may still seek medical attention, often at the expense of others.

In stark contradistinction is the view that gender identity disorders represent a wholly physical problem, either in that every organ bar the brain is inappropriately of the other sex, or that there has been some kind of endocrine or birth anomaly. Proponents of this view seem to maintain that hormonal and surgical approaches are all that is required, and that the feelings that necessitate these interventions cannot themselves need attention. This viewpoint appears to be that of medicalisation at the expense of even a hint of psychologisation.

It ought not to be surprising that psychiatrists support the view that psychiatry has a central role to play. I am not a trained sociologist or anthropologist. My views may be seen as risible by many, and offensively wrong by others. For this I can only apologise and suggest that nobody can please everybody. I describe in the psychiatric section of this book an approach that seems to work acceptably well, and that has a track record in many years of practice, as well as in theory.

The other sections of this book deal with other aspects of the management of disorders of gender identity. Each has also been written by someone expert in their field and represents up-to-date practice. The approaches they describe presume that the patients have already been screened by competent psychiatric practice. Without this screening they will have, at the very best, only limited success.

Second opinions

James Barrett

The routine use of second opinions is so fundamental to the management of gender identity disorders that it has to precede almost all else.

There is often a 'gold standard' in the world of general medicine; frequently also an associated protocol. Either the sodium is over 120 mmol/l, or it is not. Either the titre of anti-double-stranded DNA antibodies is above the relevant threshold, or it is not. Not so in psychiatry. It shares with histopathology the quality of ultimately resting solely on individual judgement, despite all attempts to operationalise diagnostic practice. And psychiatrists and histopathologists show such high inter-rater and intra-rater reliability that, despite the lack of gold standards, numerically clear cut-offs and protocols, the whole show keeps on the road at least as well as do those of medicine and surgery.

Any diagnosis carries with it an associated prognosis. Because of this, time reveals the truth or falsehood of any histopathologist's or psychiatrist's diagnostic attempt. Widespread metastases suggest that the lesion was not benign after all. The relentless progress of negative symptoms suggests that it probably was not a transient drug-related psychotic episode.

No one is perfect, including histopathologists and psychiatrists. The former group use a complex system of cross-checked quality controls, taken from cases with known outcomes, to measure whether individual histopathologists make the neccessary grade. Psychiatrists do nothing of the sort.

I would argue that psychiatrists (and perhaps physicians also) need to be more like histopathologists. This might at the very least take the form of much readier recourse to a second opinion. At the moment, such an opinion is the right of every doctor and every patient in the UK NHS, but this right is very seldom exercised. It may please the cash-conscious service managers that this is so.

The management of gender identity disorders is one part of psychiatry where it seems to me (and to the World Professional Association for Transgender Health, Inc. (formerly the Harry Benjamin Gender Dysphoria Association)) that a high-quality second opinion is not just desirable, but rather is a necessity. The diagnosis of transsexualism leads to irreversible hormonal and surgical treatment. Mistakes are, in human terms if in no other, very costly.

If each psychiatrist managing patients with gender identity disorders were to get the diagnosis right 99% of the time, they would be doing very well indeed. If they appropriately referred patients for gender reassignment surgery 99% of the time, it would be an impressive performance. Yet, even if this state of affairs were to apply, still one in every 100 of these paragons' patients would be wrongly diagnosed and correspondingly wrongly treated.

Imagine, now, that two of these superbly good psychiatrists worked together and only actively treated those patients upon whom they were agreed. The rate of misdiagnosis and inappropriate treatment falls to one patient in 10 000. It should now be obvious, if it was not before, why this is the best way to manage this group of patients. It might be a good approach to apply to lots of other sorts of medical and psychiatric problems, too.

Mathematical calculations of odds are one thing, of course, and the real world is another. This method will fail to work as suggested above if the first psychiatrist asks for a second opinion only in cases where there is diagnostic or therapeutic doubt. Personal reflection and history tell us that some of the most wrong decisions were very confidently made. Clearly, in a relatively low-volume system like a gender identity clinic, every major diagnostic and therapeutic decision deserves a cross-check.

Further, the cross-check must be just that. It cannot be simply a rubber stamp from someone who sees his or her role as that of agreeing with the first opinion. Nor can it be that of always agreeing with the patient without regard to the first or any other opinion. Rather, it has to be a frank and independent view based on data that are as unchanged as possible from that which gave rise to the first opinion.

I have worked in such an arrangement for years, and have found it both re-warding and supportive. Sometimes I disagree with the opinion of my colleagues. Sometimes they disagree with me. We are still on good terms, and I know they have saved me from making mistakes. I hope I have done them the same service.

In the case of a disagreement, a third party takes a view. If the third opinion is unable to resolve the diagnostic or therapeutic question, the patient is called for an interview with all of us at once – including the surgeons, endocrinologist, psychologist and speech therapist. This is a quicker decision-making process, which accordingly is usually more acceptable to patients. Often the patients seem surprised that we openly disagreed with each other, and more often yet they are surprised to learn that about four times in five patients get their preferred course of action after such a group interview. Usually these meetings arrive at a consensus, and a plan that everyone has agreed upon is a plan that everyone gets behind and pushes.

The World Professional Association for Transgender Health, Inc. (formerly the Harry Benjamin Gender Dysphoria Association) is clear that no one should be referred for gender reassignment surgery without a *proper* second opinion. It seems best that no one is commenced on hormones without getting the same degree of care. It seems unsatisfactory that only one person, no matter how experienced or well read, and particularly no matter how confident, should initiate hormone treatment. It is clearly even more unsatisfactory for exactly the same individual to subsequently refer the same patient for gender reassignment surgery, either unsupported or supported only by someone lacking the knowl-edge or inclination to disagree.

This approach brings with it logistical problems, of course. The need for second opinions requires either clustering of expertise or an increased amount of potentially problematic communication and patient travel. In contradistinction, from the point of view of health provision planning, it would seem better to scatter the psychiatric expertise evenly across the population.

I suspect that for very large and populous countries there might be enough patients to merit more than one clinic (east and west coasts of the USA, for example). Smaller but densely populated countries such as Japan might better be served by one centrally located clinic.

Major difficulties are faced by small and sparsely populated countries – the Republic of Ireland or New Zealand, for example. I suspect buying into the services of larger neighbours, either *in toto* or for second opinions and surgery, or perhaps teaming up with neighbouring small countries to make a joint service, might best serve countries of this sort.

For very large countries with discrete but widely separated densities of population (Australia, or Canada, perhaps) there seems, unfortunately, little alternative to the need for a good deal of travelling.

Part 1

The referral process and screening

Referrals

James Barrett

Referrals to the Charing Cross Hospital Gender Identity Clinic are accepted only if they are made by a community mental health team psychiatrist or psychologist, or the child and adolescent gender identity disorder services.

This was not always the case. Before the administration around funding referrals was introduced, it used to be that general practitioner (GP) referrals were accepted. There were considerable problems with this arrangement.

The first problem was that many GPs seemed unwilling to refer direct to a tertiary centre, no matter how insistent the patient or how appropriate the referral would have been. They might have been worried about accessing scarce resources without a supporting local psychiatric opinion.

The second problem was the reverse of the first. It was that of GPs who seemed willing to refer to a tertiary service regardless of the appropriateness or otherwise of the ensuing consultation. Sometimes the patient and assessing gender identity clinic were bemused by these sorts of referrals.

Because of these problems, referrals are now required to come from local psychiatric services and not direct from GPs. The arrangement seems to have worked. GPs seem not to be scared to refer patients on, and the frequency of bemused but otherwise contented transvestites, lesbians, gay men and acutely psychotic people has proved acceptably lower.

I suspect that since this policy was introduced there has been a generally increased awareness of gender identity disorders and the possibilities for treatment. If direct GP referrals were reintroduced, there might be no increase in inappropriate referrals. As it is, this filtration through local community mental health teams now serves also to satisfy the funding arrangements currently in force in the UK. For this secondary administrative reason, it is likely to remain in force for the time being. However, direct GP referrals might be appropriate in settings where either an even more centralised or a wholly privatised healthcare system applied.

A separate problem is that of patients who do not keep appointments, particularly a first appointment.

This had been a problem at the Charing Cross Hospital Gender Identity Clinic. Patients repeatedly confirmed that they would attend first assessment appointments and then failed to show up. Each time, they stridently asserted that the next time they would.

Of course, it was impossible properly to judge the motivation behind such behaviour without ever seeing the people concerned. From the content of the referral letters, though, it was suspected that many of these patients (who tended to be male) were mildly gender dysphoric individuals, who saw having an appointment at the gender identity clinic as a validating statement of some sort. It was suspected that their gender dysphoria might well have been so slight that simply having possession of a symbolic appointment letter was the only step they wished at that time to make.

Though such behaviour might be understandable, it nonetheless placed an unacceptable load on an overburdened system. Our response was to offer no further appointments in the event of either non-arrival or cancellation on the same day. Such patients now need to be referred again. The local psychiatric services are advised to explore the reasons for non-arrival and not to re-refer unless they are confident that the behaviour will not be repeated.

Similar approaches now apply to patients who fail to arrive at follow-up appointments or cancel on the same day. A further appointment is given only if the patient or their GP actively requests one. Two non-arrivals in a row require the patient to be re-referred by local psychiatric services as if they were a new patient, partly because so much time may have passed since they were last seen that there would be too much to cover in a single follow-up appointment.

Being a tertiary referral centre is being the last resort, as well as being viewed as a diagnostic paragon. There are strengths and weaknesses to these positions. One notable weakness is that this is definitely where the buck stops. One finds oneself interviewing someone who is six feet four and grossly overweight, ravaged by acne and looking like a nightclub bouncer. This is someone with a declared drive to change gender role and with little realistic idea of the difficulties that will be involved; someone who has already resigned from a forklift truck driving job and who has hopes of being a model ('I've got the height, you see!').

This person has already been seen by everyone else in the referral chain. Yet no one has explicitly said that there might be problems ahead. One wonders whether no one appreciated this, or whether no one had the courage to say so. Either way, it seems that it is often the role of a specialist clinic to impart mixed, if not frankly bad, news. The imparter is sometimes blamed for the unwelcome news.

Diagnosis

James Barrett

Taking a history

Taking a history in a gender identity clinic is much like taking a history in a general psychiatric setting, but with extra emphasis on sex and gender matters. What follows is my preferred practice. This is not to say that it is somehow fundamentally 'right', merely that it works for me.

Firstly, why is the patient here? What is the problem?

Responses to this can be informative, ranging from 'I don't know, my psychiatrist told me to come here' through the rather stereotyped 'I'm a woman trapped in a man's body' to 'my soul is male but my body is female'. A high degree of concreteness and fixity on hormonal treatment sets the tenor for subsequent conversation. It suggests that there will be a low tolerance for suggestions of a delay to treatment on the grounds of a need for further psychological assessment.

Family is relevant in the usual sense – serious mental illnesses with heritability, transgenerational predicates etc – but also in the sense that gender identity disorders can run in families, and may be associated with homosexuality or transvestism in other family members. Accordingly, it is worthwhile asking if any family members are gay, cross-dress, or have a gender identity disorder. Lastly, this sort of family history can help reveal a partial androgen insensitivity syndrome (*see* 'Chromosomal and hormonal abnormalities', p. 51 and Chapter 12, p. 157)

Next, medical history

This is as standard, with particular concentration on anomalous pubertal development and any earlier surgery overtly or covertly related to gender identity disorder. The latter might include having cajoled general medical services into providing a hysterectomy or bilateral mastectomy on the grounds of mennorrhagia or a risk of cancer, the provision of gonadotrophin-releasing hormone (GnRH) analogues on shaky grounds, scrotal exploration to investigate testicular pain or drain a trivial hydrocele, or a particularly feminising rhinoplasty elicited on the grounds of nasal congestion.

Often, as ever, there is a history of accidental fractures. It is worthwhile enquiring into the circumstances, as sometimes they point to an earlier period of hypermasculine protest. For example, it is worthwhile determining the cubic capacity of the motorcycle the patient was driving when they sustained their fracture – moped or overpowered monster?

Drug history is much as for any other circumstance, save that there must be a lot more attention to the use of sex steroids. The nature, dose and duration of dosing as well as the effects should be noted. Many patients get steroids from black market or internet sources, and these should be directly enquired about, always being aware that the patient may lie about such use.

Psychiatric history is particularly important. It is best to start with the very first consultations with anyone, for any reason, as many patients have seen child psychiatric services for reasons that were directly or indirectly connected to a childhood disorder of gender identity. Every treatment agency seen, the reason for each contact and the outcome of the meeting should be sought.

Earlier contact with private practitioners can be particularly troublesome if patients assume that such contact means that they will be considered to have met all the requirements for gender reassignment surgery as soon as they are seen for the first time in the NHS. In general, no patient should be assumed to have completed a satisfactory real life experience unless there is believable documentary evidence or a credible account that they have done do. Every case must be assessed on its merits.

A history of brief middle-childhood anorexia nervosa is not uncommon in male patients, but eating disorders are not common in adult patients – occasional bulimia nervosa or anorexia nervosa in model or actress patients is all that is seen. The childhood anorexia nervosa is often recognised by the patient as having been driven by a desire to defer puberty (*see* 'Coincidental non-psychotic mental illnesses' p. 101).

There is, as ever, a need for an adequate social state examination. The state of the patient's finances (debts, creditors, savings) may reveal financial stress, and may explain why they have just left the private sector for the state sector. Housing circumstances might be important if the patient has a joint mortgage with a spouse, from whom divorce seems likely.

Occupational circumstances are most important in terms of whether the patient is occupied in their preferred social gender role or, if not, whether they have any realistic plans in this regard in their current or any other occupation.

The current relationship may as well be considered in concert with previous ones – with men, women, or both? How long have they lasted, and why have they ended? If the history seems to be of relationships with one sex only, has the patient *ever* had a relationship with the other?

Sexual matters require a lot of attention. What is the quality of the sexual content of the current and previous relationships. In patients seemingly attracted to one sex only, is there any history of sexual relations with the other (perhaps unwillingly)?

Forensic history needs to be brief, to avoid lengthy descriptions of allegedly trumped-up offences and the manner in which some injustice or another occurred. It is best simply to ask what the charge was, and what the penalty incurred. Theft of opposite-sex clothing is important enough to merit more detailed exploration.

A cross-dressing history is specific to disorders of gender identity. I have found it useful to ask the following questions for male patients:

- at what age do you recall having worn female clothes of your own accord? This avoids accounts of having been cross-dressed by parents or others, or participation in school theatricals. Histories of having been cross-dressed by parents are rarely confirmed and often refuted

- were you caught cross-dressing? What was the response? An exceedingly negative response can lead to a long inhibition of cross-dressing even though the urge to do so has been strong, sometimes with a display of ostentatiously masculine behaviour
- at what age did you first buy your own female clothes?
- was your cross-dressing ever associated with excitement, sexual arousal or masturbation? Is it now? If not, when did this stop?
- have you ever tried to stop cross-dressing? How many times? How long was the longest you managed to stop? When did you last try to stop?
- when was the first time you went out of the house so dressed? Where did you go? (A typical answer might be 'for a solitary walk or drive at midnight)
- when was the first time you went out so dressed and met other people? (A typical answer might be that the patient went to a club or a pub. It should be established whether this was a 'TV-friendly' venue or not)
- when was the first time you went out so dressed and met people who weren't expecting that sort of thing – shopping, for example?
- when was the last time you were in a male role, for whatever reason? (This might be a work appointment, family reunion, funeral or whatever).

The following questions have proved useful for female patients:

- did your school have a girls' uniform? How did you cope? (Some patients refuse to comply until they are expelled; others singlehandedly change the rules, either for them alone or generally. Some unwillingly comply)
- when was the last time you were in a dress, for whatever reason? (Often this is work, school or a family wedding)
- how did it feel? (Like drag? Like being dressed up as a doll?)
- what were you wearing under it? (Often boxer shorts)
- how long after the event did it stay on? (Usually as short a time as humanly possible)

Biography is an area where there is great inter-rater variation in the amount of detail recorded. I find the following necessary but by no means always sufficient:

- parental occupations (to determine social class of origin).
- schooling record, in both academic and social terms: was the patient regarded as gay at secondary school? Did the patient regard him or her self as gay? Were there friends, and what sex were the friends? How did they occupy themselves in their free time – gender neutral pursuits, sex-stereotyped, reverse sex-stereotyped? What age did the patient leave school? Did they pass any exams?
- higher education or vocational training: were any such endeavours completed or dropped? If dropped, why?
- occupational history of sex-stereotyped jobs: reverse sex-stereotyped jobs? No job at all? Often fired or resigned? If so, for a recurrent reason?

This last point is often tied up with a shifting pattern of making and breaking relationships, the course of which might as well be charted in parallel with the changing occupations.

More than in any other aspect of psychiatry (save perhaps forensic psychiatry), gender identity disorders require collateral history and confirmation. The general model in psychiatry is to believe what one is told. This applies also in gender identity disorder, but with the proviso that it should be confirmed. As Soviet Premier Mikhail Gorbachov said, 'trust, but verify'. Confirming things does not imply distrust or disbelief.

This latter point is particularly true of claims of occupational and military service. The former is fundamental to the real life experience (*see* Chapter 8), so it has to be verified. The latter is important because military medical records often provide a refreshingly frank set of opinions about the patient recorded at a well-defined time in the past (and so not subject to recall bias). The military keep wonderfully good records, and their promptitude shames the NHS. They require a patient's consent for release. Sometimes patients are unwilling to provide this, or claims of military service turn out to be bogus. Claims to have served in Special Forces, with their mystique of being mysterious supermen, is a special feature of what Baggaley has termed 'military Muchausen's'.[1] Bogus claims cast grave doubts, of course, over the whole of the rest of the history the patient has given.

The most common motivation for falsehood is a desire to present a story designed to elicit from the interviewer the responses the patient desires. These desired responses are usually those the patient honestly believes will provide the best for him or her. This story may be invented, or may consist of only those parts of the true story that the patient feels will be viewed in a manner liable to elicit the desired response.

Falsehood in these circumstances causes problems because, if it is detected immediately, it casts doubt upon the whole content of the patient's statement. The interviewer then feels a pressure independently to verify all the other parts of the patient's statement. Paradoxically, it often happens that the true state of affairs, which the patient had been keen to conceal, would not have caused the interviewer any great problems, and if the patient had been honest things would have progressed a lot faster without independent verification having to be sought. Effectively, the patient's ability to produce a worrying history is usually less than the interviewer's ability to fear or imagine one.

Rather than inventing a 'better' history or selecting the 'best' parts of their true history, some patients present only those parts of their story that they feel to be important. The distinction between this and a selective history is subtle, but a true distinction is present because the second is not motivated by a desire to deceive, but by a genuine belief that all relevant information has been imparted.

Patients who present only what they feel to be important do themselves a disservice because limiting the information they give in this way will, of course, limit the ability of the interviewer to make a properly informed decision – just as someone who presented to a chest physician and who failed to report smoking because he was quite sure he had tuberculosis would get his lung cancer diagnosed later. This attracts a worse prognosis.

Factitious stories are sometimes suggested by the attitude and demeanour of the patient. This is hard to describe but can be likened to the patient attempting to have the sort of conversation which used to pass between benefits agency staff and claimants at a time of very high UK unemployment in the 1980s. The agency worker would ask the claimant whether he had done any work since his last visit (the 'right' answer was 'no'), and whether he had been actively seeking work (the 'right' answer was 'yes'). Both agency worker and claimant knew that the real answers were 'yes, a bit of cash in hand' and 'why would I bother? There's been no proper jobs round here for years and besides I am 53 and have no formal qualifications'.

Under these circumstances, it seems worthwhile reminding the patient that this is not the intended nature of the interview, and that the interviewer seeks to know the truth of the patient's situation. If the texture of the interview remains unchanged, there is an even greater call for collateral history and verification than would ordinarily be the case.

Examination

Mental state examination in a gender identity clinic is as with any psychiatric assessment, in so far as mood and thought form are recorded. Usually, these will not be disturbed. More pertinent than is usually the case is the question of appearance.

Firstly, it is worthwhile noting the physical composition that nature has provided the patient with. This is what they have had to work with, after all.

Secondly, it is worth noting how well the patient manages to pass as the other sex, purely in terms of appearance, and as an overall impression.

Thirdly, it is useful to scrutinise for created features. These would include tattoos, and the presence of fetishistic elements such as leather, chains, dog collars etc. They might be quite slight, but still a clue to the route by which the patient arrived at the current position. Does the patient look sexualised in a fetishistic sort of way, or more mundane in a manner more in keeping with dual-role transvestism? Are they dressed appropriately for their age and circumstances?

Lastly, does the patient manage the trick of wearing clothes that are technically all those of the other sex, yet still achieving an overall impression of their biological gender?

Mannerisms and demeanour are particularly important. A good way to measure whether the patient comes across as female or male is to see which pronouns are used when subsequently dictating a report about the patient. Have they been she, he or a mixture of the two? Having to concentrate on other aspects of the content gives the subconscious a free choice of pronoun.

The patient's talk is important not simply in terms of form and content but also in terms of whether the vocal pitch and quality is masculine, feminine, neutral, falsetto or whatever. The threshold for a speech and language therapy referral should probably be low (*see* Chapter 11).

Physical examination

This should be as thorough as any general physical examination, and may already have been performed by the referring service. Of particular interest are the following:

- cardiovascular status, particularly any history of thromboembolic disease or abnormal clotting (for example, prolonged bleeding after dental extraction)

- weight parameters, particularly body mass index
- testicular examination
- cervical cytology: this should be confirmed as up to date, if it is indicated.

In addition, all patients should have the following serological investigations, as well as any others that seem to be indicated by their history:

- follicle-stimulating hormone
- leutenising hormone
- sex hormone-binding globulin
- testosterone
- dihydrotestosterone
- estradiol
- prolactin
- bone metabolic parameters
- lipid profile
- prostatic-specific antigen (for those with a prostate).

Reference

1 Wessely S. Risk, psychiatry and the military. *British Journal of Psychiatry* 2005; **186**: 459–66.

5

Categorisation and differential diagnosis

James Barrett

Overview

There is a public and, to some extent, general psychiatric perception that transsexualism is the only or at least the main disorder of gender identity. That this is probably illusory has been pointed out by Levine from an analytical perspective,[1] but the illusion persists, in part because most dual-role transvestites do not come to the attention of psychiatric services.

Certainly, transsexualism is the diagnosis for which most treatment evidence is available. There is little research into dual-role transvestism, nor much into dysmorphophobia or autogynephilia *per se*, or into autogynephilia presenting as or relating to a gender identity disorder, even though these and related areas such as gynandromorphophilia are important differential diagnoses and there is the suggestion that non-transsexual disorders of gender identity are more associated with psychopathology.[2-4] This is unfortunate, given that it seems an increasing proportion of dual-role transvestites are migrating toward full-time living as a woman.[5] These differential diagnoses may require different management to transsexualism.[2]

Currently, disorders of gender identity are classified as disorders of adult personality and behaviour in the *International Classification of Diseases* version 10 (ICD-10), and comprise the following:

- F64.0: transsexualism
- F64.1: dual-role transvestism
- F64.2: gender identity disorder of childhood
- F64.8: other gender identity disorders
- F64.9: gender identity disorder, unspecified.

Whether transvestism is contiguous with transsexualism or distinct from it is a debate that has endured over the decades, being reported, for example, by Buhrich and McConaghy as early as 1977.[6] The current diagnostic position reflects this uncertainty since it includes dual-role transvestism but not fetishistic transvestism as a gender identity disorder.

Transsexualism is described in the ICD-10 as a desire to live and be accepted as a member of the opposite sex, usually accompanied by a sense of discomfort with one's anatomical sex. For the diagnosis to be made, transsexual identity should have been present for at least 2 years, and must not be a symptom of another mental disorder, such as schizophrenia, or associated with any intersex, genetic, or sex chromosome abnormality.

This last stipulation implies that there is never a genetic or hormonal element in transsexualism, and that any such abnormality, if present, would always account for the cross-gender identity. Either or both of these implications may be without foundation.

In clinical work, it has long been the practice to subdivide referred people into a number of discrete groups. These subdivisions have clinical utility, and in some cases may reflect valid underlying natural divisions.

The most obvious division is that by birth sex. There is the growing impression that transsexualism may be different in males and females, and this is not reflected in the current classification system.[7] There have been many clinical observations that male and female patients differ in their clinical presentations and trajectories, and the physical aspects of treatment are rather different. This division seems particularly sensible.

A second reasonably widely accepted division is that between primary and secondary transsexualism. Primary transsexualism has also been called 'core' or 'true' transsexualism.

Those with an early age of onset, low sexual activity, lack of any history of sexual arousal with cross-dressing, sexual interest in the same biological sex and some degree of gender identity disorder in childhood have been viewed as 'core' or 'primary' transsexuals. They have been thought to have a better prognosis. This pattern was found by Verschoor and Poortinga to be more frequent in female patients.[8] A note of caution is sounded by Blanchard et al, who noted that it is possible that the differences in the histories produced by transvestites and heterosexual transsexuals are exaggerated to an unknown degree by the motivation of the latter to obtain approval for gender reassignment surgery.[9] They emphasise that this does not diminish the importance of distinguishing between these groups, but they do suggest caution in interpreting the self-report data that have frequently been used in comparing them.

Male patients, especially those sexually attracted to women, tend to present later in life. There is the suggestion that this late presentation may relate to number of earlier marriages and number of children fathered.[10] Many male patients (almost always those sexually attracted to women) would first have been identified as fetishistic transvestites, as noted by Buhrich and McConaghy as early as 1978,[10] and later as dual-role transvestites, before meeting the diagnostic criteria for transsexualism.[11] These patients, and those female patients with a similar history, are sometimes said to display 'secondary transsexualism'.

Another distinction that can be made is that of the sexual orientation of the transsexual person, felt by some to be important.[12] There is the suggestion that female patients attracted to females differ quite markedly from those attracted to males,[13,14] who are said to be more akin to gay men.[15] Male patients who would earlier have been seen by themselves and others as very feminine gay men are also classed by some as displaying secondary transsexualism.

Female transsexuals

Female patients represent a minority in a gender identity clinic, but a large one. They are popularly perceived as being few in number. This popular perception is distorted because fewer female patients seek media attention.

There is a clinical impression that transsexualism may be different in males and females. This is not reflected in the current classification system.[7] It seems that female patients display closer ties to their parents and siblings, establish stable partnerships more frequently, usually solely with the same biological sex, and are more satisfied sexually. This is not connected to whether they have undergone surgery.[16,17]

Female patients seem to be qualitatively different from male ones, although no such distinction is made in the ICD-10. The origins of their transsexualism seem mostly not to lie in transvestism, but rather to be of a primary sort, or arising out of an earlier masculine lesbian identity. The majority are gynaephilic. Unlike male patients, most have either no history of sexual relations with males, or report a single episode of such sexual interaction. This may have occurred while intoxicated, at the instigation of others, 'as an experiment' or against the patient's will. Usually not enjoyed, it has rarely been repeated.

Female patients have usually not been pregnant nor had a child. When they have, it may have been in the context of an earlier identity as a very masculine heterosexual or homosexual woman. More rarely, it may have been because of rape or sexual assault. In this upsetting circumstance, the patient may have presented too late for a termination of pregnancy, not accepting that it was possible that they were pregnant.

In the course of their relationship histories, female patients may recount relationships with males. Often they say that these started (and even more often ended) more like friendships. They often tell of having been more attracted to the masculine possessions and lifestyle of the man in question than to the man himself.

Relationships with other women can be subdivided into those with heterosexual and homosexual women. The latter may occur either when patients have been through a period where they self-identified as being lesbian or where they have been widely identified as such by others, and as a consequence moved in lesbian social circles. These relationships seem to prosper for a time but eventually to fail when the lesbian partner reports that being with the patient is uncannily like being with a man. Sometimes when the partner had a significant degree of interest in the opposite sex the relationship seems to survive, even through a change of gender role on the part of the patient. More often, though, there is a pattern of several relationships with lesbian women, all of which founder because of the masculine psychological attributes of the patient.

Relationships with heterosexual women are common, especially in patients who do not experience a phase of being identified by themselves or others as lesbian. These relationships are often initiated in circumstances where the partner believed the patient to be male. They may be sustained through the partner discovering the truth about the situation. There is sometimes a brief period of separation where the partner accommodates to this realisation and reconciles her own heterosexuality with the superficially lesbian nature of the relationship.

Female patients characteristically give a history of childhood revulsion to stereotypically female clothes and activities. Usually, there is a history of having had to be bullied, coerced or bribed into wearing female clothes for family social gatherings, school or work. Often at such events male clothes were worn beneath, and the female clothes were worn for the shortest possible time. Patients may recount having been astonishingly active in changing school rules to allow girls to wear trousers, and having gone to extraordinary lengths to avoid stereotypically female sports or other activities at school.

Female patients' choice of male clothing may be of some significance. Some choose exceedingly 'macho' clothes and often augment these with tattoos, cigarette or cigar smoking and exaggerated masculine gestures. Others employ formal three-piece suits. Both styles may prove curiously less evocative of masculinity than less extreme or formal male dress, perhaps because the contrast between the clothes and the wearer is more marked and causes the latter to be examined more closely. It has been suggested (Mark Morris, personal communication) that extreme or formal choice of male appearance is associated with poorer prognosis, but as yet no evidence supports this clinically based suggestion.

It was once held that female patients were shorter than average women from their communities. There is no evidence to support this supposition, but its previously widespread acceptance reinforces what can be a striking contrast between masculine appearance and feminine height – incongruity making the height seem less than would otherwise be the case.

Although few female patients have children, many make relationships with women who do. Fewer make relationships with childless women, and then as a couple seek artificial insemination by donor. This has been done in the past and has led to the creation of families that seem to function in a normal way, although not many of these families have children old enough to ask penetrating questions about the nature of their parents. It should be noted that the paternity and maternity of patients' children is a complex legal matter. (*see* 'Legal issues', p. 259).

The nature of sexual relations between female patients and their partners differs strikingly from that which might be seen in a lesbian couple. Patients usually do not wish to have their feminine attributes touched or appreciated. Breasts and genitals are described as 'no go areas'. Prostheses mimicking a penis are very often employed. Lesbian partners become increasingly dissatisfied with the inflexibility of such sexual arrangements. They may eventually terminate a relationship on these grounds. Heterosexual partners seem to find the situation easier to tolerate.

Female patients find menstruation particularly distressing, and sometimes give a history of having attempted at first to simply ignore their periods. Others report having never used conventional sanitary towels or tampons, favouring more makeshift arrangements. These worked less well but they were preferred because they were fabricated from gender-neutral items and not manufactured specially for women.

Female patients show a complex relationship with the social label of lesbian identity. While some patients report having earlier socially identified themselves as lesbians, they tend to claim that this identity was adopted because it was one that was imposed on them by others and one that was accepted because it allowed access to a more tolerant sector of society. It is often claimed that the identity was tenuous from the start, and became more so as experience in lesbian social circles grew. The relationship history in such patients' cases tends to support such claims.

Some female patients have earlier adopted a stridently politicised lesbian identity, in some ways analogous to the hypermasculine compensatory behaviour seen in some male patients.

A slight majority of female patients seem to have refuted the suggestion of a lesbian identity from the outset, having always been at pains to emphasise that they felt themselves to be male, even if those they were addressing had difficulties with this concept. Continued suggestions of lesbianism despite this explanation seem often to have angered such patients, and one has (while intoxicated) murdered a male friend who made such a suggestion.

Uncommonly, female patients report sexual attraction to men, experienced as male homosexual arousal. These patients differ quite markedly from those attracted to males.[13,14] The desired men are gay, the nature of the desired contact is also seen as gay, and the patients to be akin to gay men.[15] It seems that if a sexual relationship does form in this context, anal rather than vaginal intercourse is preferred.

Male primary transsexuals

Those with an early age of onset, low sexual activity, lack of any history of sexual arousal with cross-dressing, same-biological sex sexual orientation and some degree of gender identity disorder in childhood have been viewed as 'core' or 'primary' transsexuals, and thought to have a better prognosis.

Almost all are androphilic, and most have a low libido. There is usually a history of being mistaken for female in childhood and of not being bothered about it. Almost all have a solid history of gender identity disorder of childhood or, more rarely, a phase of it followed by a hypermasculine protest.

The extent of childhood femininity in such patients, and the degree to which they can come across as female at a first appointment, can be quite staggeringly great.

Case report: male primary transsexual

GB presented for a first appointment in a female role, before any hormone treatment, looking exceedingly feminine. She gave a lifelong history of feminine behaviour.

It seemed that GB had attended a mixed comprehensive school and that at the age of nine the other boys had attempted to articulate a problem with sharing a PE changing room with her. It seemed that her presence made them feel uncomfortable, somehow, even though she was anatomically like them.

GB had an almost exclusively female circle of school friends. These girls, in contrast to the boys, were very much at ease in GB's presence. They would chat animatedly with her, and their conversations would continue if they went to the toilet; they were quite happy for GB to follow them in and talk to them whilst they were in the toilet cubicle.

GB worked at a call centre. She reported that she was usually taken as female by clients. She had to give her name when complex matters were referred on to her supervisors, and her unequivocally male name always caused confusion. She admitted that the problems were such that she no longer bothered to tell routine callers that she was not a woman, finding it easier to let them assume she was a woman with a man's name.

> Before presenting to the gender identity clinic, GB had thought that she would have to remain in a male social role until a supportive second opinion was obtained. She was relieved to learn that she could change her social gender role before this, saying that she was having the greatest of difficulty functioning as a man.

Not all such patients have quite such a benign school experience. Sometimes imaginative answers to their educational problems have to be found.

Case report: educational problems in primary transsexualism

DS presented at the gender identity clinic having already changed social gender role to female. She gave an account of a very troubled childhood, having been steadily bullied at secondary school because of her extreme femininity. It seemed that her attendance had declined to such an extent that the educational authorities had become involved.

The educational authorities had considered DS's situation in some detail. They were at the point of considering whether state-funded home tutoring would give DS some sort of education. It was felt that this would be better than nothing, although inferior to attendance at school.

Eventually, it was decided to send DS to a drama school. It seemed that the school offered a good education, as well as dramatic training. In this environment DS prospered. The other students seemed to be much more tolerant of her femininity. She changed social gender role while attending the drama school, with no problems.

DS had no great dramatic talents, as it happened. Nonetheless she enjoyed the last part of her time in education and left with both some formal academic qualifications and able to sing, dance and act to a rather better than average extent.

Heterosexual male secondary transsexuals

Heterosexual male secondary transsexuals can be described as those in whom the transsexualism has arisen after a preceding history of fair or good function in a heterosexual male role.

It is usually preceded by dual-role transvestism. This in its turn is often preceded by a period of fetishistic transvestism. Libido in such patients is often low, a typical finding being the diminution of sexual drive within a heterosexual relationship after an initial few years of apparently normal libido. Sex is characteristically described as 'boring'. This pattern was reported as long ago as 1978 by Buhrich and McConaghy.[10] It was reiterated by Tsoi in 1992.[11] A note of caution is sounded by Blanchard *et al* who noted that it is possible that the differences in the histories produced by transvestites and heterosexual transsexuals are exaggerated to an unknown degree by the motivation of the latter to obtain approval for gender reassignment surgery.[18] The findings do not diminish the important distinction between these groups, but they do suggest caution in interpreting the self-report data that have frequently been used in comparing them.

The decrease in heterosexual libido is not inversely proportionally accompanied by any increasing homosexual drive, although some patients report a very slight awareness of (or increase in) sexual drive towards men. This is, however, rarely translated into action.

Heterosexual male secondary transsexuals sometimes report a lifelong sense of insecurity in a male role. Some have reacted to this by engaging in ostentatiously masculine behaviour, such as aggressive sports or bodybuilding. They may have joined the armed forces (*see* 'Patients in the police or armed services', p. 117). Their subsequent change of gender role may come as a great surprise to those who knew of their hyper-masculine behaviour but did not know them very well.

Fetishistic transvestism is seen in such patients as an initial phase. It typically commences at puberty, and at first features cross-dressing in underwear rather than socially visible outerwear. Often a sibling's or mother's clothes are employed at first, although sometimes underwear is stolen or obtained from jumble sales. Patients can often recall this clothing in detail. Their rich descriptions of the nature and texture of the clothes seem sometimes to have the feel of erotic memories.

As childhood progresses into adolescence, such patients usually progress to buying their own female clothes. An idea of the progression of the condition can be gained by asking at what age the patient first cross-dressed of their own accord, and at what age they first bought their own female clothes.

It often seems that the clothes first bought were those that the patient would have found sexually attractive if women around him had worn them. Cross-dressing at this stage is usually accompanied by sexual arousal and either masturbation or heterosexual intercourse. Patients often describe a feeling of revulsion and a sudden cessation of the desire to cross-dress after orgasm. Patients in this phase sometimes feel guilty. They may have episodes where they resolve never to cross-dress again, particularly if they do not have a relationship in which the behaviour is validated. They may throw their entire female wardrobe away in such a state, or donate it to a charity shop. These episodes of attempting to give up cross-dressing are often repeated many times, with successive attempts getting shorter in duration until attempts are no longer made. Patients may find themselves having to buy another wardrobe of clothes or having to buy their own clothes from the shop to which they earlier donated them.

Obtaining a history of these episodes of attempting to stop cross-dressing may give an idea of the intensity of the drive to cross-dress and the stage at which it became so overwhelming that it was no longer resisted.

Many patients describe reaching a phase where they no longer resist their urge to fetishistic cross-dressing, and do so whenever both the urge strikes them and the circumstances permit. This situation is often accompanied by a decrease in the associated sexual excitement, a loss of both the feelings of guilt, and the habit of removing the clothes after orgasm. Patients seem to evolve into a situation where their cross-dressing is no longer purely sexual. Instead it assumes a 'relaxing' rather than 'exciting' effect. At this stage, it may no longer be regularly accompanied by masturbation or sexual intercourse. Instead, for increasing periods, the patient may engage in ordinary activities in a cross-dressed state in the privacy of his own home. These periods may come to replace masturbation as a stress reliever. If the patient has a female partner she may find this change hard to come to terms with, having earlier been able to accept the cross-dressing solely as a part of the couple's sexual life.

Another judgement of the progression of this sort of secondary transsexualism can be made by asking at what stage the cross-dressing stopped being primarily sexual in motivation.

At this stage, patients' choice of clothing and interest in clothes tends to change from being centred on underwear and slightly sexualised garments, to social outerwear with a less sexualised presentation. An increasing amount of time is spent in a female role. Patients at this time qualify for a diagnosis of dual-role transvestism and may be inclined to join an organisation for dual-role transvestites, such as the Beaumont Society. Patients with partners may be supported in this. Wives or girlfriends may accompany them on outings, or their partners may join the 'Women of the Beaumont Society' adjunctive group. Partners who are not supportive may find the transition from fetishistic transvestism into dual-role transvestism traumatic. They may refuse to see the patient in a socially female role, even when they had earlier been prepared to tolerate a sexually circumscribed feminised appearance. Such partners sometimes reach an accommodation that allows the patient to spend a fixed period in a female role, out of their sight but with their knowledge. There is sometimes a fear (usually unjustified) that the patient will seek other sexual contacts when in a female role and out of their sight.

Many men seem to move from a fetishistic transvestite position to that of dual-role transvestism, and thereafter firmly to remain dual-role transvestites. Some, though, experience an increasing sense of their own femininity and begin somehow to feel 'a fake' when presenting in a male role. Coincidental with this feeling of fraudulence may be an increasing loss of communion with others in the Beaumont Society, sometimes expressed as a feeling that the others somehow do not 'take it seriously' or are 'just blokes dressed in women's clothes'. After some time, this feeling seems to grow until patients (often under pressure from partners) seek psychiatric help. It seems that partners often hope that the psychiatrist can somehow restore an earlier position of dual-role transvestism or even fetishistic transvestism. They may be annoyed to find that instead the patient seems to want to discuss how further to advance a change of gender role, and disappointed that the psychiatrist accepts this agenda. Sometimes the presentation to a gender identity clinic seems to be precipitated by the loss of a relationship with a partner through death or divorce, or by the departure of dependent children.

These patients are sometimes termed secondary transsexuals. The changes in their relationships with the women in their lives are outlined in Chapter 9 and will not be covered further here. What follows are remarks about their individual prognoses.

Secondary transsexualism of this sort has a very variable outcome. Some patients settle very well into a female role and remain happily in that role for the remainder of their days. Others have a much stormier course.

A good prognostic factor seems to be more advanced age. Older patients seem to move into the role of a late middle-aged woman with relative ease. A supportive partner or newly single status, the financial and occupational stability attending retirement, and the much less sexually distinct roles of older people seem to be helpful. One thinks of couples in their mid to late 60s, in nearly identical fleeces and bobble hats, walking their dog. Their social roles and appearances seem potentially quite interchangeable.

Most secondary transsexuals report a low libido. Certainly their libido will be lowered yet further by hormone treatment. Some vaguely talk of wanting to make a relationship with a man. Most either continue the relationship with any existing female partner or stay single. Despite the high likelihood of either a chaste relationship with a woman or no relationship at all, many are very insistent on a full vaginoplasty. The impression is that if this is provided the neovagina is often not maintained and its capacity is lost (though not its liability to prolapse). It appears that the neovagina was wanted as much for a sense of being 'a full woman' as anything. The patients seem indifferent about whether they continue to have a functioning vagina, so long as they once had one.

A more guarded prognosis is that seen in patients whose relationship arrangements are more complicated. Some make a relationship with a much younger man. They may seem very insistent on gender reassignment surgery with a full vaginoplasty, feeling that it is essential in order to maintain the relationship. The male partners seem sometimes to be somewhat financially or emotionally dependent on the patients, as in the case that follows.

Case report: relationship pressure for gender reassignment surgery (1)

FP presented to a gender identity clinic in his mid-50s, with a history of initially fetishistic and later dual-role transvestism. He was divorced with two adult sons, but had no contact with his ex-wife or children and very little with his family of origin. His wife had been wholly unsupportive of his change of gender role. He felt that his marriage would probably have ended in any case, because after their children had left home he had grown apart from his wife.

FP changed gender role with relative ease. He settled into the role of a late middle-aged woman very well. She made no pressing demands for gender reassignment surgery. She seemed to accept that if all want well it might be offered, but felt that a change of social gender role had been her most significant step. It was suspected that FP might never want gender reassignment surgery or might prefer a cosmetic vulvoplasty to gender reassignment surgery featuring a vaginoplasty.

FP presented some months later with a pressing demand for full gender reassignment surgery. She had formed a relationship with a much younger man. The relationship was complex in that for most social purposes she presented herself as the man's friend, although in truth the relationship was also a sexual one.

It was suspected that the relationship lay behind FP's sudden demand for gender reassignment surgery, although she denied this and the man concerned would not be drawn on the matter. There was also an impression that the relationship might not have good prospects for longer-term stability.

Case report: relationship pressure for gender reassignment surgery (2)

CB presented with a story strikingly similar to FP's, but made a relationship of sorts with a rather younger man who had a successful career in banking. She also pressed for gender reassignment surgery after having earlier seeming relaxed about whether or when this might occur.

On closer inquiry, it appeared CB's boyfriend seemed reluctant to make any great commitment to her. He had declared deep affection but would not agree to cohabit with CB. He had at times been violent towards her. His work was said often to take him away for considerable lengths of time.

Conversation with CB revealed that she had doubts about her boyfriend's fidelity, despite his protestations of affection. She had attempted to put out of her mind what were, in truth, persisting concerns about both this and his occasional violence towards her.

Over time, CB grew increasingly distrustful of her partner. As she did so, her pressure for gender reassignment surgery decreased. The relationship eventually failed, and CB returned to her previous state of mind about gender reassignment surgery.

Sometimes a seemingly unremitting insistence on gender reassignment surgery in a secondary transsexual is entirely dropped if the patient makes a new relationship with a woman. There may be a wholesale return to a male role and denial of any drive to change gender role. This reversal seems to last as long as the relationship, which is possibly for some considerable time. Clingy, dependent patients who seem unable to stay single and who always seek a relationship are a worry, because their desire to have a relationship with a woman may outweigh their desire to change their gender role (*see* Chapter 10 dealing with reversion to former gender role).

Homosexual male secondary transsexuals

A rather smaller proportion of male patients report a lifelong sexual preference for men, with an earlier fair to good function in a male gender role. This has been thought to have a better prognosis. This pattern was found by Verschoor and Poortinga to be more frequent in female patients.[8]

These patients would earlier have been identified both socially and by themselves as feminine gay men with a liking for cross-dressing. It seems that such patients have a fairly low libido combined with a lifelong moderate sense of femininity. This last feeling grows as time passes.

These patients often show a history of contact with a gender identity clinic that is characterised by being at first intermittent, with many missed appointments and droppings out of treatment. Presentations seem to have been coincidental with emotional crises, and well spaced in time.

Later presentations seem to be more closely spaced and less clearly associated with crises. Sometimes, though, there is no change of social gender role despite these more frequent appointments – simply increasingly expressed dissatisfaction with a role as a gay man and a growing sense of femininity. It sometimes seems that an emotionally or financially dependent relationship with a man inhibits expression of femininity. Patients sometimes present living in a female role, but not wanting to undergo genital surgery because of the lack of support from a partner.

Often, after some time (which may amount to years), such patients do change social gender role and commence hormone treatment. Loss of an already low libido is usually viewed with relief, and function in a female social role is often very good indeed. The relationship with a gay male partner usually deteriorates, despite ostensible support. The partners often leave after a change of gender role, when feminisation becomes marked or when the patient has gender reassignment surgery. Several patients' previously 'supportive' boyfriends have dumped them while they were still inpatients recovering from gender reassignment surgery. The patients seem not to have been wholly surprised and one suspects that both patients and partners knew, deep down, that this was on the cards.

The reverse can apply. Sometimes the ending of a gay relationship by death or departure of partner can be the change that allows a sudden and usually rather successful change of gender role and subsequent gender reassignment surgery.

I have heard of one case in which the whole situation was inverted. The patient had lived in a female role for over a decade with a rather older male partner (who had never known the patient in a male role). The patient had never had gender reassignment surgery because neither patient nor partner wanted this. When the partner became elderly he was cared for by the patient for many years, and upon his death the patient reverted to a late middle-aged male role and subsequently made a successful relationship with a woman.

A common story in these circumstances is one of insidiously advancing femininity on a background of feminine homosexuality, as the following case report illustrates.

Case report: insidiously advancing femininity

SA presented to a gender identity clinic in his early 30s, claiming to have already changed gender role from male to female. He presented in female clothing, but came across as a feminine gay man.

SA gave a history of lifelong feminine homosexuality. He had a brief adolescent experimentation with heterosexuality, but found it not to his taste, and thereafter made relationships only with men.

SA had a fairly low libido, and formed a long-term relationship with a gay male partner. In the course of the relationship, SA took a very feminine role. Sometimes he went out socially with SA in a female role, with his partner playing a masculine 'boyfriend' role. SA was said to have seen himself as more female than most feminine gay men, citing his low libido and monogamy as being atypical.

The relationship lasted for about a decade. It developed sexual problems when SA increasingly desired a permanent female role with a vagina, and his partner was oppositional – especially to the last desire. After the relationship had ended, SA presented to the clinic.

As time passed, SA began increasingly to come across as female rather than as a feminine gay man in women's clothes. This occurred despite the choice of clothing style remaining the same.

SA continued to move in the same social circles and reported that while formerly gay men had treated her as a feminine gay man, after her relationship had ended and she had adopted a permanently female role she had been treated as a friendly 'drag queen-like character'. This was described as someone who would not be seen as a potential partner, but still decidedly part of the gay male crowd nonetheless.

As time passed, SA came to give an increasingly female (as opposed to feminine) impression. She reported that in gay male circles she came to be treated as a woman might. This was described as being viewed by gay men with a friendly familiarity but accompanied by her sensation that she was no longer accepted as part of the group, but rather more as a respected visitor to it.

References

1   Levine SB. Psychiatric diagnosis of patients requesting sex reassignment surgery. *Journal of Sex and Marital Therapy* 1980; **6**: 164–73.

2   Blanchard R. The she-male phenomenon and the concept of partial autogynephilia. *Journal of Sex and Marital Therapy* 1993; **19**: 69–76.

3   Blanchard R. Clinical observations and systematic studies of autogynephilia. *Journal of Sex and Marital Therapy* 1991; **17**: 235–51.

4   Miach PP, Berah EF, Butcher JN and Rouse S. Utility of the MMPI-2 in assessing gender dysphoric patients. *Journal of Personality Assessment* 2000; **75**: 268–79.

5   Docter RF and Prince V. Transvestism: a survey of 1032 cross-dressers. *Archives of Sexual Behavior* 1997; **26**: 589–605.

6   Buhrich N and McConaghy N. The discrete syndromes of transvestism and transsexualism. *Archives of Sexual Behavior* 1977; **6**: 483–95.

7   Landen M, Walinder J and Lundstrom B. Clinical characteristics of a total cohort of female and male applicants for sex reassignment: a descriptive study. *Acta Psychiatrica Scandinavica* 1998; **97**: 189–94.

8   Verschoor AM and Poortinga J. Psychosocial differences between Dutch male and female transsexuals. *Archives of Sexual Behavior* 1988; **17**: 173–8.

9   Blanchard R, Clemmensen LH and Steiner BW. Gender reorientation and psychosocial adjustment in male-to-female transsexuals. *Archives of Sexual Behavior* 1983; **12**: 503–9.

10 Buhrich N and McConaghy N. Two clinically discrete syndromes of transsexualism. *British Journal of Psychiatry* 1978; **133**: 73–6.

11 Tsoi WF. Male and female transsexuals: a comparison. *Singapore Medical Journal* 1992; **33**: 182–5.

12 Clare D and Tully B. Transhomosexuality, or the dissociation of sexual orientation and sex object choice. *Archives of Sexual Behavior* 1989; **18**: 531–6.

13 Chivers ML and Bailey JM. Sexual orientation of female-to-male transsexuals: a comparison of homosexual and nonhomosexual types. *Archives of Sexual Behavior* 2000; **29**: 259–78.

14 Dickey R and Stephens J. Female-to-male transsexualism, heterosexual type: two cases. *Archives of Sexual Behavior* 1995; **24**: 439–45.

15 Coleman E, Bockting WO and Gooren L. Homosexual and bisexual identity in sex-reassigned female-to-male transsexuals. *Archives of Sexual Behavior* 1993; **22**: 37–50.

16 Kockott G and Fahrner EM. Male-to-female and female-to-male transsexuals: a comparison. *Archives of Sexual Behavior* 1988; **17**: 539–46.

17 Fleming M, MacGowan B and Costos D. The dyadic adjustment of female-to-male transsexuals. *Archives of Sexual Behavior* 1985; **14**: 47–55

18 Blanchard R, Clemmensen LH and Steiner BW. Social desirability response set and systematic distortion in the self-report of adult male gender patients. *Archives of Sexual Behavior* 1985; **14**: 505–16.

6

Dealing with the differentials

James Barrett

Transvestites

Whether transvestism is contiguous with transsexualism or distinct from it is a debate that has endured over the decades, being reported, for example, by Buhrich and McConaghy as early as 1977.[1] The current diagnostic position including dual-role transvestism but not fetishistic transvestism as a gender identity disorder reflects this uncertainty.

The *International Classification of Diseases* version 10 (ICD-10) divides transvestism into fetishistic and dual-role types. Both in their ordinary form would probably be reasonably familiar to any general practitioner (GP) or psychiatrist. There will be only a very brief description of uncomplicated fetishistic transvestism and dual-role transvestism. More problematic are atypical presentations and the evolution of dual-role transvestism into secondary transsexualism. These will be discussed below.

It should be remembered that in some men, situations of high stress elicit a transvestism that is usually repressed. At the height of the second World War, in the Western Desert campaign, the psychiatric consultant to the Middle East force came across transvestism practised by a considerable group in a unit in 1940. It could not have been entirely harmless as officers, sergeants and other ranks were involved. The military work of the unit was at a high level and there was very little drinking. The 'girls' and their partners were particularly contented people though the opportunities to dress up became increasingly difficult and this created unhappiness and irritation. The moving spirit was an officer with a splendid fighting record and the group was left alone as very few people knew of its activities which took place under the guise of 'rehearsals for a play'.[2]

Fetishistic transvestism

Fetishistic transvestism is cross-dressing in a sexual context. It may feature eroticised clothing styles. Often there is accompanying masturbation, and post-orgasm is often accompanied by a cessation of the urge to cross-dress and a sudden revulsion for cross-dressing. The choice of female clothing is often inappropriate to the subject's age or the social setting. It is apt to be the sort of clothes that a man of that group would find erotic on a young woman rather than the sorts of clothes women of the same group or age would wear. Elements of other fetishes may creep into the presentation, so one may see leather miniskirts and ankle chains, or dog collars worn as necklaces.

Uncomplicated fetishistic transvestism usually remains stable with time. It very rarely presents in a gender identity clinic, as it is familiar to most psychiatrists. It may, however, take a less overt form and be fetishistic transvestism nonetheless. The following is such a case.

Case report: less than obvious fetishistic transvestism

C presented with an urge to live as a woman, reporting that he found it exciting when he passed as one. Closer enquiry over the course of several appointments determined that he was interested only in passing as female with young women who he found sexually attractive. Passing among men, or older less attractive women, proved of no interest to C.

C spent increasing amounts of his spare time in a female role. In the course of this he obtained a part-time retail job. Over the course of time the sexual excitement associated with his cross-dressing decreased. There was an accompanying increase in quiet satisfaction and contentment. C seemed to be drifting from an initial fetishistic transvestism towards dual-role transvestism.

Dual-role transvestism

Dual-role transvestism is a disorder of gender identity. It is much commoner than transsexualism. Dual-role transvestism may represent a stable way of life. Accordingly it ought, in theory, rarely to be encountered in a gender identity clinic. In fact it is seen fairly often, which may simply reflect its high prevalence.

Men are said to display dual-role transvestism when they spend a significant portion of their life in a female role, valuing the expression of female feelings this allows. It is not sexually driven, but might have evolved from a previous fetishistic transvestism. Men displaying dual-role transvestism tend to dress in clothes appropriate to their age and the social setting, and sometimes to an age greater than their own.

The proportion of time spent in a female role varies between individuals, but may be over half of the available time. No matter how much time is so spent, though, the men concerned do not feel as if they are truly female. They view their male personas, and particularly their genitals, as valuable.

Dual-role transvestites are mostly heterosexual, as are most males. They are usually easily identified by themselves and psychiatrists as transvestite. This does not preclude confusion, though, as the following case illustrates.

Case report: fairly simple presentation of dual-role transvestism

SP was referred to a gender identity clinic when in his late 20s. He was divorced, but his marital breakdown seemed unconnected to his cross-dressing – which had always successfully been incorporated into the marital sexual relationship as 'role-play'.

At the time of referral SP complained, 'I feel as though I am in the wrong body'.

SP recalled having worn two pairs of 'fascinating shoes' that his mother owned, when he was aged 5 or 6. His mother had caught him doing this and had expressed mild displeasure.

At puberty, SP's cross-dressing became rather more sexual and he recalled feeling more sexy in a female role. SP first went out cross-dressed when in his early 20s, going for a walk around the block at midnight. His first daytime outing was a year later, to a shopping arcade in an adjacent town. At referral SP was in a female role when at home, but in no other circumstance.

When asked what he wanted SP said, 'my life is not right; I live in two different worlds. When I am Sarah, I am a lot happier. I tend to forget S's problems when I am Sarah'.

SP was advised to consider joining a society for dual-role transvestite men. He failed to attend further appointments.

Transvestites (both fetishistic and dual-role) are not necessarily heterosexual, as the following case history illustrates.

Case report: homosexual dual-role transvestite

H was initially presented by his community mental health team as what they thought to be a clear case of transsexualism. He had been noted to be sexually attracted only by males, and to be requesting treatment with female hormones. He was said to spend much of his time outside work in a female role.

It emerged that H had an exceedingly anankastic and narcissistic personality. He was sexually rather energetic, in a receptive way, and greatly feared ageing and losing his looks. His mirror gazing took up a substantial part of every morning. He had twice crashed his car through using the rearview mirrors to check nothing other than his own appearance.

H had associated a feminine appearance with being young and fresh looking. He sought a female social role partly as a means to avoid masculine ageing. He dressed casually as male at home, when there was no one to see him. Once H had understood that estrogens would not delay ageing and might also erode libido, he did not want them. He had never wanted gender reassignment surgery.

H's life did incorporate much time in a female role. This had seemed at first to be wholly connected with sexual attractiveness. H reported distress at being easily taken as male, but delight when he initially passed as female and was a sexually attractive object to heterosexual men. His pleasure was only complete, though, if the heterosexual men realised after a time that he was male and that they had desired another man. H would shop and go about other business solely to encounter handsome heterosexual men.

This flirting aside, H reported no sexual activity in a convincingly female role. Sexual contact seemed mainly to happen when he was in a male role.

As a man, H would sometimes pretend to be much older and less attractive, sometimes using particularly unflattering older men's clothes to enhance this fiction. In these situations he would provide fellatio for younger males who favoured such partners. The motivation seemed to be a mixture of never being *justifiably* thought of as unattractive, and of gaining sexual attention by deceit. In what he felt was a related way, H sometimes took particular care to present himself as less convincingly female, seeking an 'ageing transvestite' look. He saw this persona as the older and unattractive man in drag, and was aware that it was similarly motivated.

H initially presented in turmoil, demanding the immediate provision of hormones and subsequent provision of facial cosmetic surgery. Hormone treatment was precluded by his dual-role transvestite status, and he was offered group psychotherapy.

Group psychotherapy proved very helpful. Over the course of about 18 months, H determined that he was quite unlike the transsexual members of the group. They, in their turn, identified him as 'a happy transvestite' who happened to be homosexual rather than heterosexual.

H continued to ruminate about living his life in a female role. He suggested that he might take a female role in a weekend job in a chain store. He remained psychologically and sexually male.

H remained preoccupied by thoughts of himself in an attractive female role. He saw himself as always being 'male underneath' and wanted others also to be aware he was male, eventually if not initially. He gained relief from his urge to cross-dress by taking his holidays in a nudist colony. There, he found that the universal nakedness led to a cessation of any urge to present himself in a female role save on occasions where a naturist evening event had allowed women partially to dress. At this time H had been seized with the intrusive thought that he could look more attractive to the heterosexual men than could the women.

As time passed, H's time in a female role came to be less associated with sexual attractiveness. Instead, life in a female role was seen as more vibrant and enjoyable.

Dual-role transvestism often follows fetishistic transvestism, and may precede transsexualism. The change from dual-role transvestism to transsexualism tends to be steady and even in pace. It often features an increasing dissatisfaction with a sexually compartmentalised lifestyle, and a sensation that life in a female role is somehow more real and vibrant. This change in feeling is often accompanied by a loss of empathy with dual-role transvestites, and a feeling that they are somehow not serious, or are just dressing up. After a while, a male role begins to feel somehow fraudulent, an act, not 'the real me'.

At this stage many dual-role transvestites change social gender role permanently. Sexual orientation rarely alters, and there is often no desire to lose a penis and gain a vagina, although libido is often low and the penis has become an object of indifference rather than strong positive or negative feeling. *See* 'Patients who choose not to have gender reassignment surgery' (p. 134).

Autogynaephilia

Autogynaephilia is a disorder of sexual object. It is being aroused by the thought of oneself as female, or with female primary or secondary sexual characteristics. This disorder is a major differential in a gender identity clinic. It may present as or relate to a gender identity disorder.[3,4] There is little research into autogynaephilia *per se*,[4] nor into autogynaephilia presenting as or relating to a gender identity disorder,[3,4] even though these and related areas such as gynaendromorphophilia are important differential diagnoses of transsexualism,[4,5] and there is the suggestion that non-transsexual disorders of gender identity are more associated with psychopathology.[6]

There may well be a greater measure of autogynaephilia in male patients attending a gender identity clinic than might at first be thought. Sometimes the autogynaephillic drive is rather clear, as in the following case.

Case report: patient with clear autogynaephilia

SM presented in his mid-40s. He had a stated desire to change gender role, and aggressively pressed for hormonal treatment. He was upset to learn that this would be dependent on a change of gender role. SM's demeanour was unequivocally male. He had no history of childhood unmasculinity, let alone femininity.

On review, SM had not changed gender role. He became annoyed when hormones were not prescribed, arguing that he had been attending the gender identity clinic for longer than others who had been prescribed hormones. It was pointed out that they had changed their gender role, and that it was this and not length of attendance that mattered in the initiation of hormone treatment.

At a third appointment, SM presented in an aggressive male manner. He wore jeans and a T shirt in combination with three-inch heels, large false breasts and nail varnish. He looked embarrassed, and became annoyed almost immediately. SM confessed that at his masculine, manual work he had taken to wearing clear nail varnish, but that this was as far as any change of role had gone. He admitted that his appearance at interview sent very mixed signals, and that he had been taken as male throughout his journey to the appointment. SM became very angry and freely admitted that all he wanted from the gender identity clinic was treatment that would allow him to grow breasts. He said he had no idea why, and then left the interview never to return.

Sometimes the presentation is not so clear-cut. Patients may state that they seek to change their gender role and request hormonal support in so doing. Further enquiry reveals that they have the firm view that they do not support stereotypical roles for men and women, and claim that they have a more modern and enlightened view. This transpires to be a belief that their own feelings of femininity are all that count, and that the views of the rest of the world are an irrelevance to them. When asked what, in practical terms, they are requesting, they go on to describe what amounts to a fundamentally unchanged life, in a male social gender role. In this setting they would anticipate the prescription of estrogens.

Sometimes autogynaephillia is yet more tangentially presented, as illustrated below. The sometimes transient nature of an autogynaephillic drive also features.

Case report: patient with less clear autogynaephilia

DW presented in his mid-40s. There was a childhood history of cross-dressing in his mother's and sister's underwear, with sexual arousal, at age 9 years. Sporadic cross-dressing occurred after the age of 12 years. There had been no features of femininity when DW had attended school. DW had been married for 14 years, but there had been no sexual activity between the couple for the last four.

Before DW's marriage there had been a fetishistic transvestite phase of about 2 years, but this was described as having been 'explored to the fullest degree'. At the time of presenting, DW owned only four items of female clothing, and wore these every 3 months or so. There was still some sexual arousal with DW's cross-dressing, but the main motivation was pleasure at the thought of imagining himself to have female genitals and breasts. This had affected the latter stages of the sexual relationship with his wife.

DW sometimes took illicitly sourced estrogens for about 4 days at a stretch, and very occasionally took cyproterone acetate. These tiny amounts of hormone were said by DW to produce femininity but were always stopped after a few days because he perceived his face as being 'too female'.

Sometimes the autogynaephillic element becomes apparent only after some time, as the following shows.

Case report: less obvious autogynaephilia

DM presented in his mid-60s. He was a bank manager who had taken slightly early retirement. He gave a history of lifelong episodic cross-dressing with a sexual element that was said to have decreased over the years. He presented with a stated desire to change gender role. There was no history of childhood femininity, but some suggestion of mild unmasculinity. DM had been married for very many years and had grown up children.

DM initially described his wife as supportive, but as appointment followed appointment it seemed that his marriage stood in the way of his changing gender role. Financial co-dependence and failing health on his wife's part were cited as two of many reasons why divorce would be no easy matter. It seemed that his wife did not want the social stigma of a husband who had changed gender role.

Eventually, DM quietly but firmly suggested that he thought gender reassignment surgery without any role change would be quite satisfactory to him. He said that it would give him quiet satisfaction and secret pleasure to be aware of himself as 'a covert woman'. There was the strong impression that this was probably what DM had wanted all along. Not long after, DM wrote a letter relinquishing all requests for treatment of any sort, saying that he thought he was too old, and that the opportunity for such things had passed him by.

Patients who change gender role but do not greatly prosper sometimes show flashes of thinking that seem rather autogynaephillic. An example is a patient's statement that she was sure all other women were envious of her breasts, and that men lusted after them.

Autogynaephilic patients seem to attempt to fulfil the letter of the law but not the spirit. They wear entirely female clothing, but choose clothes where the overall impression is one of masculinity. This is often accompanied by a willingness to exaggerate or frankly lie about their degree of acceptance in a female role. Sometimes this dishonesty is readily admitted if it is suggested that they are generally still perceived as men. Sometimes it is necessary for this to be elicited by asking about which public toilets are used, and which pronoun is employed by work colleagues. Occasionally, mystified or frankly unsupportive communications from employers are needed.

Autogynaephilia is important because it may not be stable, as the case of DM shows, and as is shown more clearly in the case of EF (*see* 'Sexual deviance' p. 60). The impression is that when males present at a gender identity clinic, the prognosis is inversely related to the autogynaephilic component.

Dysmorphophobia

Dysmorphophobia is a well-known condition. When it is concerned with the nose, ears, lips, or whatever, it is usually easily recognised by psychiatrists and very often detected by surgeons – who are reluctant to offer surgical intervention. Some view it as a sort of delusional disorder, others as more akin to an obsessive rumination.

If dysmorphophobia is concerned with primary or secondary sexual characteristics there is a good chance that the person displaying the dysmorphophobia will be referred to a gender identity clinic, because the complaint will seem akin to transsexualism.

Sometimes the distinction can be easily drawn, particularly when the patient seeks no change of role and is concerned only with unwanted genitals. This teasing apart can be more difficult when it is the effects of sex steroids that elicit the phobic response, and not the organs that produce them.

Most challenging of all are those in whom the search for iatrogenic cosmetic perfection seems to have become an unachievable goal, the search often eclipsing what had earlier seemed to be uncomplicated transsexualism. The psychological picture in such cases may slowly come to resemble dysmorphophobia more than transsexualism.

The first group is those whose phobia is concerned solely with their primary sexual organs. Whilst diagnostically least challenging, this group presents great challenges in terms of management, as the following two cases show.

Case report: dysmorphophobia directed against male genitals (1)

MT, in his 20s, presented requesting amputation of his penis and scrotum. He was disappointed to learn that the gender identity clinic usually required that a real life experience be completed. He said that he had no desire to change his gender role. MT suggested that he might perhaps do so in order to satisfy the clinic requirement, obtain the amputation he wanted, and then revert to a male role.

MT also quite independently contacted urological surgeons in his home town, requesting penile and scrotal amputation, making it clear that he wanted this without any change in his lifestyle. He was annoyed to be told to obtain a referral to the gender identity clinic.

After a time, MT came to the gender identity clinic and suggested that he had now decided to change his gender role, saying he had become enthusiastic about living in a female role. A few days before he had contacted the urological surgeon reporting that he had tried changing his gender role and had concluded that he absolutely could not do so. He told the surgeon he still wanted penile and scrotal amputation.

Case report: dysmorphophobia directed against male genitals (2)

DB presented with nothing other than a profound dislike of his penis, which he saw as an ugly and unnatural growth on his lower abdomen. He showed neither psychological femininity nor any desire to live in a female role. Married with three children, his sexual life had been, in his view, purely procreative. Once his family had been completed it had ceased. His wife complained that he was always preoccupied with his penis and was almost intolerable to live with, so great was his constant irritation and distress. He felt that his life would be greatly improved if he were to be rid of both penis and scrotum, having a smooth perineum with a small, simple orifice from which to pass urine. He requested post-operative treatment with androgen depot injections to protect his bone mass, but was not concerned whether he lost or retained other male physical or psychological sexual characteristics. Despite lengthy and multiple interviews, there was never any sign of any psychosis in DB's case. Neither did psychodynamic factors seem to play a significant part in his presentation.

DB was assumed to display dysmorphophobia concerned mainly with his penis and, to a lesser extent, with his scrotum and its contents. He showed no response to full-dose antipsychotic agents. These he described as being experienced as nothing other than sedative. He did not alter with cognitive behavioural therapy. The therapist said that he could not co-operate with treatment.

Cognitive behavioural therapy might have failed because current effective cognitive therapeutic approaches have been devised for people concerned that their body parts are the wrong size or shape. The treatment often consists of asking the patient to defend the normality of the parts concerned in a debate against the therapist, who espouses the patient's usual point of view. This approach might not be suitable for patients who complain of the mere existence of a body part rather than its dimensions or appearance.

Eventually it was accepted that no other treatment seemed to have made any inroads into what was experienced as a great and growing source of distress to DB and his family. After several individual assessments with three psychiatrists and a group meeting, it was decided to accede to his request. There was to be a moratorium on any further surgical consideration of such patients until after a lengthy period of follow-up in DB's case, and then only if the initial relief was maintained, without supervening psychosis.

In the event, DB left the surgery ward the night before his penile and scrotal amputation, having stated that coincidental acute physical health problems had prevented him going through with surgery he would otherwise have wanted.

In all dysmorphophobic presentations there is, of course, grave underlying doubt about whether acceding to the initial request produces long-term psychological benefit or merely proves to be the first in an unending series of requests for bodily alterations. These in DB's case might include vaginoplasty in the absence of any desire for a change of gender role.

The second group is those people who are more phobic about the effects of sex steroids than about the organs that produce them, although the genitals may initially be of lesser concern also. Men in this group often describe an inner psychological turmoil that they attribute to androgens.

Many of these patients have earlier taken prescribed or illicit anti-androgens or estrogens, both of which decrease androgenic effects. They generally report an associated increase in well-being. Most of these patients request orchidectomy, even those whose inner distress had earlier been partly or wholly relieved by chemical means, seemingly because the loss of their testes is seen as more permanent and certain than chemical treatment. These patients do not show any other features of transsexualism and do not seek a female role. Some may make a half-hearted attempt to change gender role, in an attempt to persuade a gender identity clinic to undertake the surgery they request.

The best approach to these patients is unclear. Some come across as probably mildly gender dysphoric. One suspects that if their wishes were acceded to they would in time return in a female role requesting vulvoplasty or vaginoplasty. Others come across as much more clearly dysmorphophobic. One suspects that they seek unmasculinity rather than femininity.

Treatment presents potential physical complications in that were these patients to be deprived of all sex steroids, they would be at a greatly increased longer-term risk of osteoporosis.

It seems sensible to maintain the principle of reversible steps before irreversible ones. This principle could be followed if such patients were first treated with a gonadotrophin-releasing hormone (GnRH) analogue to quell all endogenous sex steroid release. This would temporarily achieve the same effects as an orchidectomy, causing a post-orchidectomy hormonal milieu to prevail. It tests whether the postulated state of well-being would actually happen. Such a test could be sustained for at least 6 months without unduly threatening bone mass.

If it does prove as beneficial as hoped, the question arises of whether this should be continued indefinitely. If so, consideration would have to be given to protecting bone mass in the longer term. The patients would need to be given sex steroids of some sort. Estrogens would seem to be the best choice. Careful endocrine workup is needed to calculate a dose of estrogens that would be bone protective but minimally feminising, because these patients have no demonstrated ability to cope with feminisation, and many are not requesting feminisation in any case. It seems best to avoid orchidectomy, because it is not clear whether the dysmorphophobia will always be directed to the effects of androgens or whether it will wane or transfer to some other physical attribute. Chemical treatment leaves possible a restoration of previous gonadal function.

It should be noted that the above treatment plan is not acceptable to many patients. They seem to have set their hearts on orchidectomy, and a chemically derived equivalent, even as a temporary arrangement, seems not to be acceptable. It may be that this intolerance of a non-surgical approach, even as a temporary measure, is indicative of a fundamentally different substrate to their complaint – perhaps a dysmorphophobia directed to male genitals rather than to the effects of male hormones.

The following case is one in which a GnRH analogue proved very helpful. Although a dysmorphophobia both to male genitals and to the effects of androgens was the initial problem, the former resolved when the latter was addressed.

Case report: GnRH analogue for dysmorphophobia of androgenic effects

ST was a 57-year-old man, living with his daughter and employed by a commercial organisation. He was divorced, his marriage having ended because of his cross-dressing. He initially requested gender reassignment, but gave a history more in keeping with dual-role transvestism than with transsexualism.

Further exploration over the course of several appointments revealed that ST was more troubled by the presence of a penis and testes than anything else, and particularly that his sexual drive was experienced as unwanted and troublesome. He was said to have a strong urge to castrate himself, but equally to have recognised that to do this might be life-threatening.

ST was advised that to be a candidate for gender reassignment surgery he would be required to complete a real life experience. Iinitially he seemed enthusiastic to do this. It was thought by the psychiatrist, though, that it might be difficult for him to transfer his enthusiasm into action.

This turned out to be the case. ST did not change his gender role, citing worries about the reaction of his employers and fairly limited social circle as the reasons. It was suspected that the fundamental problem was that his drive to change role was relatively weak.

He persisted in articulate expression of his distress at having male genitals, and a diagnosis of dysmorphophobia was considered.

At a panel meeting it was felt that there was a high likelihood that he would end up without his testes, either as a consequence of self-castration or because he would persuade someone to undertake this surgery. If this were to happen, it was concluded, he would experience a hormonal milieu almost entirely free of androgens. It was felt important that he experience such a state prior to any surgery, and as an investigation into what role, if any, androgenic drive had in the causation of his feelings. He was commenced on a GnRH analogue.

The GnRH analogue served dramatically to improve his state. He returned very pleased with the result, and saying that he was no longer tormented day and night with an intrusive desire to lose his genitals. His libido had entirely vanished, and he was very pleased with this, describing the treatment as giving him 'a new lease of life'.

The remaining problem was that of avoiding osteoporosis in the setting of a low sex steroid state. There was a choice between non-steroid-based bone protection of the sort used for post-menopausal women with a history of estrogen-sensitive tumours, and estrogen therapy at a dose high enough to protect bone but low enough not to be grossly feminising. The patient was very happy with either suggestion.

The last group are those in whom the search for iatrogenic cosmetic perfection seems to become an unachievable goal, the search often eclipsing what had initially seemed to be uncomplicated transsexualism. These are the most challenging of all. In this group, initially straightforward-seeming transsexualism is flavoured with an unusually strong desire for the maximal use of surgical procedures to create femininity. In many cases, this represents nothing more than an enthusiasm for surgery, but in a proportion the drive for cosmetic surgery grows until it assumes the form of a dysmorphophobic preoccupation and eclipses the initial impression of transsexualism. By this stage the patient may already have undergone a number of cosmetic surgical procedures, and one is left with an uneasy feeling that these may have exacerbated rather than relieved an underlying dysmorphophobia that should have been spotted earlier.

Case report: emerging dysmorphophobia

DP initially displayed what seemed to be straightforward transsexualism: a history of marriage and children, with covert cross-dressing increasing over the marital years. Divorce followed and a change of gender role was easily undertaken, soon followed by enthusiastically received treatment with estrogens.

DP was enthusiastic about cosmetic surgical intervention from the start. She agreed to wait until estrogens had elicited whatever natural breast growth was possible. She frequently requested increased doses of estrogens. Before long, DP had obtained a generous augmentation mammoplasty without the agreement of the gender identity clinic.

Numerous unsanctioned facial and bodily surgical procedures followed, until DP's funds ran out. Despite these, she seemed, if anything, less satisfied by her appearance, and requested very many further procedures at the state's expense. All were deemed ineligible by her funding authority.

DP declined gender reassignment surgery despite being eligible by virtue of having completed a real life experience. She argued that there was no point until the rest of her was perfect. The provision of breast implants seemed retrospectively to have been a rather negative first step, and should perhaps have been viewed (perhaps always be viewed) as a late rather than an early procedure.

Dysmorphophobia may present mixed with mild gender dysphoria, which makes the formulation of a management plan much more difficult, as the following illustrates.

Case report: dysmorphophobia mixed with mild gender identity disorder

CP presented in his mid-20s in a female role. He passed fairly poorly, wearing a dress. It would seem that he wore the dress partly to reassure himself that such things were possible, and partly in order to impress the clinic with the seriousness of his intentions.

He related first having cross-dressed at the age of 13 years, wearing mostly dresses. There appeared to have been an element of sexual excitement to this cross-dressing. Personal circumstances prevented further cross-dressing for some years. When it restarted, the cross-dressing was described as having become deeper in some way.

CP had first bought his own female clothing some 2 years earlier. He had first gone out cross-dressed 18 months earlier, going to the local town.

CP explained that what he would want more than anything would be to lose his facial hair and additionally to lose his male genitals. It was clear, however, that he did not want to live in a female role, and never had done.

CP's presentation was a curious mixture. There seemed to be dual-role transvestism, seemingly evolved from fetishistic transvestism, with a weak heterosexual drive. Present also was a much more prominent dysmorphophobic sort of desire to be rid of his primary and secondary sexual characteristics, rather than acquire a female social role. This last aspect seemed never to have been present.

'Third sex'

Very occasionally, patients without psychosis refer to themselves as being 'a third sex', or sometimes 'neutral'. These patients do not seek physical and social membership of the opposite sex by virtue of hormonal and surgical treatment. Rather, they seek treatment (usually surgical) to ablate their secondary sexual characteristics to be in a position where others cannot tell if they are male or female. This is qualitatively different from transsexualism or dual-role transvestism, and would merit a diagnosis of gender identity disorder not otherwise specified.

These patients are very uncommon, and accordingly remain mysterious. They seem mostly to be female, and to have either a poor ability at (or perhaps a low interest in) interpersonal relationships. Certainly, there seems not to be any sexual motivation behind what they seek.

Patients of this sort have nearly all had rather cold, schizoid, personalities. They have tended to lack humour. Two have been fluent in psychological-sounding jargon, yet were unable to draw abstract meaning from a common proverb.

It is unclear whether there is benefit in acquiescing to these patients' requests. Certainly, the numbers are so small that there is not even a clinical impression of prognosis. It might perhaps be best to comply with the wishes of a group of four or five such patients (on the strict understanding that they accept that a good outcome can be in no way guaranteed), and then to declare a moratorium on all others until the first four or five have been followed up for at least 5 years.

Psychosis

Psychotic patients present particular challenges in the context of a gender identity clinic. In some cases, the referring person seems unaware of the psychosis. In others the referrer is aware of the psychosis but seeks an assessment nonetheless, sometimes rather apologetically.

It is crucial to determine whether there are present both a psychotic illness and a separate (but not necessarily unconnected) gender identity disorder. If there are not clearly separate illnesses, the suspicion is that a psychotic illness is presenting with gender dysphoric symptoms.

Gender dysphoria as a symptom of psychosis is probably commoner than is usually thought to be the case. Bizarre ideas about bodily change and odd ideas about men and women are usually classified under the more general rubrics of somatic delusions or paranoid ideas. This classification having been made, the exact content is usually not noted or attended to. This is not to suggest that there is any particular significance to such content. Rather, it is suggested that less obvious forms of such delusions might accordingly be fairly common. Because of their mild degree and superficial similarity to disorders of gender identity they are not recognised as delusions. People with these signs and symptoms are consequently referred to a gender identity clinic.

History, and the texture of consultations prove the sharpest instruments in the dissection of psychosis from gender identity disorder. The second, in particular, may prompt suspicion of psychosis. Such suspicions are valuable and ought not to be ignored.

History may be revealing, particularly if the declared cross-gender feelings occurred abruptly, *de novo*, later in life or in clear association with psychosis. Often, though, patient-derived history is scant, oddly unrevealing or may feel factitious. In such cases an informant history is invaluable – from the family, GP, or anyone else who has been close to the patient. If none such is to be found, one is prompted to wonder what manner of person the patient is, to be unable to provide it.

Coincidental gender identity disorder and psychosis can be distinguished chiefly by the way in which they seem to run in parallel, rather than being part of each other. Although sometimes intertwined, they remain always separate.

At times the psychosis can be in relative or absolute remission, while the gender identity disorder remains as prominent as ever. The gender identity disorder does not seem to wax and wane as psychosis does, although the extent to which it is behaviourally expressed may vary with social or psychological circumstances.

Detecting the difference between psychosis and gender identity disorder is always hardest when the psychosis is active and problematic. At these times the separate skeins may be so closely bound that their distinct identities may be hard to discern. At times like this it may be the manner that the patient presented earlier in life, which suggests comorbid pathology. When even this clue is absent or unclear, it is still sometimes possible to disentangle the pathologies by vigorously treating the psychosis. Doing so may relieve it and thus unmask the discrete gender identity disorder.[7-9]

The following cases illustrate the difficulties encountered, and range from clear-cut cases to exceedingly challenging ones. A wide range is presented because this is a particularly difficult area.

Case report: clear psychosis presenting as gender identity disorder

PM was referred by a community mental health team with a suspected diagnosis of gender identity disorder. When he arrived he was found to be a caucasian man in his 30s, dressed in slightly unkempt but clearly female clothing, featuring a blouse, short woollen skirt and matching jacket. His head was entirely shaven, and he wore a matching hat.

PM insisted that he was female, taking pains to point out that he did not simply feel female, but actually was so. He additionally provided a statutory declaration stating that he had changed his name to one that looked decidedly oriental.

PM went on to explain that he was Singhalese, and produced a large number of documents covered in hand-written characters that might have been Singhalese. He insisted that his features were classically oriental, and was amazed that it was not immediately apparent to others. He insisted that he was Singhalese born, and that his UK birth certificate was a fraud of some sort, provided by the state as part of his adoption by his UK parents.

PM was annoyed to find that he was not going to be immediately provided with hormone treatment. He left in some dudgeon. Contact with his parents revealed that his ideas of Singhalese identity had come abruptly and coincidentally with his ideas of female sex, and that his behaviour had been a source of great worry to them.

In this case it seems quite clear that PM had a psychotic illness – probably schizophrenia – which had led to delusions concerning both his gender and his ethnic identity. This formulation was communicated to his community mental health team. It seemed an acceptable explanation to them. He was not re-referred to the gender identity clinic.

Sometimes the distinction between gender identity disorder and a psychotic illness is less easily made because there is less in the way of positive symptoms of the psychosis, as the following vignette illustrates.

Case report: psychosis mistaken for gender identity disorder

MK, aged 22 years, was referred by a local community mental health team, who felt that he had a gender identity disorder. It seemed that he had rejected a male role, and that he insisted that he be addressed by a name that was not gender-specific. The problem seemed to have started soon after he had dropped out of sixth-form college. It was said to have led to him falling out with his former circle of friends. It seemed that he spent most of his time in the parental home, and was under-occupied. His mother was said to be in despair, wanting him to move out into separate accommodation.

When seen, MK presented as a thin and slightly ill-kempt young man. He was irritable and lacked a sense of humour. He was dressed in androgynous clothes, but had made no attempt to present himself in a feminine manner. He was accompanied by his aunt and a support worker from the local community mental health team.

On mental state examination MK insisted that he had no particular gender at all. He additionally insisted that the way that society classified people as male or female was somehow wrong and deeply objectionable. He became annoyed when his aunt was referred to with a female pronoun. She reported that this annoyance with gender-denoting terms was applied to everyone. The support worker reported that the linguistic contortions that had been required to avoid the use of sex-specific pronouns had exhausted all who dealt with MK. It was said that this, among other things, had driven his former friends away. Another leading contribution to their departure was said to have been his increasingly odd behaviour and poor ability to engage in social interaction.

The support worker and MK's aunt were keen that something be done to address what they repeatedly referred to as MK's 'gender identity disorder'. It seemed that the community mental health team had thought that the situation would be improved by some sort of psychotherapeutic input from a gender identity clinic.

MK proved to have no great interest in any sort of psychotherapeutic input. He was convinced that all would be well if everyone around him could accommodate themselves to his idea that he and everyone else ought not to have any kind of sexual determination or differentiation. He saw no need to live in a female gender role. Rather, he thought that all forms of sex role were a mistaken concept.

It was felt that MK's history of social and educational decline, in combination with his beliefs, suggested psychosis rather than a gender identity disorder. Particularly out of keeping with a gender identity disorder was his insistence that it was others as well as he who ought to be treated differently in some way, along with his desire to be rid of all social gender role for himself, rather than to assume a female role. This view was communicated to the community mental health team.

MK was referred again about 5 months later, and by this time he was residing in a hostel for young people with chronic schizophrenia. He seemed to fare better in this environment, but was upset because he had been gently but firmly told that it would not be possible for everyone else to accommodate themselves to his view of the world. It was notable, though, that he still attracted a diagnosis of 'gender identity disorder' from the community mental health team. He had not yet received treatment for schizophrenia.

Sometimes it is possible clearly to distinguish psychosis from gender identity disorder after only a short period of observation, as described below.

Case report: clearly separate psychosis and gender identity disorder

FP presented at a gender identity clinic when in his late teens, with a history of childhood femininity and a sexual attraction to males. His social circumstances were chaotic, as were those of his family.

When next seen, FP had left his parental home and moved in with a drug-using relation. In this context he had changed social gender role to female.

FP proved very able to live in a female role. Although her social circle was still chaotic, her place within it was unequivocally female. She was widely perceived as female, and at one point got into a fight with an associate of her relations when she refused to prostitute herself as he suggested. The associate had no knowledge of her male anatomy.

FP presented for a routine follow-up appointment, grossly psychotic. She had auditory hallucinations and a related paranoid delusion. Although floridly mentally ill, FP remained psychologically and behaviourally female. FP was formally admitted under the Mental Health Act (1983). A period of observation indicated that this was probably a drug-related psychotic episode. It settled over the course of a fortnight.

The relationship between psychosis and gender identity disorder can sometimes be hard to establish. This is all the more true if the psychosis is so mild it might be viewed by some as eccentricity, and would not be viewed by anyone as being severe enough to make the patient liable to compulsory treatment. In these circumstances, antipsychotic agents are not likely to be taken, and thus a trial of antipsychotic treatment (which might have teased the two apart) never happens. The gender identity problems still have to treated, and are addressed in the setting of a possible psychosis. Such a situation is described below.

Case report: psychosis and gender identity disorder, possibly related

MM presented to a gender identity clinic late in life, in his mid-60s. He had a history of marriage and grandchildren, as well as of homosexual relationships. He seemed unusually concerned with the proper functioning of his penis.

MM managed to change gender role, functioning at a low level in voluntary work. A persisting problem seemed to be over-valued odd ideas about her body.

MM additionally held strong beliefs about clairvoyance. She insisted that her abilities in this regard enabled her to know that spiritual guidance was being covertly employed in the assessment of patients at the clinic.

An additional odd belief was MM's conviction that she had anal menses – something that was refuted on examination.

The nature of MM's beliefs seemed stable with time. They seemed only sometimes to reach delusional intensity. She had otherwise satisfied the clinic criteria for suitability for gender reassignment surgery, and after much careful thought and multiple opinions was advanced as a candidate for surgery. In the event, MM declined surgery, for reasons that sounded to be delusionally based.

Although abrupt, *de novo* onset of a gender identity disorder should lead to suspicions of psychosis, sometimes prolonged follow-up seems to reveal no further signs of any psychotic illness. Hormone treatment and eventual gender reassignment surgery in such a setting becomes increasingly indicated by the patient's state, but the earlier suggestion of psychosis provokes anxiety nonetheless. Such a case is described below.

Case report: Gender dysphoria with uncertain origin and some features of psychosis

HP presented to a gender identity clinic at the age of 20, saying that he wanted to be a girl. His childhood circumstances seemed unremarkable. He did about as well at school as might have been expected.

HP had no history of childhood femininity at all. He had first experienced problems with his sense of gender identity in his mid teens. He was described as having woken up feeling that things had changed in some way, and said to have looked at how other people dressed and interacted with much greater intensity than he had before. Soon after, things were said to have felt as if they had crystallised, and HP felt that he was female and wanted to live as a girl. When initially seen, HP was not sure if he wanted his body or his state of mind changed. He certainly did not wish to wear female clothes.

When first seen, HP had a weak sexual drive directed towards women, accompanied by a fear of any sort of relationship curiously combined with a strong sense of wanting one.

At this stage, there were concerns that this history might represent a delusional mood rapidly followed by a delusional perception.

Six months later, HP had quite successfully changed his social gender role to female. She continued in the same job. If anything her social and occupational functioning had improved. HP was keen to be treated with estrogens, but also worried that the feelings of femaleness might vanish as quickly as they had arrived.

Over the next 2 years HP continued to show an ever-improving occupational and social functioning. She remained free of any other suggestion of psychosis. The possibility of a psychotic origin to her sudden feelings of femaleness seemed to recede. Insight-oriented psychotherapy was instituted, on the hypothesis that a previously unconscious femininity had abruptly entered the conscious arena.

Psychosis may not initially be apparent to either referrer or assessing clinician. If it is subsequently revealed and treated, management may be made very much easier. Such a case is described below.

Case report: late diagnosis of psychosis clarifying diagnosis and treatment

AP, described as having a diagnosis of Asperger's syndrome, presented in a female role. Her father seemed to have been interested in numerology, and to have been somewhat violent. There was a subsequent poor relationship with her stepfather. The presenting relationship was with a 23-year-old woman. This partner was not happy with the patient's cross-dressing, but tolerated it. AP described her partner as being wholly content with the arrangement.

AP had considerable history of deliberate self-harm. She had briefly worked in data analysis. She asserted that this sort of work had dried up, but from the referrer's letter, the problem seemed to have been more one of difficulties in relating to others. AP had a history of methylene dioxy-metamphetamine ('ecstasy') use, but had cut off all her former friends because they were drug users. At initial assessment AP was taking estrogens illicitly, liking the effects.

AP presented with a history of having difficult relationships with others. Notably, she could not judge whether others were angry or upset. Impaired judging of social signals had caused her to leave court half-way through a hearing, and inappropriately to overstay other sorts of event.

AP stated that she had first cross-dressed at the age of 6 years, but this was not verified in her extensive child psychiatry notes. It may have been unrecorded, as the least of the worries at the time.

AP's schooling was described as 'horrible'. She developed sudden and irrational aversions to people and maintained that her peers went to college for no reason other than to persecute her. The referring psychiatrist thought she had taken to behaving particularly well purely for legal reasons, and felt she did not have insight into her behaviour and its associated problems.

At initial presentation, AP had been living in a female role for 6 months. The impression of femininity was visually impressive, but curiously came across as mimicry. At interview, she seemed to have a fair range of feelings (possibly not including affection), but very limited ability to express them. She deployed the same weak and socially unconvincing smile for all occasions, including when she felt like crying.

Six months later, AP returned. In the intervening period, she had suffered a frank paranoid psychosis and had developed the delusion that a Burmese female employee in a local chip shop was trying to poison her. She had racially abused the woman, been arrested, had attracted a diagnosis of schizophrenia and had been treated with antipsychotic agents.

On this treatment, AP's general demeanour and appearance were markedly improved. She had an emotionally warm demeanour, and talking to her was more pleasant and rewarding. She reported her thoughts as being clearer, and noted that her ability to socialise had improved.

It seemed that many of her symptoms, previously ascribed to Asperger's syndrome, had probably been due to emergent schizophrenia. On treatment with neuroleptics, what remained was a much milder, barely Asperger's-like state. AP was still entirely in a female role, and prospering. She had two or three friends, with whom she seemed to engage in ordinary social activities. Her relationship continued intact and she was making a realistic attempt to seek work.

Affective disorders

Affective disorders may be coincidental with a gender identity disorder or may present with enough features of a gender identity disorder to be mistaken for one. It is most common for depressive disorders to be coincidental, and for manic illnesses to cause diagnostic confusion.

A large proportion of those referred to a gender identity clinic have a history of treatment for depression. Often, there is no great genetic loading for affective disorder. The patient may recount a lifelong problem with gender identity that caused distress, upset or sometimes frank depression, and which was not revealed to the person treating at the time. The treatment given in these circumstances seems usually to have been that for a depressive disorder. The response to treatment is usually recorded in the medical notes of the time as having been somewhere between average and disappointing.

Patients with this sort of history seem to do well with a change of gender role. Their dysphoria usually remits, and there is often no longer any question of a depressive disorder. The subsequent rate of depressive disorder seems no higher than that of the general population, and the response to antidepressant treatment seems to be better than it was before a change of social gender role.

Patients with a genetic loading for affective disorders may also experience a gender identity disorder. They also usually arrive with a history of recurrent depression and standard treatment for depressive disorders. Their response to treatment is sometimes recorded as having shown an initial improvement but never having reached a euthymic state.

Patients with this sort of genetic loading seem to continue to experience affective instability after a change of social gender role. They do seem, though, to cope with each episode rather better and to make a more nearly complete recovery between episodes.

Depressive disorders (whether arising in a context of genetic loading or not) make any aspect of a depressed person's life more difficult. This includes a real life experience. Given the frequency of depressive episodes in the general population it seems sensible to assume as a default that depression in the context of a real life experience is coincidental, and to apply standard treatment via a GP or community mental health team. Depressive disorders in the context of a real life experience seem usually to be responsive to such treatment. Failure to respond, or the hunch of the local community mental health team psychiatrist that this is not a straightforward depressive episode, should merit particularly intense attention at a gender identity clinic.

Very rarely, a community mental health team may refer a patient with a primary depressive disorder as a primary disorder of gender identity.

Case report: depression referred as a gender identity disorder

BP was referred to a gender identity clinic by her local psychiatric services. She had a history of recurrent moderate depressive episodes, but was referred because in the latest episode she had complained of 'feeling unfeminine'. BP had a history of premature menopause, although she was stable under the treatment of the local endocrine services.

At interview, BP showed generalised feelings of low self-esteem consistent with a depressive disorder. Her 'unfeminine feelings' seemed to relate to guilt at her femininity having to be maintained by the provision of exogenous hormones. She reported neither identification with a male role, nor feelings of masculinity. Her sense of femininity recovered along with her mood. It was suspected that she would not have been referred to the gender identity clinic had she lacked the separate endocrine diagnosis.

Manic states may cause diagnostic confusion, whether or not a disorder of gender identity is present, as the following cases demonstrate.

Case report: mania referred as a gender identity disorder

GC was referred by her GP to a psychiatrist, having become convinced, after watching a television programme, that she was male and needed gender reassignment to be 'seen'. She had just moved to a new area. Her referring GP had not seen her before and had not yet received her general practice notes. She had a long history of depression, and was at that time being treated with fluoxetine.

GC was interviewed by the psychiatrist, and despite not having changed social gender role was commenced on androgen treatment. It seemed that the psychiatrist had not made much enquiry into her background or investigated any family history of mental illness. It was established that she was sexually attracted solely to women.

Two months afterwards GC was detained in hospital under the Mental Health Act (1983), a diagnosis of mania being established. She responded well to treatment. Once euthymic she lost any feelings of masculinity.

She remained well on mood stabilisers but regretted the permanently masculinised voice that resulted from the androgen treatment (*see* 'Homosexuals', p. 56)

Case report: mania causing diagnostic confusion where transsexualism is present

FC, aged 42, managed a high street bank in a medium-sized town. After a life of moral rectitude that had featured 18 years of untroubled marriage, he developed a clear manic illness. The illness built slowly, and was at first mistaken for uncharacteristically high spirits by FC's colleagues.

FC's wife was disturbed when his elevated mood was accompanied by a keen interest in cross-dressing, at first in their home but later on day trips to the adjacent town. FC became increasingly annoyed when his wife refused to accompany him on such trips. Eventually his wife elected to stay with her sister.

Alone at home, FC drank more and his mood elevated further. He presented at work in flamboyant female attire. Not long afterwards he was admitted to hospital.

FC's mood disorder quickly came under control, but his cross-dressing seemed not to recede as did his irritability and expansiveness. For some months it was viewed as a persisting manic symptom until closer enquiry revealed FC had a lifelong gender identity disorder, the expression of which had always been controlled by the rigid social mores instilled by his parents. It seemed that the mania-driven violation of these mores had broken their power, even when FC had returned to a euthymic state. This had allowed him to express what had long been repressed.

Chromosomal and hormonal abnormalities

As the ICD-10 is currently constituted, chromosomal or endocrine disorders exclude a diagnosis of transsexualism. Instead, a diagnosis of gender identity disorder not otherwise specified would apply.

This approach implies that where a chromosomal or endocrine disorder is present, the disorder should be held to account for the gender identity disorder. It also implies that transsexualism is not caused by any endocrine or hormonal disorder. Either or both of these implications may be baseless.

In practice, treatment is the same, although there is a heritability issue with partial androgen-insensitivity syndrome that needs separate attention.

Claims of chromosomal or hormonal abnormality are common, and may be supported by the GP or referring psychiatrist. They should always be subjected to confirmation, as often the apparently solid support offered to the diagnosis by the referring doctor turns out to be wholly based on the vehemence of the patient's assertion.

These assertions often include statements that the patient had 'female parts at birth', which 'had to be removed', or 'male and female chromosomes'. If followed up from general practice or local hospital records, these assertions often dwindle to accounts of surgical treatment for torsion or undescended testes, explorations of an uncomplicated hydrocele or simply genital investigations which showed a normal result, the investigations sometimes being initiated by the patient's insistence that the they were needed.

Any claims of chromosomal abnormalities in a patient investigated prior to 1980 cannot mean much more than the finding of some sort of balanced translocation, XYY syndrome or Kleinfelter's syndrome. Certainly, the level of genetic investigation required to unmask partial androgen-insensitivity syndrome was not available until quite recently.

Dementia

Dementia can present to a gender identity clinic, particularly if there is a preceding history of dual-role transvestism, as the following illustrates:

Case report: dementia

WD, aged fifty-five, presented at a gender identity clinic, pressing for the early provision of both hormone treatment and gender reassignment surgery.

He was still living in a male role, but had significantly feminised his appearance with jewellery and make-up. He was a stockbroker, and rather successful in his field.

It seemed that WD had a long history of dual-role transvestism, but that only much more recently had he decided he wanted to change gender role.

WD's history was given in an expansive manner, and he seemed highly relaxed – perhaps to the point of mild disinhibition. This seemed out of keeping with stereotypical perceptions of stockbrokers.

WD was advised that nothing irreversible would be likely to happen unless he were to change gender role first. Somewhat annoyed by this he assured the gender identity clinic that he would have done so by his next appointment.

At that next appointment WD had indeed changed role. This was said to have caused some disquiet at his work, but not as much as had his new practice of urinating in the waste paper basket. His presentation was a little more disinhibited and it was said that this disinhibition extended to all other areas of his life, much to the concern of his family. There was concern about an underlying neurodegenerative process.

These concerns turned out to be well placed, and WD went on to attract a diagnosis of presenile dementia, predominantly affecting frontal lobe function. Issues around a change of gender role became secondary to concerns about his general cognitive functioning and he dropped out of follow up at the gender identity clinic.

Sometimes dementia seems not to have been noticed or taken into account, and in these circumstances the patient can present with the consequences of such an omission, as the following illustrates:

Case report 2: dementia

AE presented to a community mental health team with symptoms characteristic of a dementing process. She had changed gender role and undergone
gender reassignment surgery no very great time earlier, and with as much
haste as possible. The assessing team suspected that her dementing illness
would have been apparent at that time, but could not be sure on this point.

It proved very difficult, in the face of rapidly advancing dementia, for AE
to continue to maintain her neovagina and her quality of life was lowered
by the development of a prolapsed neovagina as well as by advancing
cognitive decline.

References

1 Buhrich N and McConaghy N. Can fetishism occur in transsexuals? *Archives of
   Sexual Behavior* 1977; **6**: 223–35.
2 Shepherd B. *A War of Nerves: Soldiers and Psychiatrists 1914–1994*. London: Jonathan
   Cape; 2000.
3 Blanchard R. Partial versus complete autogynephilia and gender dysphoria.
   Journal of Sex and Marital Therapy 1993; **19**: 301–7.
4 Blanchard R and Collins PI. Men with sexual interest in transvestites, transsexuals,
   and she-males. *Journal of Nervous and Mental Disease* 1993; **181**: 570–5.
5 Blanchard R. Varieties of autogynephilia and their relationship to gender dysphoria. *Archives of Sexual Behavior* 1993; **22**: 241–51.
6 Miach PP, Berah EF, Butcher JN and Rouse S. Utility of the MMPI-2 in assessing
   gender dysphoric patients. *Journal of Personality Assessment* 2000; **75**: 268–79.
7 Puri BK and Singh I. The successful treatment of a gender dysphoric patient with
   pimozide. *Australian and New Zealand Journal of Psychiatry* 1996; **30**: 422–5.
8 Caldwell C and Keshavan MS. Schizophrenia with secondary transsexualism.
   Canadian Journal of Psychiatry Revue Canadienne de Psychiatrie 1991; **36**: 300–1.
9 Commander M and Dean C. Symptomatic trans-sexualism. *British Journal of
   Psychiatry* 1990; **156**: 894–6.

7

Challenging patient types and circumstances

James Barrett

Patients in forensic settings

Forensic settings can be divided into either prisons or secure hospitals of one sort or another. The assumption is that those incarcerated in the hospitals will have a mental illness, either alone or combined with a personality disorder. It is hoped that those in prison will have nothing more than the last of these.

Considering first those in a secure hospital, the diagnostic problem is much as in assessing anyone with both a mental illness and what seems to be a disorder of gender identity. The issue is to distinguish the two, or establish that the illness causes the patient to present with confusing signs reminiscent of a gender identity disorder, as is discussed earlier (*see* 'Coincidental psychosis', p. 102). The forensic environment makes this harder because patients may be less forthcoming in such a setting, for fear of incriminating themselves in some way, or otherwise incurring further limits to their freedom.

A further problem in a secure hospital setting is that group of patients with multiple sexual deviance, including autogynaephilia. Their admission to forensic psychiatric services has often been caused by behaviour associated with another of their deviant drives. They are not allowed to express most of their deviant drives, and indeed may conceal many. Their autogynaephilic drive, if presented as a disorder of gender identity, causes the authorities in the psychiatric setting to be under great pressure to allow and even support the provision of hormone treatment and a change of social gender role. A change of gender role driven by autogynaephilia has a very guarded prognosis (*see* 'Autogynaephilia', p. 35), particularly in such a setting and when wilfully presented as 'transsexualism'. It should be noted that the other deviant drives will remain present and that dangerousness will not necessarily be reduced by the provision of hormone treatment.

Case report: deviance unaltered by a change of gender role

AP was admitted to a secure hospital after having been convicted of multiple rapes. After some time in this setting, AP spoke of a desire to live as a woman, this being said to have been a lifelong preoccupation.

After much deliberation, AP changed social gender role and lived with some success in a female role in a secure hospital setting. Sexual orientation remained towards women.

In time, AP was thought to represent a reasonable candidate for gender reassignment surgery, and this was performed. After this, whenever sexually segregated circumstances were directed by the authorities in the secure setting, she was allocated to female areas.

AP's psychological and social functioning was thought to have improved after a change of social gender role. The improvement was sustained after gender reassignment surgery. Of note, though, was that before and after both social gender role change and subsequent gender reassignment surgery, AP continued to behave in a sexually predatory manner. She simply moved from male heterosexual to lesbian sexually predatory behaviour.

Role of the prison medical service

The UK Prison Medical Service is part of the NHS. Accordingly, there is a duty to recognise and subsequently to provide (or allow to be provided) assessment and treatment of disorders of gender identity. This duty seems not to be discharged in the case of short-term or remand prisoners, possibly because time would not allow much to be done.

Longer-term prisoners do obtain attention from a gender identity clinic, although their management is greatly complicated by their incarcerated status (*see* 'Forensic patients and the real life experience', p. 113).

Homosexuals

It used once to be quite common to see gay and lesbian patients referred to a gender identity clinic. They were usually rather feminine gay men or masculine lesbians who turned out, on interview, to have no desire to function in the other social gender role and had no more dissatisfaction with their appearance than anyone else might – certainly nothing as fundamental as dissatisfaction with their biological sex.

This is no longer frequent in the UK. Few gay men or lesbians are so unaware of their nature and the nature of human sexuality as to misattribute an erotic liking for their own sex as a feeling of being of the opposite sex. This can still occur, particularly if there is coincidental mental illness (*see* 'Coincidental non-psychotic mental illness', p. 101), although sometimes in the absence of such illness. Very occasionally, gay men and lesbians briefly change gender role before reverting to their former role. Physical problems arising from this can be limited by not initiating irreversible treatment unless strictly necessary (*see* Case report: relationship issues and reversion to former role in 'Reversion to former gender role', p. 258).

Community mental health teams may refer gay men and lesbians because they say they want to 'change sex'. Their referrals fall into two groups, in the main.

The first, all men, are people who seem to be gay secondary transsexuals, having previously seen themselves as homosexual dual-role transvestites. One such is described on page 27 (insidiously advancing femininity).

The second group, composed of men and women, come from cultures or subcultures where being gay or lesbian is unmentionable or even unthinkable. In these cases, the reasoning behind wanting to 'change sex' seems to be the belief that this logically follows if one experiences an emotional or sexual interest in the same sex. In some of these cases there is an added religious component, the patients seeking some sort of biological 'proof' that they are really of the opposite sex, in order religiously to legitimise emotional and sexual drives which would otherwise be utterly unacceptable.

As a rule, these latter patients fare well after being referred to a low-key group for people unsure about their sexual orientation, such as London Friend.* They often fail to return for follow-up. Those who do return usually look excited and pleased. They say that they have met some quite fascinating people and are thinking of how they might extend their stay in the UK.

Those presenting for these sorts of cultural reasons need not necessarily come from outside western Europe, as the following shows.

Case report: European cultural presentation

CP, a Spanish man, came from a society where he saw the macho elements of culture as personally repressive. He felt he was kept as a prisoner in his own house 'as if I was a woman'. A sensitive child, he experimented with cross-dressing when he was in his early teens. Early sexual arousal was to the sight of women, but first sexual experiences were with other males his age, in the form of mutual masturbation. The other males identified themselves as straight. CP had a small penis and felt inferior. He began to wonder whether it would be 'better to have the operation to be a woman'. This was encouraged by some of the men with whom he was having sex, who said 'if you were a woman you could have full sex'. His cross-dressing was encouraged by these acquaintances, who might themselves have had feelings of guilt about their own homosexuality.

CP's family found out about the sexual contacts and were disgusted. He moved to another city and lived with a transsexual friend who encouraged him to take hormones, and consequently he grew breasts. CP formed the idea that if he were fully female he would be happier.

Moving to London, CP made many sexual contacts, but rejected the thought of any emotional intimacy. He identified himself as bisexual but seemed chiefly interested in men. He lived wholly as a man. He became embarrassed by his breasts (which were later removed). CP still had fleeting doubts about whether he would really like to be a woman, but said that if he had wanted this he would have gone further earlier, when it was more easily possible. CP hid his breasts and was no longer pleased but rather annoyed when sexual partners (men) paid attention to them.

Religious reasons, often in concert with deep involvement with a religious subculture, may cause western European lesbians and gay men sometimes to present to a gender identity clinic with complaints of a gender identity disorder, as the following illustrates.

---

* London Friend, 86 Caledonian Road, London, N1 9ND. Tel: 0207 837 3337/0207 833 1674 (lesbian)

Case report: religiously motivated presentation by a lesbian

LP presented looking like a lesbian woman, with a partner who looked similarly feminine. She had a history of marriage and a son, and had left her husband with help from the gay Christian movement. She had changed her name, but to a name where male and female forms are homophones if not the same in spelling. Her personal mannerisms were more characteristically female than those of her partner. Sexual relations were reported to be no problem to either.

LP had changed her work registration to that of a male employee and wore a male work uniform. Despite this, she was regarded by her colleagues as a woman who wore a male uniform.

At interview, LP's partner referred to her throughout as 'she'. LP reported meeting people who remarked on her name being spelt in the masculine way, and said that she responded by saying that this was becoming commoner among women. She did not correct their having apprehended her as female. Her view was that this was her private concern, and that telling everyone of her aspiration for male status would constitute an invasion of her privacy.

LP had managed to be referred for a bilateral mastectomy, on the grounds of positive family history of early breast cancer. Outside work she wore clothes that, although technically male, gave an overall impression of femininity. Her hairstyle was unmistakably female, if short, and it emerged that she had not changed her hairdresser or informed the hairdresser of her change of status.

Her partner understood that she might be regarded as not living in a male role rather better than did LP herself. LP seemed to see any such suggestion as implying that she was not taking the matter seriously. She seemed to feel that if she underwent treatment with hormones she would somehow be taken as male, without the trauma of having to tell anyone.

A major factor preventing LP from clearly changing social gender role seemed to be her belief that if she did so she would be drummed out of her religious community. Throughout interviews she referred to herself as a woman, and indeed said that she was – 'albeit technically'.

LP had a personal theory proposing a biological explanation of transsexualism. She applied this to herself, and felt it divorced her from any choice or personal religious responsibility for how she felt. She had no such theories for homosexuality, which she viewed as sinful. It seemed that her parents were wholly disapproving of both homosexuality and transsexualism.

Religiously concerned patients can usefully seek guidance from their faith leaders. They often find their faiths are less condemnatory than the lay religious community think they are, or than the patients imagine they will be. Knowing that the strictures of their faith are broadly supportive seems often to help those who earlier saw themselves as being trapped between the dictates of their nature and what they wrongly understood to be the rules of their faith.

Sometimes, personality structure can make it difficult to distinguish between a gender identity disorder of some sort and homosexuality. Such a case is described in the section devoted to personality disorders (*see* p. 65)

Social responses to homosexuality vary considerably across the world. A negative view of homosexuality may, as above, cause homosexual people to present to a gender identity clinic. While the cases described above have involved the patient voluntarily presenting, this has not always been so.

The South African Defense Force received conscripts from the white community of Apartheid South Africa. The society was one that viewed homosexuality very negatively. It seems that the Defense Force's response to homosexual recruits was to attempt to 'cure' them of their homosexuality. Those who were not 'cured' were, it seems, forced on occasion to undergo forced gender reassignment surgery. Not much is known of the subsequent trajectories of the individuals so treated.[1,2]

Prostitute patients

It is not common for people seen in a UK gender identity clinic to have worked or still be working as prostitutes, though it may be more common elsewhere.[3,4] It poses problems when it is encountered, and is suggested by the patient as something that should count as an occupation for real life experience purposes.

As with any other service occupation, those who work as prostitutes do so with varying degrees of competence. One sometimes encounters a highly organised patient with a regular clientele, a secure and specially rented working environment, reception arrangements and staffing, and discreet but effective security. It is hard to see this as anything other than an occupation.

Equally, one sometimes encounters those who work alone from their own homes, who have been robbed and beaten up by their clients. The impression is that of desperation rather than any sort of workable occupation.

Either way, prostitution is highly problematic as an occupation for the purposes of a real life experience. The main problem is that no matter how well organised the patient is, the clientele are paying for the services of a pre-operative transsexual. There is no reason to suppose that when post-operative the same individual will be able to make a living. She will be in a much more competitive market, having born females as competition.

Accordingly, prostitution ought probably not to be accepted as an occupation for the purposes of a real life experience. This makes no comment on whether prostitution should be considered as an occupation in any other context.

A sexually transmitted disease clinic's staff reported that transsexual people are a concern to them. It seemed to them that there was a tendency for the clients (almost all male-to-female) to show a low rate of barrier contraceptive use. The impression was that the individuals were very glad to have been treated as female in a sexual context, and were unwilling to jeopardise the sexual encounter by insisting on condom use. A further complication seemed to be the patients' reluctance, if infected with a sexually transmitted disease, to consult a sexually transmitted disease clinic. This seemed to be based in both a reluctance to attend to any sort of pelvic sensation or symptom, and to a reluctance to be in an environment where one's penis gets particular attention.

Sexual deviance

Transvestism is the commonest sexual deviance seen in a gender identity clinic, being either fetishistic or dual-role. Autogynaephilia also presents with some frequency. Both are covered separately (*see* Chapter 6 p. 31). Both may be present with other forms of deviance, and these and the others may not be disclosed.

Other sorts of sexual deviance may be seen in a gender identity clinic, examples of which follow.

Case report: rubber fetish presenting as a disorder of gender identity

TQ presented in an unremarkable male role. He was dressed in casual clothing, with a shaved head. He gave a history of rubber fetishism of many years' standing.

TQ had made a relationship with a woman, but had found sexual expression impossible unless his partner wore skin-tight rubber clothing. The relationship had fared well at first, but after a time his partner had developed the feeling that he was more sexually interested in the rubber clothing than in her. The relationship had become increasingly strained, and after a time had broken down altogether.

After the separation from his partner, TQ had developed the idea that he would be better off if he were to live as a woman. He was quite sure, though, that he would be a woman with a shaved head who always wore a red rubber dress.

TQ discussed his aspirations, and was reluctantly forced to conclude that his aspirations would be unlikely to be realised. He concluded that a shaved head in combination with an initially male appearance would make it so difficult for him to pass as female that no amount of additional hormonally mediated feminisation would enable him to achieve a satisfactory degree of social acceptance. He thought that the rubber dress would be likely to hinder rather than help him in being accepted as female.

Whilst the above fetish is a disorder of sexual object, as is transvestism, sexual deviance of other sorts may also be seen, as illustrated below.

Case report: sadomasochism presenting as a gender identity disorder

LD, a plumber, presented requesting 'a sex change'. It quickly emerged that he wanted to be a woman in order that he might 'become a lesbian'. He thought that a lesbian identity would make it possible for him to be manacled to a table while two women had sex with each other and refused to let him join in.

Discussion with LD led him to conclude that even were he to achieve a female social role it would still be unlikely that this fantasy would be realised. He began to wonder whether it might be more possible if the other participants were paid performers, and thought that the experience would be just as satisfactory if they were.

Sometimes sexual deviance is concealed, there remaining just the hint of it from the patient's conduct, as below. It is not clear in these circumstances whether the sexual deviance is coincidental to the gender identity disorder, or stands alone and has caused the patient to present with claims of a gender identity disorder, the true motivation being otherwise.

Case report: possible sexual deviance

HB was an older male patient who changed gender role with difficulty, but did manage to sustain a female role as a middle-aged woman. She had speech and language therapy, and in the course of this was noted to have stolen the speech and language therapist's hairbrush. Both before and after this she had often remarked on hairstyle as a social marker for femininity, and had commented favourably on the speech and language therapist's own hair and its styling.

Fetishes congregate together, and may wax and wane so that as one diminishes another seems to grow in its place. The following account demonstrates this. It is important also because in this case autogynaephilia was one of a series of sexual disturbances, each of which waned with time and was replaced with another.

Case report: progressively shifting pattern of sexual deviance

BS first presented in her late 20s, in a male role, and requested hormone treatment and a change of gender role. At this time, she gave an account of early fetishistic cross-dressing, but suggested that it had developed into a more dual-role sort of transvestism. She changed gender role with relative ease and lived with some success in a female role.

In due course, BS had completed 2 years' life in a female role and was considered to be a candidate for gender reassignment surgery. At this stage, she said that she did not want gender reassignment surgery, and was happy to continue as she was.

As she was followed up, BS's appearance became slightly more androgynous with each appointment. Finally, she presented wearing a surgical arm support of the sort that was once used to brace the limbs of people with a polimyelitic paralysis.

BS at this stage disclosed that at her original appointment she had concealed an earlier history of a fetishistic interest in leather clothing. This fetish had begun to decline in intensity and had been replaced by an increasing autogynaephilia. This had motivated her initial appointment, although she had chosen to conceal it.

It seemed that BS's autogynaephilia had in turn waned, and had come to be replaced by an erotic arousal at the thought of having a mutilated and deformed arm.

BS said that she now felt very much less female than once she did, and that she was indifferent about whether she was perceived as male or female. She suspected that in time she might revert to a male role, and had in any case stopped taking estrogens.

BS had thought of putting her arm under a moving train or lorry in order that it might be mutilated, but had concluded that sexually attractive though the prospect of mutilation was, to do so might be foolish in the longer term because, she thought, the mutilated arm fetish would probably wane, just as had the leather fetish and the autogynaephilia.

BS was glad that she had not had gender reassignment surgery. She added that, had it been offered earlier than it was, her state of mind at the time would probably have been such that she would have accepted the offer, only to regret it later.

Gender reassignment surgery with no role change

It is rare for people to undergo gender reassignment surgery without first living in their preferred gender role. When it occurs, the results are often unhappy. The following describe the sort of circumstances in which this might occur, and the associated outcomes.

Case report: no gender identity disorder with gender reassignment surgery prior to role change

TP was an impulsive and narcissistic man, married, in his 40s with three children. He had a lifelong history of fetishistic cross-dressing. This provoked considerable feelings of religious guilt. After masturbating, TP had often wanted to throw all his clothes and make-up away. He also made frequent use of transvestite and transsexual pornography, again with accompanying guilt. Sexual relations with his wife had dwindled to mutual masturbation.

TP wanted 'help'. He formed the view that he would be best placed to decide what sort of help would be needed. He was initially interested in orchidectomy or anti-androgens, and was said at the time to be ambivalent about gender reassignment surgery. He sought, and obtained, treatment with estrogens. These worked to produce relief from his emotional tumult by lowering his libido and removing the sexual element from his continued domestic cross-dressing. TP drew from this relief the inference that he must be transsexual.

TP began occasionally to frequent transvestite clubs. He formed the view that he would be better off living as a woman. His views were reinforced by those transvestites to whom he spoke, and were further supported by the opinions of others, with whom he corresponded on the internet.

TP concluded that the World Professional Association for Transgender Health, Inc. (formerly the Harry Benjamin Gender Dysphoria Association) criteria for gender reassignment surgery were 'hurdles' put in patients' way, and that it was not reasonable to expect someone who was biologically male to live as a woman without surgery. He felt that such a man would become a laughing stock. TP's wife supported him in these views because he seemed so sure he was right.

TP went abroad to have gender reassignment surgery. He had doubts about his plans the night before the surgery, but felt he had travelled too far in psychological, geographical and financial terms to back out at that stage. He regretted the surgery the moment he regained consciousness, and rang his wife immediately saying he regretted it and was suicidal.

TP returned to his own country and made contact with a gender identity clinic. He pressed for an unusually urgent assessment in view of what he felt was the seriousness of his case. He was in a torment of regret at the situation he found himself in, but without regret that he was architect of the situation. Psychotherapeutic services felt that if he felt a sense of his own responsibility for his plight (probably inevitable) he might develop serious suicidality.

Gender reassignment surgery without role change does not work out well even if there is a disorder of gender identity present, as the following illustrates.

Case report: possible gender identity disorder with gender reassignment surgery prior to role change

RY had a lifelong belief that he ought to have been born female, and a conviction that if he were to live as a woman he would have a better quality of life and function better in most regards.

RY did not want to change his gender role prior to any surgical or hormonal treatment. He reasoned that it would not be possible for him to function in a female role while he still looked physically male. RY was impulsive by nature. He felt that hormone treatment was too slow to effect bodily change, and that the results of such treatment were not going to be as predictable as those that could be obtained by surgical intervention.

RY was reasonably rich. He elected to leave the country and have surgical treatment overseas in a country where it was both more easily afforded and also available without what he saw as the unnecessary interference of psychiatric services. He underwent gender reassignment surgery with vaginoplasty, a bilateral augmentation mammoplasty with generous implants, and a series of cosmetic procedures that altered his cheekbones, jaw line and other features of his face. In essence, RY had everything that it was surgically possible to undergo.

Having recovered from the surgery, RY returned to his own country. He found that despite the earlier procedures, and being utterly clean-shaven, those he met still apprehended him as being his old self. They remarked that he looked a bit different and was wearing some sort of false breasts.

RY tried moving in areas where he had not previously been known. He found that despite never having known him before the people he met still apprehended him as male, but with large breasts.

After a time RY paid a considerable sum in his own country to have the generous breast implants removed, and as much as was technically possible of the earlier cosmetic surgical effects reversed. At this stage, he sought a referral to a gender identity clinic to discuss his position. He still wanted to live as a woman but was very shaken by his earlier experience.

Bilateral mastectomy without role change

Bilateral mastectomy without role change is sometimes requested in a gender identity clinic. Those requesting this seem to fall into two main groups.

The first are patients who come across as lesbians with a mild degree of gender dysphoria, but not enough to make them want to change their social gender role. Many of these have earlier tried to elicit a bilateral mastectomy on the grounds of a family history of breast cancer, or of having awkwardly large breasts.

As a rule surgeons are reluctant to offer a bilateral mastectomy on the grounds of cancer risk, preferring instead to offer increased surveillance if a truly increased risk of cancer is confirmed.

Patients who request bilateral mastectomy on the grounds of having awkwardly large breasts do sometimes elicit a reduction mammoplasty, but the resulting smaller breasts are still identifiable as breasts and, accordingly, still troublesome to the patients.

Bilateral mastectomy provided to mildly gender-dysphoric lesbians is little researched, and there are no reliable data concerning outcomes. It may be that many such requests come from patients whose mild gender dysphoria will go on to increase in intensity, and for whom a bilateral mastectomy will be a first step towards eventual social gender role change. Whether a bilateral mastectomy has an effect on the rate of progression of the gender identity disorder is not clear.

The second group of patients requesting a bilateral mastectomy without a change of gender role are those who are more deeply gender dysphoric but have a long-term relationship with a lesbian partner. They want a bilateral mastectomy because it is the most their partner would tolerate and the least they would accept by way of addressing their psychological discomfort. Such a case is described below.

Case report: request for bilateral mastectomy without role change

LM presented alone, looking like a very masculine lesbian. She requested a bilateral mastectomy.

LM had a long-term relationship with a lesbian partner of similar age. They functioned as a couple, and had a joint bank account.

Conversation with LM revealed her to be profoundly gender dysphoric, but also very much in love with a partner upon whom she was financially and emotionally dependent. She saw a bilateral mastectomy as 'all I would want', but almost immediately after stating this added that her voice was a problem as she found it distressingly feminine.

A subsequent interview with LM's partner was illuminating. The partner was an unremarkably lesbian woman with a preference for masculine partners. She said that LM was more psychologically masculine than any of the equally mannish looking lesbians in their social circle. She added that although she was attracted to masculine women she was not attracted to men, and that she was disturbed by LM's increasing desire to masculinise herself.

Conversation with the couple revealed that a bilateral mastectomy was felt to represent a compromise between their desires. Further exploration exposed LM's profound gender dysphoria, and LM admitted that it was likely that in no great time she would be unhappy with the compromise of a bilateral mastectomy and seeking treatment with androgens. It was agreed that a bilateral mastectomy would probably be a step resented by both.

Both LM and her partner decided to seek help from Relate to establish whether their partnership had a long-term future. The clinical impression was that it would be preferable for LM to make a discrete change of social gender role and if this worked, later undergo hormone treatment and bilateral mastectomy. An initial bilateral mastectomy seemed likely to become just another part of the drawn-out decline in the relationship being caused by LM's ever-increasing psychological masculinity – an accompanying inch-by-inch physical transformation being rather less effective by being done piecemeal.

Personality disorder

It is hard to make definitive statements about the rate of personality disorder in the setting of a gender identity clinic. Levine reported that although female patients were significantly healthier than the males, 92% of the males and 58% of the females had psychiatric diagnoses, apart from gender dysphoria.[5] Most of the abnormalities in both groups were character disorders, but 8% had schizophrenia.

More recently, Hepp et al reported a 42% rate of personality disorder.[6]

These sorts of findings have not been seen in larger studies in adults. Haraldsen et al found 86 transsexual people generally scored slightly higher on a Symptom Checklist 90 rating scale than healthy controls, but that all scores were within the normal range.[7] Cole et al studied 318 male and 117 female patients.[8] Less than 10% had problems associated with mental illness, genital mutilation, or suicide attempts. Overall, results supported the view that transsexualism was usually an isolated diagnosis and not part of any general psychopathological disorder. Similar results were found in adolescents, which supported the idea that major psychopathology was not required for the development of transsexualism.[9,10] It seemed that the findings of smaller studies might have represented a sampling bias.

Gender identity disorders may be seen coincidentally with personality disorders. Personality disorders may also cause patients to present either with claims of having a gender identity disorder or seeming as if they have a gender identity disorder. An example of the first follows.

Case report: schizoid personality and probable mild gender identity disorder

AP presented at a gender identity clinic in her 30s, with a clearly schizoid personality. She had always lived in a slightly masculine female role, and had always wished that she might be more masculine still. She had always been socially isolated by her own choice and had never made any sort of relationship. She was said to fantasise about a relationship with a woman, she herself taking a male role.

AP described childhood gender problems, with masculine behaviour from her earliest years. The expression of her feelings of maleness was said to have been inhibited by her general social awkwardness. She was about as masculine looking as this limitation had allowed her to be.

AP had a history of securing and preferring solitary jobs. She seemed clear that she would never be in a position to change her social gender role. Her primary complaint was menstruation, with secondary dislike of her breasts. She sought a hysterectomy.

It was concluded that AP was hard to assess because of her personality style. It was thought that she probably had a disorder of gender identity, but that it remained possible that she might be a rather masculine lesbian woman. Either way, it was thought, a relationship seemed exceedingly unlikely, and a desire for fertility even more so. In the circumstances, there seemed to be no sensible reason to resist her desire for a hysterectomy.

The following illustrates a more problematic personality disorder, again in concert with a probable genuine disorder of gender identity.

Case report: borderline personality disorder (impulsive type)

DD presented to a gender identity clinic in his mid 30s. He came from a family with a clear history of impulsive as well as self- and socially destructive behaviour.

DD appeared to be angry from his very first consultation. The referrers noted that this seemed to be his baseline emotional state. He immediately denigrated the clinic, and refused to comply with any conditions regarding smoking or weight loss and refused to wear female clothing before it was ever asked of him. He said that the request, were it to come, would be part of an attempt to brainwash him and to make him look foolish.

Over time, DD's attendance was erratic, although she did start to live in a clearly female role. Smoking cessation was followed by the prescription of estrogens. This prescription was rapidly followed by a resumption of smoking.

DD continued to show socially destructive behaviour. A local hospital refused to provide care because of violent behaviour. She spent some time in a male prison, in a female role.

It was felt that DD had a gross disorder of personality, but that she also did have a disorder of gender identity and that her functioning was better in a female role, if still very disordered. After many consultations she was advanced as a candidate for gender reassignment surgery.

DD did not undergo gender reassignment surgery because she refused to be examined by the surgeon, or to turn up to appointments on time, and proved unwilling to lose the weight necessary for her to be a safe candidate for such surgery, and to stop smoking. Her increasingly sporadic contact with the surgical services caused the funding approval for her surgery to lapse.

Personality issues causing a presentation resembling a gender identity disorder need not always be of classical and enduring types of personality disorder. More transient disturbances in personality and sense of self may also present in this way, as the following illustrates.

Case report: abnormal grief reaction

LS presented to a gender identity clinic in his late 30s. He presented in female dress, and having changed to a female name. He came across as decidedly male nonetheless.

LS's desire to live as a woman clearly dated from the death of his sister, to whom he was described as having been very close. Her death at a relatively early age from cancer was said to have devastated him. He cried copiously in the clinic when relating her slow decline.

LS had a history of mid-adolescent fetishistic transvestism. It seemed to have become less intense until the death of his sister, when he had been seized with a desire to live in a female role.

It emerged that LS had informally adopted his sister's name (although he had made no formal legal change) and was wearing her clothes. His hair was 'styled in her same way'. Informants disclosed that the resemblance was striking and rather disturbing, and that the illusion that his sister lived again was only broken when he moved or spoke.

It was suggested to LS that he might be experiencing some sort of grief reaction. Indeed, he seemed to have partial insight into this. A referral for insight-oriented psychotherapy with particular attention to bereavement was thought to be the best course.

References

1 Kaplan RM. Treatment of homosexuality during apartheid. *British Medical Journal* 2004; **329**: 1415–16.
2 Kaplan RM. Treating homosexuality as a sickness: psychiatric abuses during apartheid era have not been brought to account. *British Medical Journal* 2004; **328**: 956.
3 Lombardi EL and van Servellen G. Correcting deficiencies in HIV/AIDS care for transgendered individuals. *Journal of the Association of Nurses in AIDS Care* 2000; **11**: 61–9.
4 Zaccarelli M, Spizzichino L, Venezia S, Antinori A and Gattari P. Changes in regular condom use among immigrant transsexuals attending a counselling and

testing reference site in central Rome: A 12 year study. *Sexually Transmitted Infections* 2004; **80**: 541–5.

5   Levine SB. Psychiatric diagnosis of patients requesting sex reassignment surgery. *Journal of Sex and Marital Therapy* 1980; **6**: 164–73.

6   Hepp U, Kraemer B, Schnyder U, Miller N and Delsignore A. Psychiatric comorbidity in gender identity disorder. *Journal of Psychosomatic Research* 2005; **58**: 259–61.

7   Haraldsen IR and Dahl AA. Symptom profiles of gender dysphoric patients of transsexual type compared to patients with personality disorders and healthy adults. *Acta Psychiatrica Scandinavica* 2000; **102**: 276–81.

8   Cole CM, O'Boyle M, Emory LE and Meyer WJ 3rd. Comorbidity of gender dysphoria and other major psychiatric diagnoses. *Archives of Sexual Behavior* 1997; **26**: 13–26.

9   Smith YL, van Goozen SH and Cohen-Kettenis PT. Adolescents with gender identity disorder who were accepted or rejected for sex reassignment surgery: a prospective follow-up study. *Journal of the American Academy of Child and Adolescent Psychiatry* 2001; **40**: 472–81.

10 Cohen L, de Ruiter C, Ringelberg H and Cohen-Kettenis PT. Psychological functioning of adolescent transsexuals: personality and psychopathology. *Journal of Clinical Psychology* 1997; **53**: 187–96.

Part 2

The real life experience

8

The real life experience: introduction

James Barrett

Waiting lists (particularly the shortening of waiting lists) have been a recurring theme in the semi-socialised UK NHS. Patients have to wait for routine surgery, and the government determines the maximum time they should wait and the degree of consistency in such waiting times across the country.

Gender identity clinic patients seem sometimes to feel that the provision of gender reassignment surgery is governed by the same rules. So it is. What they often fail to grasp, though, is that as the NHS currently works, any waiting time commences only after a surgeon has accepted them as a candidate for gender reassignment surgery. Instead, many patients feel that simply attending the gender identity clinic for a sufficient length of time ought to qualify them for gender reassignment surgery. I have often heard such remarks as 'I've been coming to this clinic for over 5 years now, so why haven't I got my surgery? I know someone who only came here for 3 years and she got her surgery. It's not fair!'

The point, of course, is that suitability for gender reassignment surgery is not determined solely by the length of time the patient has attended a gender identity clinic – although a certain minimum time must apply. Rather, it depends upon whether the patient has been seen to be or to have become a suitable candidate in the time that they have attended.

For some, this might be settled after the minimum period. For others grave worries might persist even after years of attendance. The question is whether the patient has demonstrated a satisfactory adjustment to a new gender role in a real-life setting. This might be termed a 'real-life test' (of suitability for surgery).

A real-life experience is the experience of living in a new gender role, and is very likely to last the remainder of the patient's days. Although the terms 'real-life test' and 'real life experience' are sometimes used as synonyms it would be fairer to say that for patients who want surgery, particularly genital surgery, a defined first part of a real life experience might constitute a test, while the rest will not. For patients who do not want surgery, the real life experience contains no defined test period at all. It is to be noted that there is usually demonstrable psychological benefit to a change of gender role alone, as the following illustrates.

Case report: benefits of a change of role

FP changed gender role to female in her mid 30s. She was employed by a large industrial manufacturing company. Some time after her change of role she applied for promotion within the company.

> By chance, FP was interviewed by exactly the same panel of people who had earlier appointed her in a male role. They granted her promotion. Later, they remarked how much better she had interviewed in a female role. She was described as having been more animated, and somehow sharper minded and more confident.

Any psychological benefits seen with a change of gender role are usually enhanced by subsequent gender reassignment surgery. It is assumed that if there is no benefit from a change of role alone, subsequent gender reassignment surgery is, if anything, likely to be detrimental.

The 'real-life test' is thus a period in which the patient is required successfully to live in the chosen gender role. Its length is arbitrary but not capricious. Success in this setting is a condition to be met before a referral for gender reassignment surgery. At Charing Cross Hospital, a period of 2 years is used, rather than the internationally accepted absolute minimum of 1 year. Several patients who have seemed to be good candidates at 12 months have seemed very much less so at 18. The same observation has been made in other gender identity clinics. This gives some support to the strategy. Furthermore, dropouts from the post-referral waiting list are known. This again suggests that there would be no advantage in decreasing the duration of the real life experience. There is, however, research that suggests postponing surgery too long also carries with it increased psychopathology, suggesting little merit in much increasing the duration of the real life experience.

There are regrettably few reports answering whether making the requirements of a real life experience more rigorous would carry any advantage. What follow-up studies exist tend to concentrate on surgical outcomes, and tend to conclude that gender reassignment surgery is of benefit in carefully selected subjects. There are few reports on exactly how these subjects who do so well were selected. There are some reports outlining features common to patients whose surgical outcome was less good, which might help with the exclusion of the less suited. They do not advance the inclusion of the more suited though.

The question immediately arises of what constitutes 'success' in a chosen gender role. In essence, 'success' amounts to occupational, sexual, relationship and psychological stability. Of these, the first can be measured by whether of not the patient can manage to hold down a full-time (or equivalent part-time) occupation in the chosen role for a year, in the course of the real life experience. A second question arises, namely what constitutes an 'occupation'?

An occupation can be defined as almost any job, with a few exceptions outlined below; it includes almost any government training scheme and any educational course, provided it is not 'distance learning'. Any voluntary work would also prove acceptable.

Unacceptable occupations would include work in a purely transvestite or transsexual environment, because others may be supranormally accepting. Also included would be prostitution, because prostitute patients are working not as women but as 'transsexuals'. It is unclear whether they would continue to find work once they looked like other women rather than clearly transsexual.

'Success' in an occupation is achieved if the patient is treated by most others **as if** they are of the assumed sex. It is not necessary that those around the patient believe that they *are* that sex. Few patients pass this well in their new role, and many work with others who knew them before they changed gender role. Rather than being believed to be the assumed sex, the goal should be being taken as and treated as that sex. It is essential that the patient feels confident that this is occurring and is comfortable with their new role. Someone tormented by daily doubts about whether they are accepted in their new role, however well they objectively pass in that role, is living under a great stress which might prove unendurable in the longer term. It will in no way be altered by surgery to their genitals.

A frequent problem concerns dress. Patients seem often to have been advised that they should wear a dress, skirt or (for female patients) man's suit for appointments at a gender identity clinic. It seems that they have been advised that anything else will in some sense count against them. This is wholly untrue.

It is not the function of a gender identity clinic to operate as some kind of style council concerning what does and does not constitute feminine or masculine dress. After some years of seeing a very wide range of sartorial presentations, the judgement of gender identity clinic staff is likely to be very far from the norm.

All that is required is that those around them accept patients in their new gender roles. Provided this is achieved, it does not matter what sort of clothing is worn. In an occupation such as driving a forklift truck, for example, wearing a Laura Ashley frock would be seen not as feminine but as foolhardy. Better acceptance as female would probably be achieved if dungarees were worn.

Rather the reverse problem is seen in patients who seem to their psychiatrists to pass very poorly, who are without verifiable occupation, and who claim to be living their life in the new gender role. Such patients may sometimes base their claim upon wearing the appropriate underwear, proudly stating how long they have been in this habit. More often, they state that every item of their clothing is appropriate to their new gender. Often this is technically true, but the final combination that has resulted seems not to be so. A good psychological check is to ask whether a non-gender-disordered person of the same build and biological sex could wear the clothes up the high street without drawing a second glance. If this is the case, it seems to be fair to say that the clothes are taken to be those of the birth sex, despite having been purchased in the other sex's clothing store. This can usefully be pointed out to such patients.

Another test is that of asking patients whether strangers would address the patient as male or female and, if they asked where the nearest toilet was, which sex's toilet would be suggested to them.

Some patients fiercely maintain that they do not care what others think of them, and that their own conviction of their gender is what matters. This position is at odds with the philosophy of a real life experience and if followed seems not to be predictive of a good longer-term outcome. Carried to a logical conclusion, this argument leads to the view that no change of social gender role is necessary before gender reassignment surgery. This might be philosophically sound, but is associated with a poor outcome (*see* 'Gender reassignment surgery with no role change' p. 62).

The real life experience should be considered to have started on the day the patient was last in their biological gender role, for whatever reason. Reverting to the original role for a special occasion carries with it a poor prognosis, suggesting as it does that the patient sees the change of role as essentially reversible.

9

Common issues

James Barrett

Occupational matters

See also 'Legal issues', p. 259.

An 'occupation' can be defined broadly or narrowly, and the most practical definition will depend on the prevailing social circumstances, particularly with regard to the availability of paid work. It seems best to define an 'occupation' widely at a time when paid work is less available, and more narrowly when it is.

Patients commonly assume that a change of social gender role will require a change of occupation, particularly if their occupation is stereotypical of their birth sex. This assumption is not well founded for the following reasons:

- frequently workmates have suspected something and may react with rather less surprise than the patient expects
- it is easier to avoid being fired by bigoted employers (or successfully to sue them if one is fired) than it is to gain new employment from other bigoted employers (or successfully to sue them for an unfair failure to appoint)
- changing from a skilled or professional occupation, however stereotypical of the birth sex, to another for which one is less trained or experienced is likely to entail a considerable drop in income for some time – possibly permanently
- one's assumption that one's employer would not tolerate a change of gender role may be wrong. Trying to change role but losing the job leaves one no worse off than simply leaving without trying. Trying and managing to keep the job may enable one to continue in a rewarding occupation as a valued employee.

Some employers have a particular acceptance for transsexual employees. Usually this is because they have successfully employed others in the past. Such employers include the commercial bus companies, the Police Services, the Benefits Agency, Marks and Spencer, the Civil Service and WH Smith. Other employers may favour transsexuals because they will be sure not to require maternity leave or because the employer will be seen to be unprejudiced.

There are particular problems with self-employment because it can be hard to verify. One solution is asking for advertisements and references from clients. Occupations that are said to preclude the revelation of clients, such as 'private detective' might be confirmed by asking for tax documentation suggesting that income has been earned as self-employed.

Military service is a particularly specialised form of occupation. It is easy to confirm, and sometimes subject to bogus claims (*see* 'Taking a history', p. 11 and 'Patients in the police or armed services', p. 117).

Further complications ensue in the case of those occupied with those artistic endeavours that sometimes or always pay very poorly. These include many musicians, most poets, novelists and visual artists. As a rule of thumb, any artist making a living from sales of their work or obtaining exhibitions in independent galleries might be considered to be occupied. Poets and novelists who have had work published at the expense of anyone but themselves, or who have secured an advance, can be considered to be occupied. Jobbing musicians who can produce multiple flyers for gigs are occupied, as are those with a recording contract or session bookings. Conversely, songs written but not sold, or a possibly epoch-making novel not yet published or subject to an advance, do not constitute employment. These would better be described as hobbies.

A great many patients seem to work in information technology. The proportion so occupied seems far greater than chance would allow. The same has been observed in a variety of national settings. It might be suspected that people with gender identity disorder are skilled in this regard because of the appeal of communicating by a medium as instantaneous yet disembodied as email. This attractive theory is weakened by the observation that patients with gender identity disorder who have never so much as turned on a computer seem often to have a natural flair when encountering one for the first time often in the setting of a government training scheme.

People with disorders of gender identity who display a talent with computers seem often to gravitate into teaching others how to work or repair computers. Internet service provider helpdesks or commercial intranet helplines are often-reported occupations. It seems that those patients who are skilled with computers often also display an ability easily to communicate with others much less skilled. This combination of talents is much rarer than either ability with computers or good communication skills occurring alone.

Incapacity benefit and employment

See also 'Physically disabled patients', p. 108.

A number of patients at first presentation are in receipt of incapacity benefit. Many suggest that because of this it would be both unrealistic and unfair to expect them to seek or obtain occupation as part of the real life experience.

I would advise a close examination of those patients who are incapacity benefit recipients. It is illuminating to ask what incapacitates them. Often, they say they do not know, and cannot imagine what. Sometimes the supposedly incapacitating condition clearly no longer applies, and the patient admits this. Sometimes it is freely admitted that the Benefits Agency suggested eligibility for incapacity benefit without the patient ever learning the nature of the incapacity. Most curious of all are those patients in receipt of incapacity benefit where the incapacitating illness is supposed to be transsexualism.

A person has a disability if he or she has a physical or mental impairment that has a substantial and long-term effect on his or her ability to carry out normal day-to-day activities. This would include learning disabilities but exclude most mental illnesses (Disability Discrimination Act 1995 Code of Practice).

Unless there seems to be a genuinely incapacitating illness it seems best that every patient capable of occupation is occupied. Supposedly incapacitating illnesses should be investigated and confirmation sought (*see* 'Physically disabled patients', p. 108).

A common problem is how to inform employers and colleagues of an intention to change gender role. There are two distinct potential problems. The first is that of senior managers insisting that immediate colleagues will not accept a suggested change, and the second is that of the colleagues not doing so. Each needs a different approach.

The first approach is the 'bottom up' method. It is needed when it is anticipated that senior management will resist a change of gender role because 'it will upset immediate colleagues'. It consists of first consulting on a private and personal level with the colleagues in question, seeking confirmation from each that there will be no problem with a change of gender role. Once such confirmation has been obtained from a majority of colleagues, an approach to management can be made. Any objections based on the supposed upset that will be created among immediate colleagues can be dealt with by assurances that no overwhelming cry of opposition has been raised. This approach tends to be needed in small to medium-sized (often family-owned) companies.

The second approach is the 'top down' method. It is needed when colleagues might well not be supportive, but management are likely to be aware of their obligation to avoid discrimination. This usually applies to large industrial and state-owned concerns. The approach consists of talking to management first, negotiating any changes in working conditions that seem to be needed. The management are required then to send a memorandum to the other workers, making it clear that discrimination or bullying will not be tolerated. This needs to be carefully timed immediately to precede a change of gender role.

A common problem in both small and large companies seems to be what might be termed 'the toilet question'. In essence, what is to happen with regard to lavatorial facilities? Even otherwise very accommodating employers seem to be fazed by this question. A common solution seems to be an insistence that the patient use the disabled lavatories, often until gender reassignment surgery occurs.

This seems an odd 'solution' for a number of reasons, all of which might reasonably be put to an employer:

- firstly, the patient is not disabled, and so there is no need to use the disabled toilets
- secondly, it is likely to irritate those who are disabled that someone able-bodied has hijacked their toilet
- thirdly, male patients using women's toilets would never be in the position of exposing themselves to female employees since the design of the facilities does not allow this. Female patients would be using cubicles and thus similarly would avoid any sort of exposure
- fourthly, it is unclear how the provision of gender reassignment surgery would change these things, and accordingly unclear why gender reassignment surgery should make any difference.

Employers' concerns often evaporate in the light of practical experience. One male patient was a very senior civil servant. The government department for which she worked accommodated a change of role well, but there were problems with lavatorial facilities in that her female peers were assumed by her (male) senior managers to be unwilling to have her use their facilities. Accordingly, a lavatory was constructed especially for her. It was much more conveniently located than the existing women's facilities, and was quickly adopted by her female peers who were (and always had been) perfectly happy to share it with her.

Some patients, particularly female ones, pass so well in their acquired social gender role that they obtain employment without their employer knowing anything about their change of gender role. Those working for small employers without much in the way of an occupational health service may continue without their employer ever knowing. This can cause them problems in that they may be reluctant to join an otherwise excellent occupational pension scheme for fear of their employer finding out. This need not necessarily be the case (*see* Part 7).

Occupation is important because it is a good and verifiable test of whether the patient can manage on a day-to-day basis in their acquired gender role. Letters from employers on headed paper make fraud less likely. It is of course not necessary for the reference or other work confirmation to be addressed to the gender identity clinic. For those patients who pass so well their employers are ignorant, a 'to whom it concerns' reference or indeed a reference regarding suitability for custodianship of the church organ fund would serve perfectly well.

References are often very revealing. 'She used to be a man' suggests a current female identity, with knowledge of the patient's male background, while 'he's trying to be a woman' suggests that social identity is still male, albeit with an awareness of the patient's aspirations.

Many larger employers have specific policies regarding change of social gender role that apply in addition to their statutory obligations (*see* Part 7). Some have drawn these up in anticipation of such a situation arising and others have calmly drawn up policy as it has become necessary.

A unique set of problems faces those in personal care, paramedical or policing professions. It seems that many years ago, the UK Central Council for Nursing, Midwifery and Health Visiting (UKCC) considered a change of gender role to be incompatible with a continued career in nursing, and that 10 or 15 years ago it was suggested that although continued employment might be possible it would be necessary for a chaperone to be present with both male and female clients. More recently, transsexual people have worked as nurses, nursing assistants, physiotherapists, radiographers, physicians and surgeons. There seems to be no further concerns around chaperones, perhaps because it is no longer considered acceptable for patients or clients to be legitimately concerned about the sexual orientation, political leanings, racial origins or original biological sex of healthcare staff (*see* Part 7 'Legal issues', particularly Chapter 21, 'The Gender Recognition Act').

A persisting problem is experienced by patients who are police officers, and concerns whether they are allowed to search males or females. In practice, the issue seems largely to be avoided rather than addressed by means of a definitive policy.

Children's reactions

The reaction of children to a parent's change of gender role depends upon the ages of the child and the parent, and the quality of the relationship that existed between them prior to a change of gender role.

Pre-adolescent children whose parents change gender role and divorce the other parent are known to fare less well than those whose parents remain in the birth sex and stay together. They do *not* fare less well, though, than children whose parents have divorced for any other reason. It seems to be parental separation rather than the change of role that is damaging.

It follows from this that it would be better if people kept contact with their children after a change of gender role. Despite this conclusion, regrettably few male patients remain in proper contact with their children, and the reasons for their loss of contact seem often to include fears by their ex-wives or courts that continued contact would harm their children or put their children at risk of bullying. Sometimes contact orders stipulate that the transsexual parent presents for an access visit in their former gender role, or an androgynous or neutral appearance. There is no evidence that any such behaviour benefits children but it does distress patients and prevent them properly from changing their gender role by precluding irreversible hormonal or surgically induced bodily changes.

School-age children seem often to fare well, particularly those born to male patients whose former role had included some traditionally maternal aspects. Many such patients see their role as always having been that of a parent rather than particularly as a father, and continue to do at least as well as parents in a socially female role. Their children seem to prosper in both academic and personal terms.

Parents who change social gender role may embarrass teenage children. Often the children have never seen their parent in a new gender role and have been told of the situation by the other parent, who has gained custody. It seems that often the children imagine a more outlandish appearance or demeanour in the absent parent than is actually the case, and that anticipated embarrassments serve to prevent contact or to confine it to phone calls or letters.

The natural history of this situation seems to be a gradual re-establishment of contact, meetings sometimes initially ocurring in an area where the teenage child is not known. The longer-term outlook seems to be quite good. Late-teenage children can sometimes take advantage of their parent's drive to re-establish and maintain a relationship, extracting accommodation and other favours as the price of their continuing contact.

Family reactions

The wider family may have knowledge of a patient's change of gender role withheld from them by closer family members. The usual motivation for this is a belief that the change of role might not be permanent. That if the matter is not mentioned, the patient may have reverted to their original role before meeting the wider family, avoiding distant relations ever knowing.

Similar motivations may lie behind patients not informing their wider family, and accordingly a refusal ever directly to inform them (as opposed to planning to tell them immediately or when the need arises) is a poor prognostic sign.

Sometimes wider family members have ambivalent attitudes to the change of gender role. They may accept it in principle, but tell the patient that they would rather he or she presented in the original role if visiting or attending family gatherings. There may be great pressure on patients to acquiesce in this. If they do so it sets a precedent on which it is easy for the family to build.

A particular problem seems to be weddings. Families seem sometimes to insist on a reversion to original role for the purposes of group photographs. This is a cardinal misapprehension. The photographs will be displayed for years, leaving the family forever having to explain that the man in the back row with the ponytail is Auntie Anne. Attending in a female role might allow her to pass without comment both in life and in the group photograph.

Sometimes family opposition appears to inhibit patients from embarking on a real life experience, only for closer inspection to suggest that the patient may be perfectly happy to be able to blame his or her own inaction on others.

Case report: family opposition?

CS was a 23-year-old male presenting with a stated wish to live in a female gender role. He was slightly alexithymic, and presented looking masculine save for hair in a ponytail. He was said to have been socially isolated at secondary school (although not identified as gay or feminine) and to have gained poor exam results. After school, he worked in his father's small engineering business.

He attended appointments diligently, but his situation seemed never to change. He seemed to be waiting for the gender identity clinic to do something that would cause things to alter. CS had spoken of his cross-gender desires to his family and social circle. His friends were said to be supportive, but his father not. His father had insisted on a continued male role at work. CS said he was keen to be prescribed hormones and said he had made no moves on his own because he was waiting for this to occur – despite being told on two successive appointments that the next move must be his.

The major obstacle, as CS presented things, was that of working for his oppositional father. He ruefully agreed that were he to be prescribed hormones nothing would change save his hormonal milieu. Certainly, his lifestyle and gender role would not. Interestingly, his father would, it seemed, not have been able to employ a non-family member as the wages involved were so low, and CS could not have survived on the low wages had he not been accommodated by his parents without any need for rent. It seemed just as fair to say that CS had his father in his grasp as to say that his father controlled him.

Unbending, often irrational, family opposition can prove a very potent source of distress. Often, prolonged attempts are made to win round intransigent family members. Progress to gender reassignment surgery after a successful change of gender role seems particularly to be delayed by relations continuing to be deeply opposed, as the following shows.

Case report: unbending family opposition

MD was one of a large number of children born into an Irish Catholic family. Nearly all the male members of the family worked as unskilled or semi-skilled labourers, often in the UK. MD followed this family tradition.

In her 30s, MD presented to a gender identity clinic and went on to change her gender role. Her family was doggedly opposed throughout. They insisted that were she to want to visit the family's home village in Ireland she must do so in a male role. They further maintained that MD had ruined her life by changing her gender role, and that the level of ruination would worsen the longer she persisted in living as a woman. This view remained unaltered, despite MD's acquisition of a university degree and a well-paid civil service job with an associated pension.

Despite considerable social and occupational success in a female role, MD continued to be worried about her family's lack of acceptance of her. She communicated at length by post, hoping to influence their views, entirely without success. She changed the focus of her attention from her parents to her siblings, and later to her nieces and nephews. No generation seemed even slightly tractable. While MD moved her focus around her wider family in this way, she seemed to lose focus on gender reassignment surgery. Although still saying that it was a goal, it seemed not to be as high a priority as gaining family approval.

The irreversible nature of gender reassignment surgery seems to make it a particularly hard step to take without family support, or at the very least, no outright opposition. Attempts to gain such support often continue to the brink of gender reassignment surgery, as the following shows.

Case report: family support sought right up to the brink of gender reassignment surgery

RP came from a Jehovah's Witness family. She was well aware that her change of role from male to female was viewed by that faith and by her family as repugnant and sinful. Her family's opposition was solid and unchanging, and their contact with her, diminished as it was, seemed always coloured by their continued deep aversion to what she had done.

Over time, as she prospered in a female role, RP drifted away from her Jehovah's Witness faith and gradually lost contact with her family.

RP was referred for gender reassignment surgery, having easily completed a real life experience. After she had been admitted but before the surgery had occurred RP contacted her family to inform them of what she was about to undergo. It seemed that she had hoped they would feel that it was too late to stop her and would, given the situation, support her. They did not. They reiterated their opposition and did everything in their power to dissuade the surgeons concerned from operating. RP was upset but not surprised by their behaviour. She was surprised how great had been her continued need for parental and family approval.

Family influence need not be direct and does not always come from currently active family members. Someone who opposed any change of gender role, recently dead, may be problematic as illustrated below.

Case report: family factors and a bereavement reaction influencing presentation

TC came from a rather conventional, close and loving middle class family. His parents had always assumed from his childhood femininity that when he grew up that he would be gay. For very many years he was so identi- fied – by his family and himself. He continued to reside at home after all his siblings had set up homes for themselves.

As time passed, TC experienced an increasing sense of femininity, and tentatively raised with his family the prospect of a change of gender role. Although one parent was supportive, his three siblings and the other parent were horrified.

TC worked as a sports centre manager. He began to manipulate his appearance until it was as unmasculine as his family and employers would tolerate. He presented at a gender identity clinic seeking hormone treat- ment and claiming to want gender reassignment surgery.

TC's attendance at the gender identity clinic was exceedingly sporadic. He attended just enough to avoid being discharged, and not quite enough to persuade anyone to prescribe him hormones. There was no change of gender role, despite increasing unmasculinity, and no change of name or re- registration as a female employee.

After some 10 or more years of this pattern, TC's disapproving parent died. TC had remained very close to both parents, and was very distressed by this death. He presented at the gender identity clinic, very much more stridently demanding hormone treatment, but no further towards any change of gender role. He complained that nothing was done for him, and pointed out that parental disapproval need no longer be a concern to the clinicians who advised him.

Over the next 2 years, TC's appearance became much more con- vincingly feminine, and he seemed less and less like a gay man. After 18 months he changed his name to an unrelated female forename, and changed his social gender role in both work and private settings. As these considerable moves were made, his presentation became less rather than more strident. His demands for treatment became both less forceful and easier to accede to.

TC related having come to terms with the loss of the disapproving parent over the 2 years since the death. It seemed that at first he had been desperate to proceed, despite feeling that the dead parent would be spinning in a grave, but that later he had felt that the dead parent would not have minded. These feelings were said to have been particularly strong when TC had visited the place where the ashes were scattered. He had spoken aloud to the spirit of the dead parent. TC felt that the 2 years in which he had been more strident had been years in which, in retrospect, he would not have been ready to take hormones or change gender role. He felt that now the parental disapproval had gone he could wholeheartedly commit to a measured pace of progress, sustainable in the very long term, and free from ambivalence.

Reconciling a greatly changed life with a dead parent (or anyone else) who patients feel would have seriously objected can often be done in this way. Patients can write a letter explaining things and either bury it in the dead person's grave or burn the letter and scatter the ashes where the dead person's ashes were scattered.

Parents' reactions

Parents' reactions to younger children with a gender identity disorder are outside the scope of this book, which deals with adult disorders of gender identity.

Parents whose adult children admit to a previously unsuspected disorder of gender identity are in a different position to parents in whose children the disorder was evident but not diagnosed. Furthermore, reactions vary with the sex of the parent and the sex of the child in question.

Parents whose children appeared 'different' from an early age seem usually to have assumed that their son or daughter was gay or lesbian. In some families this is openly acknowledged and discussed, and in others tacitly assumed. Very often, this assumption has been shared or at least unchallenged by the child. It is, nonetheless, still rather surprising to parents of such children to be told that their child seeks to change gender role. Because parents have accommodated to the idea that their child is gay or lesbian, it does not automatically follow that they will just as easily accommodate to a change of gender role and physical form. In some cases the first accommodation does seem to pave the way for the second.

Parents whose child has disclosed a previously unsuspected gender identity disorder are usually more distressed. Mothers, particularly, seem to worry whether they or the child's father have in some way caused the disorder. The patient's childhood development is recalled and scrutinised both for early signs of what was to come, and for possible causes. Interestingly, parents seem often to worry greatly about 'nurture' factors but rarely to have considered that the problem might be congenital or even genetic. In those few cases where a partial androgen-insensitivity syndrome is detected, simple biology can be cited, and genetic counselling is indicated.

For male patients who have always seemed 'different', a change of role to female is usually well supported by both parents, mothers particularly. Mothers seem more distressed than fathers when female patients, who had earlier been assumed lesbian, change role to male and begin treatment with androgens. One wonders whether women experience growing a female child in their bodies as more self-reproducing than if that child is male. The subsequent rejection of bodily femininity by that child might then be felt as more personally rejecting than would a different sexual or romantic preference.

Whatever the birth sex of the patient, and whether the change of role was anticipated, suspected or a surprise, mothers seem to adapt to the new role faster than do fathers, even if their initial distress was the greater.

The main concern for most parents, whether or not their children have a gender identity disorder, is the welfare and happiness of their child. Parents learning of their child's change in gender are often tormented by worries that their child will be unemployable, destitute, friendless and without a relationship. Secondary concerns are often what other relations, neighbours and associates will think.

If people change gender role and prosper, many of these fears are assuaged. Having a good job and a wide circle of friends is hugely reassuring to one's parents. Looking more like an average citizen than a drag act calms ones parents' worries and fails to alarm their neighbours and friends.

Intimate relationship issues and outcomes

Some patients present at a gender identity clinic with a current relationship, often of long duration. Others present with a history of many short-term relationships. A further group seem never to have made any significant intimate relationships. I will consider female patients first since they have a less varied pattern of relationships.

Female patients seem more often than not to have made intimate relationships in their earlier lives, usually with women. A frequent finding is a history of many short-term relationships with lesbian women, which have all ended more in sorrow than in anger because the partner found the relationship sufficiently like that with a man as to be unsatisfactory.

A frequent problem is sexual difficulty, usually involving the patient being unwilling to be treated explicitly as female in the course of sexual interaction. Most female patients habitually take a more active or initiating role in sexual relations and prefer providing sexual stimulation for their partners. They seem often to employ a strap-on dildo. Female patients are characteristically reluctant to tolerate being the recipient of sexual attention and are particularly averse to having such female sexual characteristics as their breasts attended to or appreciated. They typically find difficulty even exposing their breasts, and may refuse to be naked in the sight of their partner.

This pattern of behaviour may not cause great problems early in a relationship, but as time passes partners appear to find the one-sided nature of such a sexual life increasingly disturbing. There is often for partners also an increasing sense of discomfort with what feels to be the fundamental masculinity of the patient. Partners who have a history of satisfactory relationships with masculine lesbians report that there is something unspecific, but very definitely, different about this biologically female person. This sometimes crystallises around a single event. One partner reported that such an event occurred when the patient refused to use her underarm deodorant because it had a pink top, and wanted another with a blue top. The partner reported thinking that this was absurd, and 'just what I would expect from a bloke'. After this epiphany, she was unable to resist the increasing impression that she was in effect living with a man.

Many female patients report that earlier in their lives others identified them as lesbians and that socially, if not always internally, they so identified themselves. These patients often report that their earliest relationships were made in a lesbian social arena, with women attracted to masculine lesbians. It seems that as time passes and such patients feel increasingly out of place in a lesbian context, relationships are more often made with women who previously self-identified as heterosexual, who have a much greater history of relationships with men, or for whom this is a first apparently same-sex relationship.

Established relationships in female patients who change their gender role tend to display two distinct outcomes.

The first is seen in patients whose long-term relationship is with a woman who is clearly a lesbian, who wants relationships only with women, albeit very masculine ones, and whose history of relationships with men is, at the most, limited. The relationship with the patient is often presented as very solid and supportive by both patient and partner, and the partner is presented as supportive of the patient's drive to change gender role. These relationships seem to remain intact with the change of social gender role, but with the increasing physical masculinity caused by androgen treatment there is often a deterioration in the relationship despite the high regard patient and partner have for each other. The relationship may change to that of a supportive friend.

The second outcome is seen in patients whose longer-term relationship is with a woman with a more extensive history of relationships with men and for whom the relationship with the patient is often the first apparently same-sex relationship. Such relationships seem equally able to weather a change of social gender role, but rather better at enduring as an intimate one despite the patient's increasing physical masculinity.

Few female patients are predominantly attracted to men, and those that are seem attracted to gay men. Few seem to have managed to contract longer-term relationships with gay men before a social role change, but more seem to do so afterwards. Such patients sometimes make relationships with each other. These seem to prosper.

Male patients can broadly be classified by their sexual preference, the larger proportion being interested in relationships with women. Generally, their libido seems to be average to low. The pattern of relationships seen in male patients is more complex than that seen in female patients.

Many male patients have a history of cross-dressing since middle childhood that started out with rather fetishistic features but which has evolved over time through dual-role transvestism into transsexualism. These patients have often had a relationship with the same woman over the course of this whole evolution. The fate of the relationship seems mainly to depend on whether the woman concerned can adapt to the evolving psychological position of her partner. A complicating factor is that often the woman has been shielded from knowledge of the fetishistic cross-dressing, and sometimes from that of the subsequent dual-role transvestism. I will deal first with women who have knowledge of the situation.

Women knowingly involved with fetishistic transvestite partners are often relatively unconcerned, providing their own social and sexual lives are unimpeded by the fetish. This is understandable, given that in the majority of such cases the fetish will either not evolve into dual-role transvestism or will move so very slowly that potential problems seem reassuringly distant.

Women knowingly living with a man displaying dual-role transvestism show a variety of responses. Many are accommodating and may assist the man in his periodic feminine presentation of himself. Problems seem to arise when the proportion of the time spent in a female role grows and when (as often eventually happens) the patient is angry and emotionally cut off when in a male role. This situation is often accompanied by a decrease in the patient's libido. The women concerned seem to grow increasingly dissatisfied, and may wrongly suspect that the decrease in sexual activity and emotional expression comes because their partner is seeking sexual or emotional contact elsewhere.

Patients whose dual-role transvestism has evolved into transsexualism may present with female partners who are said to be willing to accommodate to their partner's change of social gender role. Others present accompanied by women who are overtly angry and disappointed. Such angry partners seem to feel that they have been ever more accommodating, often over many years, but that the patient seems never to be satisfied. Either way, the patient seems to expect the woman to continue the relationship despite the change of social gender role. The longevity of the relationship, the shared interest in their children or their intertwined finances are among many factors that may be invoked as reasons to stay together.

Regardless of the apparent initial level of support from the woman concerned, these relationships may well founder. Angry women may say that they married a man, and are not lesbians. Others, although accepting in principle, may find that in practice they do not want the social stigma of being with a man who has changed gender role, or the prospect of others wondering whether they are lesbian.

Women who present as supportive at first interview and who seem also to accept the social stigma of a partner changing social gender role, may yet have particular difficulty with the cessation of sexual activity and the bodily feminisation of the man they know. One woman reported waking confused, having been dreaming that she was staying in a hotel. On waking, she remained slightly confused for a few seconds, unsure as to whether she was in her own bedroom or the dream hotel's room. In the brief moments of confusion she looked at her partner and thought 'bloody hell, I'm in bed with some woman!'. The confusion settled after seconds, but the partner was thereafter unable to shake from her mind the impression that the man she had known for years had become a woman, despite the continued presence of his (steadily atrophying) penis.

Some male patients' long-term relationships with women seem to prosper despite their social role and genital change. These may be those relationships where the sexual activity had always been rather limited or purely procreative. This is sometimes seen with female partners who have themselves a history of sexual trauma or no great liking for sex for some other reason. Another quite successful outcome may be that where the patient has married a bisexual woman. There is sometimes the suggestion in both these circumstances that from the partner's point of view the marriage might have been contracted because of the patient's soft and rather feminine demeanour rather than regardless or in spite of it.

Women who have lived for years with a man who has concealed his cross-dressing from them tend to present in a more distressed state. They may have stumbled across a cross-dressed husband or partner when returning home unexpectedly, or been told of the activity by a third party.

For women subjected to such a revelation, a source of immediate distress seems often to be the extensive deception, particularly the substantial time the behaviour has been going on and the lengths that the man has gone to in order to conceal it. A later concern may be that the man concerned might be obtaining sexual congress in association with the cross-dressing. This concern is often prompted by the observed decrease in libido.

The cross-dressing men so exposed seem often to believe that their wives had known of their habits and said nothing. Or they may feel that their wives ought to have known of their cross-dressing because they openly expressed an interest in women's clothes. Such assumptions are often unrealistic. What that man saw as 'obvious clues' seem usually to have gone unnoticed by the woman.

Such exposure having occurred, the women are usually faced with the prospect of having to accommodate both to the knowledge of their partner's cross-dressing and the prospect of a change of his social gender role. Such a great and sudden transformation of the relationship parameters is harder to accommodate, and the prospects for the relationship are correspondingly worse.

For male patients, a change of role to female with pre-operative status may render relationships, particularly sexual ones, rather difficult.

Relationships with women may founder if the partner continues to view the patient as male, despite the change of social gender role. A close relationship with a woman may develop into an intimate relationship that does not include sexual intercourse. Problems may come if the partner expects the relationship to include this. If the patient is just as keen to engage in intercourse, there may be a reversion to the former, male, role (*see* 'Reversion to former role in RLE and prior to GRS', p. 124).

Relationships between male patients and women that do not feature the desire for sexual intercourse, especially those where the partner feels the patient to be female, tend to prosper and to endure through subsequent gender reassignment surgery.

Relationships between male patients and men seem to be much more fraught. Male patients who have changed gender role to female tend to attract the attention of men who are sexually interested in people with both male and female characteristics, most often breasts and a female shape as well as a penis. These men are not likely to be a good match for a patient who has changed gender role to female, since they will mainly be interested in the one bit of the patient's anatomy that least interests her. It seems common for such men strenuously to insist that they will treat the patient entirely as a woman, only to later focus their attention on her penis.

Case report: gynaeandrophile man and male patient

CS changed gender role in her mid-30s, and prospered in a female role. She had earlier identified herself as a dual-role transvestite and still had contact with dual-role transvestites via a society for transvestites.

CS made a relationship with a man who she met via this society. He repeatedly assured her that he viewed her as nothing other than a woman. Their friendship deepened, but she warned him that if it were to become sexual, any attention to her penis would result in the end of the relationship. He readily agreed to this, seemingly indignant that she would think him likely so to embarrass her.

Their relationship did progress to a sexual level. To CS's disgust as soon as she had removed her clothes the man grabbed at her penis, seeming keen that much be made of it. Although feeling it to be a somewhat unladylike response, CS summoned up skills she had learned in her earlier male role and threw him, entirely naked, out of the door to her house, depositing his clothes on top of him via a third floor window.

Some relationships between male patients and men seem to thrive, but to fail as soon as gender reassignment surgery has actually happened (*see* 'Chapter 19', p. 251).

More rarely, male patients make relationships with men that prosper and endure through gender reassignment surgery.

Case report: successful pre-operative relationship

JP changed gender role in her early 20s and passed well as female. She had little history of childhood femininity, but did report a marked lack of childhood and adolescent masculinity. She had made no intimate relationships by the time she had changed gender role, and was unclear where her sexual interests lay.

JP had never identified herself or been identified by others as transvestite. After her change of role, she continued to mix in the same social circles as before, quickly being accepted by her friends as female.

In this social setting, JP made a relationship with a man slightly her senior. He had suspected her of a change of gender role but had been embarrassed to ask JP about it, eventually managing to elicit the truth from one of her friends.

JP at first viewed his attention with mild suspicion, but felt that he seemed genuine. Her friends reinforced this impression, and their relationship started.

The relationship proved enduring and profound. JP found anal intercourse acceptable in the context of the relationship because she felt herself truly to be viewed as a woman. The relationship prospered and endured through gender reassignment surgery, after which vaginal intercourse occurred.

Relationships contracted during a real life experience can influence the drive for treatment expressed by the patient. Reversion to original gender role can be one result (*see* 'Reversion to former role in RLE and prior to GRS', p. 124), but so can a precipitate and unwise rush for gender reassignment surgery.

Case report: relationship issues precipitating a drive for gender reassignment surgery

MP changed gender role in her early 40s, having previously been married but childless. She had a history of fetishistic transvestism and later dual-role transvestism, but seemed to be prospering in a transsexual solution with a role change. MP was about three-quarters through an uncomplicated real life experience when she began to press for gender reassignment surgery to be expedited by any means possible.

It seemed that MP had contracted a relationship with a rather younger man, and placed a high value on the relationship. The man concerned, however, seemed not to want MP to live with him. His contact with her seemed mostly to be on his terms, and at his convenience. It was also becoming ever less frequent. It seemed that MP had begun to wonder whether he was also seeing someone else, although he was said to have denied this. Rather, he was said to have implied that MP's pre-operative status troubled him.

MP accepted that the relationship seemed likely naturally to end whatever she did. On cool reflection, she thought that the man had falsely attributed the cooling of his feelings to her pre-operative state. She was pleased not to have spent money on overseas gender reassignment surgery, and decided that she wanted surgery at a less forced pace. She concluded that if he genuinely was not prepared to wait a moment longer for her to have gender reassignment surgery (which she doubted), he was not the man she needed. MP continued to nurture what she accepted was a distant chance that he would again be interested in her if she contacted him after she had undergone gender reassignment surgery.

A change of social gender role often enhances the capacity to form both social and intimate relationships, particularly in male patients. The patient may, in a male role, have been seen as cut off, grumpy, and emotionally unresponsive. In a female role these characteristics may be replaced by a much happier and interactive response.

Having said this, a poor capacity for relationships which is based on personality factors will not be altered by a change of gender role, much though patients might want or expect it, as the following illustrates.

Case report: schizoid personality unaltered by a change of gender role

KB presented extremely convincingly in a female role, having retaken some Civil Service exams. Dropping down a year meant mixing with a new cohort and fewer people recognised her as somebody who used to be working in a male role.

KB's leisure time was occupied with solitary hobbies. A flat mate had moved out to live with a boyfriend. KB was unmoved by this. KB did not herself want a relationship, describing it as being 'too messy'. She expressed vague hopes of this occurring in the future. It seemed she had a schizoid personality and it was suggested to her that it was not likely that she would ever make close relationships. She accepted that this might well be true, and was not worried about it.

KB had no friends at the time of interview. She felt she was more open and honest with others in a female role, much less trammelled that once she was. She remarked, 'things are just easier, everything just used to be an effort before'. It seemed that most people were unaware of her originally biologically male status. She had earlier made a point of telling people of her situation and reported that they were often surprised. She said she no longer bothered telling them. KB accepted that she had changed one set of anxieties for another and was still somebody with something to hide, but said that she was at least no longer required also to put on an act as a man.

Orchidectomy in a female role

People attending a gender identity clinic sometimes seek orchidectomy (that is to say, castration) as a discrete procedure. There are probably many motivations behind such requests.

A proportion of these requests come from men who have not changed their gender role and who do not intend to do so, although they may not readily admit this. Their motivation might well be dysmorphophobia directed towards primary sexual characteristics, or perhaps the effects of androgens (*see* 'Dysmorphophobia', p. 37).

Requests for orchidectomy made by those who have already changed role are probably not wholly dysmorphophobic in origin, although there might remain an element of this. A more likely motivation would be the desire to be rid of unwanted and disliked male genitals (rather than purely the hormones they make). Patients are aware that a premature request for a penectomy and orchidectomy would be declined, but may feel that a request for an orchidectomy alone might be more justifiable because it can be argued that there will be hormonal benefits to the procedure.

Orchidectomy conducted before the end of a real life experience represents an irreversible step and thus prejudges the result of what is being tested by the real life experience, and the World Professional Association for Transgender Health, Inc. (formerly the Harry Benjamin International Gender Dysphoria Association) rules forbid it. Orchidectomy after a successful real life experience would be perfectly permissible, but it would seem better to move straight to gender reassignment surgery.

In purely practical terms, early orchidectomy carries with it the risk of subsequent scrotal shrinkage. This renders later vulvoplasty more problematic. Later orchidectomy carries less risk of this sort, but if late enough to carry no risk, would be so close to eventual gender reassignment surgery as to render the separate procedure and associated extra anaesthetic rather pointless.

Case report: orchidectomy in a female role

LO, aged 44, had changed gender role to female in her late 30s. She had remained married and cohabiting with her wife. She had an orchidectomy after some years in a female role. For occupational and marital reasons, LO had long resisted the drive to change gender role, and having done so was very glad to have left a male role. She presented the value of orchidectomy as that of removing the possibility that she would remasculinise if for some medical or other reason she had to stop taking estrogens. She saw the procedure as the removal both of masculinity and the risk of masculinity, rather than a feminising procedure in itself. In addition, much was made of her stated fear of the complications and risks of more complex gender reassignment surgery.

LO's wife had accommodated to her change of gender role, but resisted her having gender reassignment surgery. It seemed that in addition to the stated motivation, orchidectomy served also as the minimum amount of surgery able to placate LO's drive to be genitally female and yet preserve the marital relationship.

Two years later, LO had settled easily into a female role and what she felt was a lesbian relationship with her wife. She reported that her remaining penis was still capable of erectile function in the context of sexual arousal, and that its behaviour in this way was oddly disturbing to both her and her wife. Rather to her surprise, LO now felt that her penis had to go. Her wife was said to agree only because the penis bothered LO, but mounted no active opposition. In addition to penectomy, a cosmetic vulvoplasty was requested.

The later procedures doubled the number of anaesthetics and admissions that were needed, and rendered the later vulvoplasty harder to do than would otherwise have been the case. LO said she was aware, and accepted, that after a cosmetic vulvoplasty a vaginoplasty would be impossible, but there were worries that her assurances in this regard would evaporate, as had her earlier ones concerning orchidectomy.

Psychotherapy for gender disorders

Mark Morris

Patients with gender disorders do not want therapy. They want surgery. So why is it that most gender reassignment clinics have a psychodynamic psychotherapist as part of the team? In this section, I hope to examine these dilemma by looking at the role of the psychotherapist with gender-disordered patients by looking at various theories of the transsexual symptom that have evolved in psychodynamic practice with gender-disordered patients, and then by looking at ideas underpinning approaches to psychotherapy with this group.

It often seems that gender-disordered patients not only have doubts about therapy, but are also somewhat dismayed by being referred to a psychiatrist by their GP or surgeon when they request treatment. Broadly, it would seem that gender-disordered people view their difficulties as a problem with their body, not a problem with their mind. In the history of western philosophy, there has been a divide between philosophers as to what can be a starting point of what is known. The continental philosophers are certain of their mind first, and then move on to consider whether they can trust their senses that tell them there is an external world, starting with Descartes' 'I think therefore I am', and on to the existentialists. The British empiricists, Locke and Hume, on the other hand ridicule this position, challenging Descartes to stop eating food, if he doubts its existence.

Gender-disordered patients come from the Cartesian tradition, 'I think I am a man/woman, therefore I am', in spite of a biological reality that evidences the opposite. My understanding of the clinical approach to reassignment treatment is more in the philosophically empiricist tradition; the gender-disordered individual is deemed to have a mental illness until proven otherwise, and therefore their first point of call is a psychiatrist. Once they have proved that their transsexual symptom is not a mental illness, following psychiatric examination and having demonstrated an improvement in social and psychiatric functioning during the 'real-life test' period, then it is sanctioned that the body can be brought in line with the sane, although transgendered, mind.

Once the transsexual symptom is diagnosed, the medical model takes over. The medical model would propose that the science of medicine has identified a particular psychosexual psychosomatic disjunction that can take place, leading to the medical condition known as 'transsexualism'. It would argue that there is good evidence that the physical reassignment of people with the transsexual symptom results in an improvement in their global functioning. The task therefore, is accurately to diagnose the transsexual symptom to identify patients for treatment. A more psychodynamic perspective would argue that the issue is vastly more complex than this; that there are may more variables that should be taken into consideration, not least of which are disavowed unconscious motivations that lead to some of the theories of transsexual symptom formation described below.

The role of the psychotherapist

The role of the psychotherapist on the reassignment team can simply be understood as providing more detail to the psychiatric examination that is required before the diagnosis of transsexualism can be made. If the psychotherapist proposes that one of the dynamics described below is a significant element in the request for reassignment, and the team agrees, further assessment and investigation might be required prior to offering physical reassignment.

I believe that there is, however, a second more important role that is illustrated by the foregoing discussion, namely that the psychotherapist develops a 'meta' perspective on the process of diagnosis and treatment that questions the assumptions on which the process proceeds; that identifies the medical model and pinpoints its potential drawbacks; that recognises the conflict between the patients' and psychiatrists' position; and that bears in mind the gravity of the actions that are being proposed.

Fundamentally, the psychoanalytic psychotherapeutic task is to help the individual come to terms with reality. The term 'shrink' for a psychoanalytic psychotherapist is quite a sophisticated epithet for a person who tries to deconstruct their patients' unrealistic, unreasonable, narcissistic, conditioned and misguided expectations, to be able to focus more effectively on their real life, and to be able to make the most of their real assets. The real-life fact is that the 'male-to-female' transgendered patient is biologically a male. The psychoanalytic psychotherapy task therefore would be to enable the person to come to terms with their biological sex, difficult though this might be, and to make the most of their life in spite of this disappointment.

If the first injunction of medical ethics is to 'do no harm', then it has to be noted that the patient starts out with a physically normal sex hormonal balance, and morphologically normal sex organs. These are then changed and altered making something pathological-irreversible masculinisation in biological females, or female secondary sexual characteristics (breast development) superimposed on a solid post-androgenised biological male. Likewise, the risks of complications from surgery carried out on healthy tissue can be challenged, as can the legitimacy of the alteration of perfectly healthy morphology.

This 'loyal opposition' to a potentially overly mechanistic medical model approach to gender disorders is significant, because it is not based in a reactionary ignorance, as is much popular criticism of gender reassignment programmes. Instead, with a training in empathetic sensitivity, and exposure to patients as part

of the programme, the 'loyal opposition' role is held with an agonising awareness of the anguish and torture that these patients suffer with feeling locked into
the wrong sexual body, being forced to play an counterintuitive social gender
role, and themselves faced with the agonising choice of the social and biological
consequences and stigma of changing gender versus the equally miserable
prospect of not doing so.

In psychoanalytic theory, this position might be understood in terms of Klein's
'depressive position'. The surgeon can castrate the patient with an omnipotent
sense of a curative procedure to rescue the patient. The psychotherapist who
agrees to sanction this does so while being much more aware of the psychological,
physical and social damage that is taking place, and of the equivocality of the
assumptions on which the decision is based, while supporting the course of action
in spite of all these, with a sense of guilt and regret. I believe that the role of the
psychotherapist is to hold an awareness of the moral and psychological dilemmas
mentioned above, and on occasion to remind the team of them. This may sound
like a rather mystical and even crazy role, but then critics of reassignment have
argued that so is the idea of playing god by turning men into women.

Psychodynamic models of the transsexual symptom

In psychoanalytic thinking, symptom diagnosis and classification is less important
than the issue of meaning. The symptom itself is seen as a symbolic representa-
tion of the mental conflict. The mind struggles with an issue or a conflict. When it
hits upon a symptom that captures the power of the conflict without the pain,
it is adopted.

Case report: Life-threatening illness precipitating change

A 27-year-old male-to-female transsexual patient gives a history of poor
social integration growing up, and of being a rather feminine boy, but he
dates his conviction of transsexualism to his recovery from a very serious
road traffic accident 4 years earlier in which there were fatalities. As a result
of his own injuries, he was briefly in a coma and required several months of
hospitalisation. Family members express surprise that he never seemed
to register the trauma, but instead began to seek gender reassignment.
Challenged with the interpretation that he had adopted the idea of gender
change instead of facing the implications of his accident, namely mortality,
he partially accepts, saying that it was when he realised that the thread of
life was so tenuous that he felt he should go for what he felt was right,
namely reassignment.

This example demonstrates the first psychodynamic theory of transsexualism – namely that it is a symptom in the classic psychoanalytic sense – that it is a
way for an individual to symbolise a mental conflict, in this case the conflict being
post-traumatic stress and survivor guilt following the road traffic accident. The
transsexual symptom combines the factors of the fantasy of his life potentially
being better if he was a woman, with the issue of mortality that he cannot face

having nearly died, leading to the conviction that he must pursue gender change 'because he's only got one life'.

A second psychodynamic hypothesis is that the transsexual symptom is a delusion, using the usual psychiatric tests of falsity of the belief, as it is impervious to rational counter-argument, and is out-with cultural norms.

Case report: Mitigation of a delusion

A 42-year-old divorced father of two presents with a transsexual belief after a lifelong history of secretive fetishistic cross-dressing, with waning sexual excitement over the past decade. He asks his GP for feminising hormones, having read an article on the internet, and is referred by his GP to the practice counsellor. To the counsellor, he accepts that he has a penis, which for years in his marriage he has used ego-syntonically, accepts that he is biologically male and has fathered two children, but even so believes that he 'really' is a woman.

From the psychodynamic perspective, the transsexual symptom passes the tests to establish whether a belief is delusional, and this position is only mitigated in the highly specialist environment of a gender clinic, and among gender disorder-friendly mental health workers, where arguably the belief is a cultural norm. Out-with this setting, the belief remains a delusion, and treatment to consolidate the delusion to collude with it is counter-therapeutic and ethically questionable.

Contributing to this position is an observation that gender-disordered people are more certain of their gender than normal. For everyone, gender identity is a complex compromise, made up of maternal and paternal identifications, of differential biological drives, of sexual proclivities and of general body perception. If I say 'I am a man', this is shot through with more doubts, insecurities and uncertainties than a female-to-male patient saying the same thing during a gender reassignment assessment. This very lack of doubt, this very certainty, is a component of transsexualism, and is more characteristic of a delusional belief than is the precarious and fluid compromise that is normal gender identity.

Case report: Abnormal certainty

A 35-year-old man has worked as an infantryman and subsequently as a scaffolding erector, has had various heterosexual relationships in his 20s, but is more asexual now, and reports gender dysphoria, although he does not cross-dress, and has not been in touch with transvestite/transsexual groups, so is not aware of the 'real-life test' process. His request is for sex reassignment surgery, 'because only without a prick, with boobs and a, you know, a vagina will I feel right . . . complete'.

A third argument supporting the hypothesis that transsexualism is a psychotic phenomenon is the concretisation of the fantasy. I have suggested that gender identity comprises a complex mix of psychological, social, sexual and occupational factors. For some gender-disordered patients, it becomes concretised and reduced to a single concrete fact the nature of the genitalia. In psychoanalytic understanding, a symptom of a more psychotic functioning is the concretisation of mental concepts, in this case, the concretisation of a feeling of femininity into the need for physical castration and creation of breasts and vagina.

Another psychodynamic hypothesis concerns the mechanism of identification in the context of loss – that the individual struggling with the loss of a figure of the opposite sex 'becomes' them.

Case report: Identification with a lost figure

A 32-year-old biological male presents passing reasonably well as a woman in her mid-50s, wearing long hair in a bun, a tweed skirt and a blouse. He reports a childhood history of preferring female company and games, an unconsummated dysphoric homosexual sexual orientation, unsatisfying because of his desire for straight rather than gay men and social isolation. Following his father's death in early childhood, he has lived with his mother. He dates his realisation of being transsexual and deciding to pursue gender reassignment to the aftermath of his mother's death 3 years previously. During the consultation he brings out a photograph of her, a woman dressed in tweeds in her mid-50s.

Case report: Identification with a lost relationship

A 24-year-old socially isolated biological male reports that his jeans, shirt and jersey are in fact from woman's ranges, so that he is technically cross-dressed. He talks at length about the one girlfriend that he has had, a sexual relationship between age 16 and 18, with a woman one year his senior. Six years later he continues to dwell on the reasons for their break-up, idealising her, clear in his view that no one else will come close. In his discussion of this relationship and of his understanding of his gender, it becomes clear that he identifies very strongly with her, that she wore female versions of masculine clothes and took a lead role in their relationship. He accepts that there is a link between his vision of his female self and her, accepts that he might be fearful of committing in another relationship for fear of beng hurt again, but rejects the idea that his solution might be to make himself into his girlfriend.

In Stoller's original hypotheses of the psychodynamics of gender disorders,[1] he hypothesised a transsexual solution to the boy's pre-oedipal developmental dilemma, that for the first year of life or so, the baby believes they and mother are one – fused – part of the same thing. As the Oedipus complex develops, babies have to accept that fathers exist, and little boys have to accept that they never were like mother in the first place, because they are male not female. Stoller sees transsexualism as the failure of this early recognition of the difference, along with the trauma and grieving that result, and argued that these difficulties are potentiated in families with the constellation of absent fathers and domineering mothers.

These examples both involve dynamics similar to those envisaged by Stoller, although with the transsexual solution to the rupturing of the fused relationship with the partner or mother happening later in life. By becoming the loved and depended upon person, the mother or the girlfriend, the patient triumphs over their dependency and vulnerability – in fantasy at least.

A further psychodynamic hypothesis regarding transsexualism is that it is a perversion. This can be conceived in two ways. Firstly, in a more straightforward way, that there is a minority of transgendered patients who are sex workers, and who fund their gender treatment privately from funds raised thereby.

Case report: Transgendered sex worker

Maxine is a 24-year-old male-to-female transgendered patient who has been living in the female role for the past 3 years, working as an escort and 'glamour model'. In her real life test, it is clear that she follows a female social role, her name has been changed, and she has been supported through the prescription of feminising sex hormones. The question now is whether she has been in gainful employment for a year, so demonstrating completion of the second part of the test that would support a surgical referral.

A classical Freudian position on perversion argues that sexual desire strays from the normal because of fear of castration and that the woman with the fetish object – the whip, the high heels – symbolises potent castration, being castrated (because they are female) but still having a potent phallic symbol – the whip, the high heels, and so on. From this perspective, the transgendered person as a fetish object is simply a less-symbolised, more concrete version of the woman with the fetish object, being a woman (with breasts) and therefore castrated, and yet still having a penis. From this perspective, transsexualism is a perverse solution for the individual to the fear of castration – becoming their own fetish object.

The second perspective on perversion derives from other psychoanalytic understandings of the term as developed by Chassequet-Smirgel[2] and others, that perversion is a denial of differences of various sorts, including the difference between the sexes, by trying to become the opposite. They also suggest that perversion involves a notion of the ideal, that gender-disordered individuals often have a notion of becoming an ideal, either an ideal woman or man, or an ideal version of themselves. Finally, it is suggested that perversion can invoke 'pseudo-creativity', where, in part object terms, the creation of faeces is mistaken for the creation of a baby – illustrated by the proliferation of self-help groups, websites, pressure groups and so on. The Freudian metapsychological explanation of perversion is that it is a result of very early confusion of the destructive and creative drives, such that destructiveness is articulated via sexuality or the erotic. From this perspective, the effort to change sex, to destroy the physically healthy sexuality and put in place a substitute can itself be interpreted as a perverse act.

Psychotherapeutic approaches to gender disorders

Having looked at the role of the psychotherapist in the reassignment team, and then some more psychodynamic understandings of the transsexual symptom, I propose to move to look at the three characteristic approaches to providing psychotherapy for this patient group, a supportive approach, a radical one, and one that I shall argue is most appropriate, namely a non-directive dialectic to develop informed consent.

The first approach – supportive psychotherapy – is carried out by all professionals working with gender disorders, and may be structured into a monthly group programme. Such groups may be unstructured, and facilitate a self-help discussion. A shared sense of purpose is allowed to develop, in which the task is making progress along the path of gender reassignment, either as a female-to-male patient or vice versa. Patients further along the path inform those less far down about what they can expect; there is much discussion of the difficulties of living in the opposite gender role, about the dilemmas of friends, family and work as one changes gender, about prejudice and being 'read' as transgendered, and how people react subsequently, and so on. At a more practical level, there is discussion of where cheap facial electrolysis is offered, about statutory rights and case law in relation to treatment being funded, about the differences between pursuing state-funded and private treatment, and so on.

As well as having a supportive and educative function, these groups can offer the clinician the opportunity to observe their patients in a slightly more spontaneous setting than the one-to-one consultation, facilitating the establishment of attitudes to treatment and their gender disorder, and observing their general development with treatment. The groups provide an opportunity for patients to vent their frustration at the structuring of treatment with the professionals in a position of power relating to the rate at which their treatment proceeds – or whether it progresses at all. The therapist's sensitive and explanatory response to these challenges will articulate the reasons and rationale for reassignment being structured as it is, which may be the most significant psychological movement for the patient to make – recognising and accepting the reassignment treatment structure as protective of their interests and appropriate.

Supportive psychotherapy groups assume that the patient is capable at the outset of making informed consent to treatment (as they are often in the stages of treatment as it proceeds); however, it is undoubtedly the case that people become better informed as they attend the groups. They will learn, for example that attaining the next stage of treatment is not the nirvana that it is built up to be – that feminising hormones can dull the edge of gender dysphoria – but that they, or even surgery, are not totally life changing. The criticism of this approach is that it might be insufficiently challenging and might be seen as collusive with patients who are requesting the prescription of medication and treatment that will produce major iatrogenic disease in their healthy bodies.

The second psychotherapeutic approach might be termed 'radical', in the sense that its aim is to enable the patient to eschew the wish for gender reassignment. The rationale is based upon some of the theories noted above, combined with an overarching position that transsexualism is a psychological disorder, and that treatment for this should also be psychological, and specifically not physical in the sense of the prescription of contra sex hormones or surgery, or social in the sense of recommending a 'real-life test' of living in the chosen gender role. Both of these would be seen as enactments of a psychological conflict, and therefore as non-therapeutic.

The justification for this therapeutic approach is several-fold: firstly, for some patients, their gender disorder is almost entirely ego-dystonic. Their request and therapeutic need is for the eradication of the symptom, and their own conception of it as a severe psychopathology is reflected in the treatment approach. A second justification is that it presents a logically coherent position, namely that gender disorders are psychological disorders and are to be understood rather than ignored, in favour of realigning the body. Thirdly, there is experience from in-depth psychological work that the transsexual symptom, when understood and explored with sufficient rigour, does melt away, as the individual becomes more aware of deeper conflicts that they have been unable to resolve, but that the transsexual symptom has adequately masked. With the exploration and partial resolution of these deeper issues, it is not that the cross-gender fantasy disappears, but rather that the heat and power is taken out of it, so that it becomes just another one of life's disappointments, rather than the life's work.

One effect of this rationale is for the therapist not to collude with the patient's 'enactments' of their psychological conflict, by referring to them by their sex-appropriate title and the use of the sex-appropriate personal pronoun, as well as only offering treatment if the patient presents in an iso-sexual gender role – dressed as men if they are biologically so, and so on. Clinics that offer and argue for this sort of approach to treatment have been subject to considerable criticism and, indeed, negative lobbying by transgendered groups.

The third approach to psychotherapy might be called 'motivational enquiry'. It combines aspects of the two treatment approaches mentioned above: the rigour of theorising that underpins the radical approach, with the non-directive discourse about the issue that is more characteristic of the supportive approach. Motivational enquiry focuses on the issue of informed consent. There is a strong argument that the treating professional has a paramount duty of care to a transgendered biological woman to ensure that her consent to being prescribed irreversible masculinising sex hormones is fully informed. The psychodynamic hypothesis of the unconscious assumes that in addition to the conscious reasons and motivations that the patient has to choose in relation to the reassignment path to manage their gender dysphoria, there will be other hidden ones of which they are not aware.

Given that there are legitimate psychological theories about the aetiology of gender disorder that might apply to them, patients have a right to be able to be informed of these in order to establish to what extent their own motivation for gender reassignment is a function of these theories. Arguably, only after establishing and exploring their own unconscious motivations can their consent to irreversible physical treatment, and to the irreversible disruption of social structures involved in social gender role change be fully informed.

The notion of expanding the field of informed consent is conceived as the central task of this third approach. As such, it is distinct from the task of psychologically supporting the patient through the arduous process of reassignment of the supportive approach, or of the reversal of the reassignment wish of the radical approach. In practice, this motivational enquiry is simply the psychoanalytic psychotherapy process taking place in a group or individual setting, but without the therapist's position being that the gender reassignment solution is a negative one.

There is an argument that it is a central tenet of a psychoanalytic therapy approach that the therapist needs to be able to remain neutral about the patient's actual choices, limiting themselves to trying to understand the patient, rather than influencing what they do. It may be worth raising a personal thought that emerges in the psychodynamic work with gender patients that I think might contribute to therapists taking up a radical position in relation to their gender patients' treatment rather than the more non-judgemental one proposed as part of a motivational enquiry approach. For the psychoanalytic psychotherapist, work with gender-disordered patients can be profoundly dispiriting and agonising. From the therapist's position, the unconscious motivational dynamics underlying the wish for reassignment are painfully clear and obvious; the patient's wish for social gender change and physical reassignment seems to be a disastrous choice that adds social and physical complications to an already very confused picture, but one that seems potentially resolvable, given its psychological understand-ability. With their detailed knowledge of the patient, the therapist comes to a clear conclusion that reassignment will compound their problems, yet has to stand by and watch this happen.

Two factors then potentiate these difficulties, firstly if the therapist becomes more persistent in their articulation of the unconscious motivational dynamics, for example by taking up the resistance (which arguably, they have a duty of care to do), and they are effective, there is often a negative therapeutic reaction by the patient. The patient, feeling persecuted, mistakes the therapist's perusal of ideas as prevention of their chosen course of gender change. The issue becomes conflated by the patient into an argument of rights to appropriate (reassignment) treatment, and the patient launches complaints about the therapist that can have real adverse professional consequences.

The second factor that reduces psychotherapeutic optimism is that even with patients who can accept and recognise the psychodynamics and motivations that underlie their reassignment wish, their expanding insight seems to have no effect on the basic wish for reassignment. The pressure of the situation is often taken out, such that patients can more patiently wait for the assessment and 'real-life tests' to take their course, but in my experience, 'post-analytic' gender-disordered patients are simply better-informed gender-disordered patients. All that has changed is that their consent to their reassignment treatment is better informed, their understanding of their reasons for making their choices is more profound, but they remain the same. This is difficult for therapists whose own belief system is based on their own experience of well-analysed gender compromise and con-fusion, but for whom reassignment would seem a crazy option. The continuation of the symptom, as strong as ever (and indeed often stronger and more stable), is profoundly dispiriting, and demarcates in a rather painful way the limits of the therapeutic potency of the psychoanalytic method itself.

Conclusions

In this section, I have tried to explore some of the issues that emerge at the interface of gender reassignment treatment and psychotherapy by looking first at the role and tensions for the psychotherapist with the reassignment team, then by looking at some psychodynamic theories about the nature of the transsexual symptom, and finally by looking at approaches to psychotherapy work with these patients. I have argued that gender patients both require and deserve psychotherapeutic input in order to be able to clarify their motivations for seeking gender reassignment treatment, but that at the same time, gender disorders present particular challenges to psychotherapists because of the patient's wish to adopt a physical solution to what the psychotherapist perceives as a psychological problem. I have argued that it is this very tension held by the psychotherapist that is an essential contribution to the deliberations of gender reassignment teams, necessary for maintaining a therapeutic balance in their work with patients being assessed and prepared for hormonal and surgical reassignment.

References

1 Stoller RJ. *Sex and Gender: The development of masculinity and femininity*. London: Karnac Books; 1968.
2 Chassequet-Smirgel J. *Creativity and Perversion*. London: Free Association Books; 1996.

10

Challenging patients and circumstances

James Barrett

Coincidental non-psychotic mental illnesses

Eating disorders

Anorexia nervosa seems to be rather more common in gender dysphoric male patients than chance would allow.[1] The rate of bulimia nervosa seems to be no higher than chance, in both male and female patients. Usually this is childhood or adolescent anorexia, and more often than not it seems not to be a currently active problem. The impression is that the motivation for the disordered eating was the desire to maintain a body weight low enough to preclude gonadal functioning.

There is not, it seems, an increased history of eating disorders in gender dysphoric female patients despite the potential delay in puberty that would result. One suspects that male patients find a frail hypogonadal frame feminine, while for female patients physical frailty is too unmasculine to outweigh the benefits of a hypogonadal menopause.

Obsessive-compulsive disorder

Obsessive-compulsive disorder has been reported in association with gender identity disorder, the treatment for the obsessive-compulsive disorder seeming to lead to remission of the gender identity disorder.[2] In general, though, the two problems seem distinct entities.

Obsessive-compulsive disorder is an underestimated complaint. It can be very disabling, and may be so in the context of a real life experience. Obsessional worries and ruminations about the side-effects of hormone treatment (especially the question of whether twinges in the patient's calf represent symptoms of a deep vein thrombosis) may rule out its use. Rituals and obsessions about make-up and dress may extend preparation time to the point that the patient never actually gets out of the house.

Patients with obsessive-compulsive disorder coincidental with a gender identity disorder need cognitive-behavioural therapy. Response to such treatment is the main determinant of their prognosis of their gender identity disorder treatment. This, in its turn, depends on whether the patient gives cognitive-behavioural therapy the best try possible. There should be a careful liaison with the cognitive-behavioural therapist, because a suboptimal effort at cognitive-behavioural therapy may represent a masked or subconscious ambivalence to a change of gender role.

Case report: obsessive-compulsive disorder

AP had quite severe obsessive-compulsive disorder, and had been treated with both drugs and cognitive-behavioural therapy, with only a partial response. Effectively housebound, she took up to four hours to wash because of the associated rituals. She reported that she and her doctors had thought that the two problems were essentially unconnected, but that she had improved with regard to the obsessive-compulsive disorder after gender re-assignment surgery. On exploration, it seemed that this had been partly because she had rather liked the sense of cleanliness that she met in hospital.

Addictions

Addictions are just as common in gender identity disorder as anywhere else. There is a tendency for the patient to ascribe the addiction to the gender identity disorder. Sometimes this seems justified, but more often, especially where there seems to be a high genetic loading for addiction, it seems a less than plausible link. Even in those cases where the gender identity disorder might be seen as the origin of the addiction often the addiction takes on a life of its own and persists even when the gender identity disorder is being addressed.

In these circumstances the prognosis of the addiction determines the prognosis of the gender identity disorder rather than the reverse. The services that one would normally suggest in the context of addiction are almost all appropriate if the addiction is coincidental with or caused by a gender identity disorder. Alcoholics Anonymous, particularly, are concerned only with their fellows' alcohol use, and make a point of not being concerned with any other aspect of lifestyle or behaviour.

Conversion disorders

Conversion disorders are a particular worry, since there is always the suspicion that the disorder reflects the expression of a strong unconscious ambivalence. They are considered in the section dealing with disabled patients (p. 110).

Coincidental psychosis

Making twin diagnoses of a gender identity disorder and a psychotic illness is a challenging business, discussed earlier in the section dealing with referrals and screening. This section deals instead with the emergence of a coincidental psychotic illness after a real life experience has commenced.

The main task in such circumstances is to review the diagnosis to decide if what was previously supposed to be a gender identity disorder should now better be viewed as a prodrome or early symptom of psychotic illness. The closer the temporal association between the first presentation of the apparent gender identity disorder and the onset of psychosis, the more seductive is this suggestion. If the two are linked, brisk treatment of the psychotic illness should result in the amelioration of both the psychotic illness and the symptoms that had earlier suggested a gender identity disorder. Should only the psychotic symptoms abate, the probability of both a psychotic illness and a disorder of gender identity re-asserts itself.

If the psychosis and gender identity disorder are thought for temporal or phenomenological reasons to be distinct, the problem becomes more one of a real life experience conducted in the presence of a disability, with the added com-plication that the psychotic illness might impair capacity to such an extent that consent for gender reassignment surgery is absent.

As with any other chronic illness, in psychotic illnesses it is reasonable to expect their patients to do everything in their power to maintain the best possible health. This would imply co-operation with whatever treatment a community mental health team offers. Failure to do this would be a very doubtful justifica-tion for relaxing those strictures of a real life experience that would otherwise apply. If patients make an honest attempt to maintain their health but none-theless shows some decline in functioning, it might be reasonable to relax the boundaries of a real life experience.

It is reasonable to advance for gender reassignment surgery patients with truly co-incidental gender identity disorder and psychosis if it is honestly believed that the patients will cope better with the psychosis, and with other aspects of their lives, if the gender identity disorder is treated with gender reassignment surgery. This would feature a psychoses under sufficient control for the patient to have the capacity to consent to the surgery.

Case report: A case of a new psychotic illness occurring while undergoing a real life experience

PL presented at 19 years old, stating that she wanted to be a woman. She had no psychiatric or medical history of note but was recorded as smoking a moderate amount of cannabis.

PL had a lower second-class university degree and still lived at home with her parents. She was unemployed, but earlier had worked in both technical and semi-skilled jobs. She once had a girlfriend, but the relation-ship had broken down on the grounds of personality differences. It seemed that the girlfriend had colluded with her cross-dressing, and that PL had taken the girlfriend's contraceptive pill throughout the relationship.

PL was reported as having first cross-dressed aged 8 years, wearing her mother's dress. This had been worn in bed, and was reported as having felt 'really nice'. Subsequent cross-dressing was said to have happened about weekly, and her mother to have been told of this when PL was aged 16 years. It was said to have been viewed as 'a phase' and not criticised. At presentation, PL reported she was cross-dressing in her own room at home in the evenings. Family were said not to have been supportive of open cross-dressing.

PL was said to have been viewed by school peers as 'sissy' and probably gay, and to have been aware of only a weak sexual interest in women. She nonetheless was said to have prospered at school, and obtained a university degree. She said she dropped out of a higher degree course and returned to her family home because her flatmates had not tolerated her cross-dressing.

Six months later, PL had assumed a more androgynous social role and still smoked cannabis. She was advised that any hormone treatment would need to follow a clear change of gender role.

Four months later PL had changed to a clearly female name, and was working under that name. It seemed, though, that she still had an ambiguous presentation and was regarded as male by her peers.

After a further 4 months, it seemed that PL had unequivocally changed her social gender role. She was dressing in an unmistakably feminine manner at work, and was treated by her peers as if she was female. Her family were said to have accommodated to this change of gender role. Hormone treatment was commenced.

PL's progress over the next 4 months seemed to be good, with further consolidation of her female role. She commenced speech and language therapy.

Five months later PL arrived late for an appointment, and related having made a relationship with a man who used cocaine on a regular basis. She admitted to using cocaine on a few occasions herself. PL continued to work at her job.

Six months later, the relationship was said to have ended, but PL continued to use illicit drugs – mainly amphetamines. Her GP had commenced treating her with a specific serotonin reuptake inhibitor-type antidepressant. PL had formed another relationship with a man who used stimulants.

Four months later PL presented with clear symptoms of psychosis. She reported hearing male and female voices speaking about her, making both positive and negative remarks, and had noticed that when she said 'relax' to herself everyone around her relaxed too. She ascribed these sensations to the voice of God, or extrasensory perception. Five months later, and despite certainly having ceased all illicit drug use, the psychosis continued, and she was being treated with risperidone. She continued in employment despite an active psychosis, the symptoms of which she ascribed to 'spirit people'. She continued to feel female and live her life accordingly.

PL's clear psychosis showed no response to any neuroleptic agent, typical or atypical. The only effect seemed to be mild sedation. She coped well with her continuous low-level hallucinations and remained in employment. Throughout the psychotic illness her gender identity disorder remained unchanged in nature and intensity, unaltered from what had been seen before any psychotic symptoms were present. She remained attractively presented and charming. In due course, she was advanced as a candidate for gender reassignment surgery, with the advice that her mental state might need examining immediately before surgery if there were the slightest concerns about her capacity to consent.

Learning disability

Daniel Wilson

This section explores the historical issues of people with learning disabilities and their struggle to be accepted within a society that thrives and promotes success based upon both academic achievement and perfection. These two areas are outside the scope of achievement for many people with a learning disability.

It is most beneficial to practitioners clearly to define learning disabilities and also to outline what needs to be considered when working with people with learning disabilities. The aim is to ensure that patients get the most appropriate treatment and that practitioners ensure their rights by understanding their individual needs – as well as safeguarding their own professional practices.

Learning disability is clearly defined in the *Diagnostic and Statistical Manual of Mental Disorder* (DSM-IV (1994)) as having an IQ of 70 or below.[3] This definition is outdated in practice. It does not reflect the needs of modern multi-cultural societies. Modern learning disability practice holds that a broader view is required, considering the increasing number of people with mild or borderline learning disability and those diagnosed with Asperger's syndrome and autism. These last two diagnoses often technically fall outside learning disability services.

Many standard IQ tests are not relevant to a large number of people within modern society. Many of the symbols and tests used would not be recognisable to those who have spent much of their upbringing within other countries or in families where an English culture is not paramount.

Accordingly, alternative assessments are valuable, particularly those that are more observational or skill based. One such is the Assessment of Motor and Process Skills assessment (AMPS) (Kielhofner (2002)).[4] This is a skills-based assessment. It can assess an individual's level of functioning and interaction. It is designed to work across cultures and can be used in conjunction with the standard IQ assessments.

This is important because in practice one should be aware of a patient's learning disability. Often one works with patients who have undiagnosed learning disabilities, or the GP or another professional will not have informed you of the learning disability. This may happen when practitioners do not use a read coding that would highlight the learning disability. The use of these codes is identified as good practice in the Department of Health document *Valuing People*.[5]

Not having a clear diagnosis for a learning disability, or not being able to recognise learning disability indicators, has profound consequences not only for the patient but also for the professional and the employing organisation.

Clinical experience has shown that where there is limited understanding of the complexities of assessing people with learning disabilities, such people often do not have their health needs correctly diagnosed. Patients without capacity may be asked to 'consent' for treatment, or wholly inappropriate people may be asked to consent in their place.

This highlights one of the more complex issues for professionals, which is that of consent. The Department of Health (2001) guidance on gaining consent for people with learning disabilities is quite clear, but still many practitioners fail to gain adequate consent.[6] Patients may have surgical and medical interventions from tooth extractions through hip replacements to gender reassignment surgery, all without a clear understanding of the whole treatment process or valid consent being obtained.

Working with patients who have a learning disability should be based upon a multiprofessional approach. It should have the patient at the centre of the treatment, along with the patient's support network. This last should include the family unless the patient refuses their involvement. It is also important to ensure the local learning disability team is involved. They can enable the process of assessment and treatment to be understood as much as possible, and promote appropriate consent to treatment.

A strategy for working with people who have learning disabilities enables a department to have the means to both improve the quality of assessment and treatment and also ensure fair access to treatment. Such a strategy should incorporate both the recognition of a learning disability and best practice guidance for those learning disabled patients within the service. Co-working with learning disability services can help patients and a gender identity clinic to manage and understand the assessment and treatment process. Many learning disability specialists might be involved, including the following:

- *psychiatrists*: for capacity to consent and judgement of whether treatment is in the patient's best interests
- *psychologists*: for diagnosis and a quantitative assessment of learning disability, and the assessment of capacity to consent
- *community learning disability nurses*: for direct support with the client to understand medical treatment and later for preparation for admission and any surgical treatment. Nurses also advise non-learning disability clinical staff about understanding the individual needs of a client with learning disabilities. Learning disability nurses, in conjunction with mainstream services, support with admission and discharge planning, and post-operative support and monitoring
- *speech and language therapists*: may work to develop communication strategies that enable the patient to better understand their condition and treatment, as well as communicate their consent or understanding of treatment
- *counsellors* (often accessed through psychology): help patients explore and understand the potential changes to their lives following their diagnosis, and to understand their treatment options. Particularly important with gender reassignment treatment is ensuring that patients understand the impact of a real life experience as well as the physical changes caused by treatment.

It is important to remember that learning disability teams vary in both specialties and skill mix. On occasion, services might be required to purchase specialist learning disability services.

Only occasionally are positive images of people with disabilities placed in the public eye. These few images are generally of individuals having stand-alone physical disabilities rather than learning disabilities. There being almost no positive images of people with learning disabilities places learning disabled people at a huge disadvantage with regard to the development of any sort of positive identity.

Society's stereotypes for men and women remain the major factor in determining what we feel is appropriate behaviour to socially express our gender, be we male or female. Developing a social gender identity is arguably harder for those with learning disability. McCarthy (1997) explored how gender socialisation affected how women viewed and valued themselves, recognising that this also affected men with learning disabilities.[7] This work was supported by Cambridge (1997), who considered the heterosexual socialisation effects upon men with learning disabilities who wanted or experienced same-sex relationships.[7]

In addition to the way learning disabled men and women are required to present, others' expectations of them are often lower than what they want to achieve. We all want what everyone else has. People with learning disabilities have exactly the same desire. They will see others in their family and social circle advancing in careers, friendships and relationships, and perhaps having a family. They, meanwhile, feel the pressure of enforced limitations and have the knowledge that they will not be able to achieve the same things to the same level, regardless of their right to be supported to have as full and independent a life as possible. This very support often requires the involvement of health and social care professionals. It may take the spark and spontaneity out of experiences, and diminish privacy in the name of safety.

These forced limitations and limited acceptance from society give negative results. Many people diagnosed with learning disabilities have diagnosed mental health and behavioural problems requiring ongoing input from both mainstream mental health and learning disability services. Access to these services has allowed the gender identity problems of people with learning disabilities to begin to be recognised.

Slowly increasing numbers of people with learning disabilities are recognised as wanting to cross-dress and/or wanting gender reassignment. For many this is not a new area, but for the first time it is being discussed openly by those professionals supporting them.

From a clinical perspective the implications are many:

- the person's understanding of what they are doing, or what they want from cross-dressing and gender reassignment
- learning disability and mental health staff understanding of the functional role that the cross-dressing has for the service user
- the service user's understanding of the implications of cross-dressing – in private, with friends and peers or within wider society
- their ability to consent to the identified risks and consequences of any treatment.

This list of issues could go on. However, the area needing most consideration is the service user's understanding of why they are cross-dressing or wanting to change gender. Having worked with a number of mostly men who cross-dress and/or want to change their sex, my experience is that the presenting issue is not always gender dysphoria.

The presenting reason for wanting to cross-dress and change sex is sometimes a desire to escape themselves and thus lose the identity of 'a man with a learning disability', or become a 'new person' to explore a desire for same-sex relationships.

Here it is essential that mainstream general and mental health services understand the complexities of both the client's gender identity and individual learning disability needs. They need to identify the point where additional specialist assessments and input is required. This will be prior to the point of commencing treatment. Taking extra time at this point is advisable. It is far easier than managing the consequences of arranging that clients have treatment and then later finding out that they either do not understand the treatment or that their reason for wanting it was not appropriate. The task is made more challenging because many people with learning disabilities, having accessed medical staff for much of their lives, have experience and skill at positively managing medical assessments.

Asperger's syndrome

This syndrome may occur in association with a gender identity disorder. The combination proves uncommonly difficult to manage, although there are reports of success with a change of role.[8]

The major diagnostic problem is the inaccessibility of the patient's state of mind. While the psychological opacity encountered is not sufficiently dense to hamper determining whether the patient is psychotic or depressed, it does greatly impair the subtle examination of the motivations behind a request for hormone treatment and surgery. One is left with the worry that the motivator might be the desire to be rid of any sexual urge (often seen as unwanted in Asperger's syndrome) expressed in a very concrete way, or perhaps be fetishistic transvestism with the sexual component somehow unacknowledged or even unrecognised by the patient.

In purely practical terms, a change of social gender role is particularly challenging for someone with Asperger's syndrome. He or she is likely to have a problem apprehending the emotional communications of others as well as difficulties expressing his or her own emotional state. This is apt to make it very difficult for someone with Asperger's syndrome to put across whatever sense of masculinity or femininity they feel.

A change of social gender role usually produces interpersonal tensions. These may be dispelled by wit or a warm, emotional approach. The ability to diffuse tensions in this way may be very limited or come across as very mechanical and insincere in Asperger's syndrome.

People with Asperger's syndrome are frequently unemployed, although often well qualified and of good intelligence. The lack of social skills that causes this serves also to make a real life experience a difficult proposition. A rudimentary social circle and adequate day-to-day functioning in the new gender role is often all that can reasonably be expected, and not very different from what would have happened had there been no change of gender role.

Asperger's syndrome and states considered to lie in the same 'spectrum' enjoyed a diagnostic renaissance in the late 20th and early 21st century. These and related diagnoses started more commonly to be made in circumstances where before nothing more pathological than eccentricity might have been imputed. The case of AP (*see* 'Psychosis', p. 48) suggests that this trend carries with it risks of missing other, more easily treatable, diagnoses.

Physically disabled patients

As in any other setting, a proportion of the patients seen in a gender identity clinic are physically disabled. As a rule, their management is not very different from routine. It is necessary to make appropriate allowances for both the disability and the social responses to the disability when evaluating the real life experience.

Disabilities affecting communication seem to make the greatest impact. Having said this, even very profound difficulties in communication seem not to stand in the way of patients whose determination to seek treatment is strong, and whose personalities are robust.

Case report: severe hearing problem

SP presented via local psychiatric services, her initial referral having been delayed while an interpreter was sought. She was an EU citizen from a non-English speaking country, and had been almost wholly deaf from birth.

SP was able to communicate in European sign language, but could only lip-read those who spoke the language of her country of origin.

Despite these barriers to communication, SP had obtained hormone treatment in her country of origin and was living in a female role when she presented to services in the UK. The occasional lack of an interpreter required the psychiatrist to relay his questions to another doctor who spoke the language of the patient's country of origin, who in turn spoke to the patient – who lip-read the other doctor and then wrote an answer in that language, which was then translated to the psychiatrist by the other doctor. Perhaps unsurprisingly, outpatient appointments had to be booked at double length to accommodate this mode of communication. Rapport and information exchange greatly improved once a regular interpreter was enmeshed into the consultations.

SP progressed well, underwent gender reassignment surgery, and thrived thereafter. Her regular interpreter accompanied her to the operating theatre and was present for a proportion of her post-operative inpatient stay.

SP became somewhat socially isolated after gender reassignment surgery. She had acquired a degree of celebrity within the small and conservative world of signing deaf people. It seemed that a majority view was one of disapproval. At first, she had been accepted as part of a gay, signing, deaf subculture. As time passed she found her circle of gay friends diminishing, she had gradually come to be seen as ordinarily female in their eyes. She experienced, though, no correspondingly increased acceptance in straight, deaf, signing, circles.

Visual handicap

Visual disabilities present particular problems for patients at a gender identity clinic. Partial sight and blindness are much as one would expect in terms of their impact on private life, but may give the added handicap of diminishing patients' ability to monitor how their new gender role looks to others. Often, people with severe visual defects have others who advise them how they appear to sighted people. When visually impaired people change gender role, they may lose the support of the person or people who used to perform this function. This may make the change much harder for them.

More subtly, mild visual defects such as an amblyopic dysconjugate gaze may prove unexpectedly handicapping. An uncertain fixity of gaze causes others to stare harder than would otherwise be the case. This increased scrutiny can be unwelcome and unhelpful. Some would argue that surgery to produce a conjugate gaze would be helpful in these circumstances, even if it were too late to allow stereoscopic sight or any other objective improvement in visual function.

Speech impediments

Speech impediments, particularly stammer, present similar problems. Stammers are more common in males than in females. The presence of a stammer seems to signal to others (in an unconscious way perhaps) that the person they have before them is not as female as they seem to be. Accordingly, if the speech and language therapist is able to offer voice work to address stammer as well as voice feminisation this is likely to be of benefit.

Conversion disorder

Patients whose disability is thought to represent a conversion disorder present a different problem. There is always the suspicion that the disorder reflects the physical manifestation of unconscious ambivalence in someone who declares utter conviction about a change of gender role. Such suspicion is greater if there is a close temporal association between the onset of the conversion disorder and the change of role.

Sometimes a symbolic link can easily be drawn between the nature of the disorder and the hypothecated ambivalence, but it is of course all too easy to imagine such links if one wishes to. Overall, a temporal association would carry more weight than seeming symbolic significance unless the latter is obvious. However, in conversion disorder chronicity usually implies permanence; the case below features a conversion disorder whose fluctuating course might shed light on a link with the gender identity disorder.

Case report: fluctuating conversion disorder

V changed gender role from male to female in her 30s. She had a history of romantic and sexual attraction to women, and had married and had children. At presentation she had a relationship with a woman who had known her in her earlier male role.

V developed a rapidly progressive upper limb weakness about 6 months after she had changed role from male to female. She had until that point continued her employment in the lower reaches of the Civil Service.

Possible diagnoses in V's case had included multiple sclerosis and a mitochondrial myopathy. Extensive and skilled investigation eventually confirmed the psychiatric clinical suspicion of a conversion syndrome.

V began to socialise in groups for the physically disabled, and to accumulate both 'cute' and 'sporty' accessories for her customised electric wheelchair. She showed some element of 'belle indifference' in that she said 'I hate this wheelchair', while smiling.

After 2 years, V's conversion disorder began to resolve when she made a relationship with a man, although she herself did not see the link until the coincidence was pointed out to her. She dropped both cute and sporty wheelchair extras as well as the disabled social circle, instead becoming a paralegal administrative worker with no special responsibility for the disabled. She reported that the strength in her arms was beginning to improve.

The relationship faltered after 6 months, and V's disability returned. Her symptoms waned again, about a year later, when V's mother made contact with her after a long period in which her father had precluded this because she would be 'too upset by the change of gender role'. V had expected her disapproval, and had been surprised to find her supportive. There seemed to be an element of 'permission from my mother' in her recovery.

Not all conversion disorders seen in association with a gender identity disorder provoke worry. Some seem easily accounted for by the circumstances.

Case report: less worrying conversion disorder

JP changed role from male to female in her 50s. She was employed as a classical singing coach at a central London drama school. Her gender identity disorder had led to the destruction of her marriage, and had been ill-received by her brother. He had suggested that were their mother (elderly, with ischaemic heart disease) to be told, she would be so shocked that she might suffer a fatal heart attack. JP had reasoned to herself that since the change or role was to be permanent her mother would have to know, despite any shock it might cause. Still, she had worried about her brother's dire prediction.

JP negotiated with her employers and secured a continued place at the drama school after her change of role. She had worries, though, about how the students would treat her.

JP's mother had retired to Scotland. JP had been driving through the north of England to visit her mother, accepting that her drastic change of appearance would make it obvious to her mother what had occurred. She experienced a coughing fit as she passed through Carlisle, which led to an acute loss of voice and an inability to speak. A visit to the Carlisle hospital casualty department replaced her visit to her mother. From there she returned home, her mother unvisited.

Speech and language therapy suggested a psychogenic cause for the voice loss, but JP was nonetheless unable to return to her job. She secured other employment soon after, and an exchange of postal correspondence with her mother revealed wholehearted maternal support.

JP's voice returned soon after. She was easily able to accept that her loss of voice might have served to prevent her undertaking a worrying communication with her mother and additionally to impel her into avoiding the anticipated conflict with her students. There were no further such problems.

Incapacity benefit

Incapacity Benefit does not always serve people with gender identity disorders well. Some of the problems with incapacity benefit are probably intrinsic to the whole benefits system, and others specific to those with a gender identity disorder.

A general problem seems to have been the tendency of the state sometimes rather readily to steer the longer-term unemployed into 'incapacitated' status. While this has served to keep unemployment figures lower than they might otherwise have been, the larger sum provided by incapacity benefit as compared to simple job seeker's allowance causes those in receipt of the former to be reluctant to relinquish the incapacitated status that allows its provision.

This problem is decreasing as unemployment reduction becomes less of a political concern and is replaced among other things by a drive to decrease taxation. Reviews of incapacitated status occur, and at least one patient has reported that her symptoms spontaneously remitted after her incapacity benefit was withdrawn.

A more specific problem has been the tendency of benefits officers to suggest that patients with a gender identity disorder ought not to seek regular employment but ought rather to be in receipt of incapacity benefit – the source of the incapacity being a gender identity disorder. This circular reasoning makes a real life experience difficult to initiate, because the patient has often become used to living on the reasonable income offered by incapacity benefit, and may argue that he or she would be financially worse of if paid work were to be undertaken. In these circumstances voluntary work can be suggested. Occasionally an incapacity benefit review goes against the patient, who may then abruptly find paid work.

Contentious disabilities

The nature or origin of a disability can be contentious. It is wise to pursue all claims of physical disability to their original source, no matter how firmly the diagnosis is presented by the patient's GP or referring psychiatrist. Very often, the unequivocal diagnosis in the psychiatrist's referral is based on the unqualified statement in the GP's referral before it, and this in turn is accepted from the notes of the previous GP, who copied it from the notes of the one before that, who based the statement on the patient's own account.

It is curious how rarely claims of surgical treatment by any psychiatric patient are accompanied by an examination for the associated scars. This seems to be just as true of patients referred with a gender identity disorder. Medically implausible procedures seem often to be reported as matters of fact by both psychiatrists and GPs.

Proven and uncontested disability can become contentious if it arises out of non-concordance with the suggested treatment plan. An example might be a smoker who was advised not to have a premature augmentation mammoplasty, but who nonetheless did so, sustaining a cerebrovascular accident in the process. She might subsequently claim to be a candidate for gender reassignment surgery without any need for the occupational part of a real life experience (on the grounds of a post-stroke disabled status). This would be a difficult matter.

HIV and AIDS

HIV seropositivity is not commonly encountered in the UK gender identity clinics' populations. It is seen mainly in male-to-female patients who might earlier have been identified by others, and sometimes themselves, as rather feminine gay men.

At the time of writing, AIDS seems to be accepted by society as a disabling illness, and as a reflection of this is accepted as a reason for the occupational component of a real life experience to be softened.

Having said this, advances in highly active antiretroviral treatment have rendered many HIV seropositive people, even those who earlier had frank AIDS, more well than would earlier have been dreamed possible. Many in this position seem keen to gain an occupation.

HIV seropositivity holds a peculiar position in that it seems to be viewed by some HIV seropositive people as clear grounds for disabled status and by others as something that should not be used as a reason to treat them any differently from those who are HIV seronegative. The very long latency of HIV infection, in combination with the increasing survival times once AIDS has manifested itself, suggests that in time the latter view ought possibly to prevail.

Forensic patients and the real life experience

A real life experience in a forensic psychiatric or penal setting is a challenging proposition. There must be understanding and co-operation from those in authority, with the clear acceptance that a proper change of role will be accommodated, rather than merely the wearing of a few items of jewellery or a full set of appropriate clothing only when isolated from others.

It is essential that the patient be treated by those around him or her – fellow patients or prisoners and staff alike – as if he or she was of the assumed sex. This is not likely to occur if the patient is in a segregated ward or prison with others of the former sex.

There is often great institutional opposition to moving the patient to a segregated place allocated to the new sex. Often, such a move is said to be dependent on the patient having had genital surgery. Such surgery will not occur unless that real life experience is completed, which in turn depends on the proscribed move. Female patients often do not undergo phalloplasty, and so the emphasis on genital surgery seems particularly inappropriate for them.

Quite apart from the institutional barriers to a real life experience, a major problem is the extent to which any sort of valid real life experience can be conducted in a prison or a secure hospital. Neither environment can be described as normal. There must be doubt whether someone who can change gender role in such a setting can manage in the new role in civilian society, or even in a less secure institutional setting.

Secure hospital settings can often be more tolerant of difference than the world outside them. Those in such a setting are likely to be unusual, and are compelled to live in extreme and prolonged proximity. Toleration of the strangeness of others is thus likely to be unusually high, in both staff and patients alike. Someone whose change of gender role is tolerated in such a setting might fare less well in a lower-security setting, less well yet in a general psychiatric ward, and not at all in a community setting. Yet it is in a community setting that the patient is likely to spend the rest of his or her days.

Prisons might be supposed to be places where difference is not well tolerated. While this might be true in some ways, those serving longer sentences are likely either to develop the ability to get on with disparate others or to spend a lot of time alone. People with a gender identity disorder who change role in prison are likely to be placed with more tolerant prisoners, or else to be segregated 'for their own protection'. Such segregation does serve to protect them from assault, but serves also to protect them from the unbridled opinion of others. This will not offer a real life experience.

Male patients may undergo a real life experience, or as close to it as the prison system will allow, and seek gender reassignment surgery. One underlying drive behind this seems to me the knowledge that, having undergone gender re-assignment surgery, they will be moved to a female prison.

Long incarceration of male patients seems to cause (or at least to fail to disabuse patients of) a strong belief in a mutually supportive sisterhood of women. There seems to be a belief that women isolated together in the absence of men behave in a particularly co-operative and pacific manner. Being told that this is not necessarily so does not seem to change the belief. The subsequent experience of hostility, manipulation and assault (including of a sexual sort) in a nearly exclusively female setting seems to cause psychological decompensation.

These problems make a real life experience in a prison or secure hospital setting particularly problematic. It might be wise to wait until those serving a short sentence or those mentally ill people who are expected to recover quickly are in a community setting, before a real life experience is considered properly to have commenced whatever the earlier behaviour in prison or hospital.

This could not be applied to those whose sentences are very long, or those whose release from hospital seems a very distant prospect. In such circumstances a real life experience might have to be embarked upon with all the concerns and caveats that such a setting imposes.

Life licence prisoners

Prisoners sentenced to life imprisonment – usually but not exclusively for murder – may under UK legislation be released from prison on life licence. They are closely monitored by the probation service. They may at any time be recalled to prison by order of the Home Secretary. No further offences need to have been committed for such a recall to be ordered.

Life licence prisoners may have problems with a real life experience, as the following shows.

Case report: a life licence prisoner inhibited by this legal status

TM had spent about two-thirds of her life in prison when she was released on life licence, having been convicted of murder. She had told the prison medical service of her desire to live as a man, but no action had been taken. It had been thought that the matter would be better dealt with when she was living in the community.

TM presented at a gender identity clinic with her probation officer. Over the course of many appointments she expressed a great desire to live as a man and an even greater fear that her initial attempts to do so might result in a public disturbance. She was terrified that if she were to be involved in a disturbance she would be recalled to prison. TM was quite sure that she would never cope with another spell inside prison. The probation officer sought guidance from the Home Office, who indicated that provided TM had no role other than as a victim, a disturbance would not be likely to result in a recall. Despite this assurance, TM's fear of recall continued to override her desire to change gender role.

Patients as victims of crime

Patients are more likely to be victims of crime than perpetrators. Within a western European setting, the crimes to which they are particularly susceptible tend to to be related to prejudice and are the sorts of harrassment one might expect. Sometimes they are victimised by institutions in ways that seem wrong but probably do not amount to a crime. An example is related below.

Case report: patient denied educational opportunities

A young female patient seen when still in a female social gender role, described having been pressured to leave her school just before sitting exams for which she had worked for 2 years. She was pressed to leave because her relationship with a 16-year-old female at her school was discovered and had been subject to a complaint by the 16-year-old's father. There would not have been the same reaction had the patient been male.

Sometimes an institutional response is odd, but does not so obviously disadvantage patients. An example is the police searching of pre-operative male patients, where the policy seems to be that areas above the waist are searched by a female officer and areas below by a male. This might become more complicated if the searching officer were transsexual (*see* 'Occupational matters', p. 75).

Patients from outside western Europe sometimes present with stories of the most gross victimisation, as illustrated below.

Case report: gross victimisation

A female patient from the Middle East related having been discovered *in flagrante delicto* by her female partner's brother. He had informed the state authorities. The local police caught the patient's partner and stood her in a freshly dug pit. They then emptied a lorry load of stones on her. The patient narrowly escaped the same fate and fled to the UK, where she had to contend with grief as well as the stigma of being seen as a refugee, and thus either a benefits scrounger or a foreign worker, driving down wages for UK nationals.

Patients as offenders

Patients in a gender identity clinic may commit criminal offences. These may be divided according to whether the disorder of gender identity played any role in the genesis or nature of the offence.

Clearly, the theft of articles of cross-sex clothing might be expected in a population with gender identity problems, and would be a clearly related matter.

More loosely connected are those offences connected with relationship problems when it seems that the gender identity disorder has either caused or aggravated the problems. For example, at least one female patient has committed a serious act of violence in the context of both intoxication and being descibed as a lesbian.

Particularly challenging are those cases where an aquisitive crime is said to have been committed in order to fund treatment for the gender identity disorder of either the offender or someone else. (This latter situation is depicted in the feature film *Dog Day Afternoon*.) The plausibility of such claims declines greatly if they are made much after the offence, and in any event should be investigated in some detail.

One offender deliberately used some degree of dual-role transvestism or other gender identity disorder to engineer an offence, as described below.

Case report: gender identity disorder as a means to offend

BW presented to a gender identity clinic in a middle-aged female role. There was a history of dual-role transvestism, which was described as having evolved into transsexualism. She gave a slightly bland but otherwise un-remarkable history at both parts of an initial assessment.

BW was provided with letters to help her obtain a driving licence and passport in her female role.

BW stopped attending the gender identity clinic. She had obtained new identity documents in a female role. She used these and her female presenta-tion in conjunction with her previous documents and previous role as a means to commit a financial fraud revolving around having two identities.

Prison placement problems

A first step in dealing with these problems, of course, is for the police and prison systems to recognise that the problems exist. This seems obvious, but does not always immediately occur. One female patient, when being arrested, told the arresting officers of his transsexualism. The arresting officers initially refused to accept his transsexual status yet refused also to examine his genitals when he suggested that this would confirm his story.

A primary question with convicted patients is whether they ought to serve a custodial sentence at all. Defence lawyers sometimes seek an opinion in such cases to see whether a custodial sentence could be viewed as a particularly unusual punishment on grounds of their client being transsexual.

If custodial sentences are applied, prison placement for people who have changed social gender role is problematic. Remand and short-term prisoners seem to be treated without regard to any actual or aspirational change of role, possibly because their expected stay in prison would be shorter than the time taken for the prison medical administration to repond to their situation. These prisoners may experience menopausal symptoms secondary to estrogen withdrawal, but seem otherwise to fare reasonably well.

The issues arising from longer sentences, particularly life sentences, have been described earlier in this chapter.

Patients in the police or armed services

There is a greater prevalence of gender identity disorders (seemingly nearly always males) inside the armed forces than outside. This is often viewed with surprise, but ought not to be.

If people have an uncertain sense of their masculinity then it can seem sensible to join an organisation that purports to 'make a man of you', or in which male roles are very well demarcated. Such organisations include the armed forces and the Hell's Angels (*see* 'Heterosexual male secondary transsexuals', p. 22).

Patients who join these organisations usually show one of two distinct trajectories. The first is that of not coping from the outset, despite their best efforts to look, sound and act in a masculine way. Those with this trajectory tend quickly to leave the armed forces with a discharge remark suggesting that they were not suited to service life.

The second and more common trajectory is that of seemingly good adaptation to a martial male role. Indeed, such individuals seem often to have had particularly outstanding military careers, with no disciplinary charges, and decorations for behaviour falling on the right side of that very fine line which lies between bravery and stupidity.

Whichever trajectory is taken, patients usually leave the armed forces or Hell's Angels without disclosing the reasons for their departure. About half of the patients in the armed forces buy themselves out, the others serving their time. Some are refused a request to extend their service, suggesting that they might have been attempting to do so in order to postpone addressing their gender identity problems.

Often, the news that an ex-service person has changed social gender role is greeted with astonishment, especially by those not personally acquainted with the person. Sometimes, though, not everyone had been persuaded by the patient's earlier performance in a male role, especially those who knew him well. Ex-Hell's Angels and soldiers who feel that they were particularly convincing may be annoyed to be told by their former chapter's or regiment's members 'we always thought you were gay, anyway'.

The UK armed services have no objection in principle to recruiting people who have changed gender role, or continuing to employ people who do so while in the services. Some such cases have reached the attention of the newspapers. It does seem that serving armed forces members who change gender role may be moved, at an equivalent rank, from one branch of the armed services to another.

On leaving the armed services, most patients change social gender role and feel very much more at ease in a female civilian role, often thriving. In a few cases, though, the decision to leave the armed forces seems to have been unwise, because the patient seems genuinely to have been temperamentally suited to service life and would have prospered better in the armed services (in either gender role) than they have fared in civilian life. One such case is summarised below.

Case example: ex-services patient

AG came from a military family, and happily joined the armed forces at a young age. Gender identity problems had been present since teenage years, but at first amounted to an easily concealed fetishistic transvestism. Over time, though, AG developed a dual-role transvestite lifestyle, which proved ever harder emotionally to contain.

AG felt that she had no choice but to leave the armed services, and asked to resign her commission. The armed forces were reluctant to lose her, arguing that she had an exemplary record and very good prospects. They could not understand why she wanted to leave. AG found herself unable to tell them.

On joining civilian life, AG quickly changed gender role to female and sought hormone treatment from a gender identity clinic. Although she prospered in civilian life, employing skills she had learned in the armed services, AG found many aspects of life outside the armed forces very frustrating. Particularly annoying were what seemed to be the chronic disorganisation she encountered, and the way lines of responsibility seemed always to be unclear.

After a time, AG sought an interview with the armed forces recruitment agency, concluding that she was better suited to service life. She hoped to rejoin the services in a female role.

It should be noted that bogus claims of military service are not uncommon, particularly if special forces training is claimed. As such claims can fairly easily be verified, they should all be confirmed (*see* 'Taking a history' (p. 11)).

The police service

The police services are employers who might be expected to attract people with gender identity disorders in the same way as do the armed services and the Hell's Angels. It seems, though, that the prevalence of gender identity disorders in the police is lower than that in these other organisations. This might be because police membership is more a job than a lifestyle, and perhaps because gender roles are less rigid in the police.

It is seemingly more common for people to work for the police service after they have changed gender role than for them to change role while a police officer. This is perhaps understandable given that the UK police services have very well-publicised policies making it plain that applications are considered without prejudice regarding ethnic group, sexual orientation or indeed anything much except intelligence, fitness, common sense and honesty. It seems that these policies are robustly applied in that several transsexual patients are serving police officers. One female patient, although born and bred in south east England, applied for training with the South Wales Police reasoning that shorter than average height in a male role would be less noticeable in a population where average male height is lower than that in England. A male patient's force appointed her to a special liaison group working with gay, lesbian, bisexual and transgendered people. Highly valuable information and convictions resulted from the increased confidence felt in the police by these groups.

The police services have more civilian employees than police officers. A number of patients have obtained employment as such civilian employees. All seem very content with how they have been recruited and subsequently treated.

Hormone treatment without role change

Hormone treatment in the absence of a change of social gender role is a common and superficially reasonable request. If it occurs, it may be a source of great problems.

The reason for the request is usually the patient's belief that he or she cannot be expected to pass in the new gender role without first being treated with hormones. It is suggested to the prescriber that once the patient has been masculinised or feminised (as appropriate) a change of role will more easily follow. Body and facial hair are often cited as particular problems; either too much or too little. In fact, the impact of estrogens on facial hair is slight, and if people do not have the genes for facial hair, no amount of androgens will make them grow some.

Providing hormone treatment at a first appointment, without a change of gender role, confuses both prescriber and patient. Any subsequent changes might be attributed solely to hormone therapy, when the process of taking a history and listening to the patient might have been reponsible for the changes. Indeed, the placebo effect of the medication is considerable. A patient prescribed hormone therapy at the first visit might reasonably infer that the prescription confirms a diagnosis of transsexualism, and might then continue with self-funded gender reassignment surgery, wrongly believing that the treating psychiatrist was convinced that this would have been the correct course of action.

For male patients, speech and language therapy cannot properly work without daily, in-role, practice. Whatever the physical successes of hormones might (very occasionally) be, male patients will be in trouble when they open their mouths.

Estrogens given before a change of role may decrease a libidinous drive that causes guilt. The patient may wrongly, and disastrously, assume that the relief from guilt confirms a diagnosis of transsexualism, and move directly to gender reassignment surgery before any change of social gender role (*see* 'Gender reassignment surgery with no role change', p. 62). More usually, estrogens serve to produce a sense of tranquillity and a mild increase in the patient's sense of well-being. It is, somehow, as if the drive to change social gender role has had the wind taken out of its sails. The accompanying decrease in libido also caused by estrogenic treatment is usually met with relief.

In such a pleasant state there is a tendency for patients to be aware of a desire to change their social gender role, but to wish to take no further active steps save perhaps for further bodily feminisation in the absence of a social role change.

This might seem desirable. However, it causes problems because it does not last. After a time, which seems to vary between a few weeks and 2 years, the dysphoria reasserts itself. The patient usually requests an increase in hormone dose. This does not fully restore the sense of tranquillity, and does not do even this for long.

Throughout this period, the patient has been exposed to the risks of thromboembolic disease. Increasing the dose increases the risk. Eventually the patient may feel just as dysphoric as they were at the start, but have had a pulmonary embolism.

If hormones are prescribed before a change of role, there is in my experience usually either a suboptimal or a frankly bad result. The following sort of development might well be played out:

- after insisting that hormones be provided, the patient takes them with much gratitude and solemnly undertakes to change role as soon as she or (usually) he has responded enough to the hormones. Some 3 months later the patient is pleased with the initial results. He says that all is on track and that he feels very much better in himself
- six months later, the patient says that development has somehow 'levelled off'. The dose is increased. Over the next two or three appointments the pattern is for the patient to report just enough development for the doctor to be unable to suggest stopping hormone treatment on the grounds of non-response, yet insufficient change for the patient to feel that he would be able to change gender role.

This last point is the kernel of the problem. The day seems not to dawn when such patients feel that hormones have done enough. Always, with eyes that have mirror gazed for decades, it is possible to discern something of the earlier appearance.

- The patient returns to the gender identity clinic and complains that the hormones have 'not worked'. Different hormones must surely be needed. Stronger hormones. Bigger doses perhaps. If only this facial hair would vanish (or appear) as hoped for and expected. By this time, the patient's manner suggests that the doctor has shamelessly misled him about the hormone treatment. It is as if the doctor had suggested the treatment, and pressured the patient into taking it. The onus seems to be on the doctor to get the hormones to effect some promised transformation. The patient behaves as if wholly justified in not changing role, as the unfortunate victim of some sort of misrepresentation. The patient may end up taking hormones for years, with all the attendant thromboembolic and other risks. There is no obvious benefit, and a role change seems ever further away. Were the patient to die of a pulmonary embolus (quite possible) it might be difficult to justify the continued thrombogenic treatment in a coroner's court.

There are, one optimistically imagines, ways that this might be avoided: setting a time-based deadline for commencing a real life experience perhaps; 'role change after no more than a year regardless of hormone effects or lack of them' maybe? It works only poorly, if at all, in my experience. With such measures, a sizeable proportion still show no sign of changing role after a year (or any other amount of time), and it is a lot harder for any doctor – GP or psychiatrist – to withdraw a drug already started. As the deadline approaches, the patients often drop out of treatment at the gender identity clinic, but may use their earlier attendance as a means to obtain continued supplies of hormones from a succession of GPs for many years afterwards. To prescribe in these circumstances would, I think, be hard to defend, but to decline is very difficult. I have often wondered whether many of the patients who so behave had, all along, no intentions other than the consumption of hormones. Many seem, in retrospect, to have arrived at trans-sexualism from a dual-role transvestism or autogynaephilic route.

Case report: hormone treatment without a change of gender role (1)

LB presented at a gender identity clinic requesting gender reassignment surgery. He was wearing denim jeans and black leather boots that might have been appropriate for either sex. Under his matching denim jacket was a purple blouse that might have passed for a shirt. The combination of the last two served well to conceal well-developed breasts. His hair was neutrally styled, and he wore a small quantity of make-up.

LB maintained he was living in a female role, but admitted that were he to ask a stranger the way to the toilet he would certainly be directed to the men's facilities. He argued that all his clothes were bought at female clothing stores, but agreed that the overall impression was decidedly male. LB said that he did wear a skirt at times, but only when he was driving his car. He had attended his appointment dressed as he was, he argued, because he had come on the train and did not know what the reaction of others might be.

LB had been commenced on estrogens and cyproterone acetate over a decade earlier, on the basis that he ought to be more feminised before it would be reasonable to expect him to change his gender role. Over the years, he had suffered from a refractory depressive disorder that had lifted when the cyproterone acetate was discontinued. It seemed that LS had lost contact with the psychiatrist who had commenced him on estrogens, and that his GP had continued to prescribe for the next decade. Throughout the 10 years LB had smoked 15 cigarettes a day, greatly raising his risk of thromboembolic disease.

Case report: hormone treatment without a change of gender role (2)

PW elicited a prescription for estrogens on the understanding that a change of gender role would shortly follow. On review 9 months later and still in a male role he remarked, 'I have not changed identity all that often'.

PW reported problems with electrolysis. He hoped, in 6 months more, 'to look like a woman who needs electrolysis rather than a woman with a beard'.

Although PW was said to have told his employers of his situation, he was still working in a male role. His wife had been persuaded but not convinced of the potential benefits of his changing gender role, and they had not yet told their daughter, aged 14, 'but will soon'. Speech and language therapy was said to be 'going well', although PW noted that he never spent long enough in a female role to get speech and language therapy practice.

Six months later, there was still no change of role. PW's daughter had been told and proved supportive, but his wife had come to find his domestic female role irritating. PW still blamed his stasis on problems with electrolysis, but conceded that there had been no problems in a female role on day trips with his wife. The main conflict seemed to be with authority figures, along with a reluctance to upset his wife and expose his daughter to teasing.

PW continued to maintain he would change his gender role at some time in the distant future. It seemed that there were no concrete plans about achieving this.

Case report: hormone treatment without a change of gender role (3)

MZ presented seeking androgens, dressed in a boyish but nonetheless feminine manner, but declaring that she presented in a very masculine way.

MZ had a history of relationships with both men and women, although it was those with straight or feminine gay women that seemed to have persisted the longest and meant the most to her. All her relationships were said to have been dilatory. It seemed that if she became emotionally involved with people she became warmer and more traditionally feminine.

MZ sought male hormones. The worry was that however masculine she might initially appear, any progressively deepening relationship that she formed with a straight woman would be one in which she would come across as increasingly feminine, and which would consequently fail with the passage of time. MZ seemed to hope that androgens would masculinise her emotional style as well as her body.

At further review, MZ had been seen at a different gender identity clinic and had been approved for a bilateral mastectomy she had not been able to afford. She was still in a female role, and was irritated at the refusal of the clinic to countenance hormones.

MZ failed to attend the next two appointments and then presented in an androgynous role, with an androgynous name, having had a bilateral mastectomy performed abroad, and taking hormones from a private doctor. These had been started when she had not changed gender role. Acne was proving a problem, possibly related to the very high doses suggested. It was not clear what MZ sought from the appointment, but it did seem that her tendency to be feminine in the context of meaningful relationships remained unchanged.

Role change without hormone treatment

It is rare for someone to undertake a change of social gender role without cross-sex hormone treatment. It might occur in the following circumstances:

- the patient has changed role without medical assistance, having had no access to hormones, but would have wanted such assistance
- the patient has changed role without medical assistance, had no access to hormones, and never saw the need for them anyway
- the patient has changed role with medical assistance but had no hormone treatment because the risks outweighed the benefits.

Sometimes patients arrive at a gender identity clinic having changed gender role without hormone treatment that they would ideally have wanted. It is rare for them to be European residents since in a western European setting hormones can usually be obtained from somewhere. An exception would be the case of those blocked from access to black market or other sources of hormones by being institutionalised, or disabled with conditions grossly impairing their ability to communicate (such as a sensory, neurological or intellectual handicap).

Most patients who have changed role without access to hormones have done so outside Europe. Several have come from Gulf states.

Some patients change role without any support and without hormone treatment because they do not feel it is necessary. This group includes primary male patients and some secondary patients coming from a gay male background. They seem to pass very well as female (some have been mistaken for female since childhood), and have managed perfectly well without hormones.

Female patients may manage to change role without medical assistance if they happen to have polycystic ovary syndrome. This condition may make them masculinised enough to pass as male with ease.

A more difficult group of male patients are those who present having 'changed role' without any hormone treatment and for whom the veracity of a role change is gravely in doubt. These often pass poorly, and have either no record of employment or occupation in a female role, or a record of an occupation in so sheltered or supportive an environment (working from home, or a relation's business for example) as hardly to count. They often take the view that it is their conviction of their own femininity that matters, and that non-acceptance by others amounts to an unacceptable prejudice that ought not to be allowed to influence the opinion of a gender identity clinic. These patients may wear an outfit bought entirely in female clothing shops, assembled so that the general impression is nonetheless masculine. They may insist that they are widely accepted as female but more often than not when no evidence supports this and the 'public toilet test' is put to them,* they either openly admit that this is not the case, or conduct themselves thereafter as if they had made such an admission. These patients tend to be gynaephilic secondary transsexuals from a transvestite background, or patients with autogynaephilia.

---

* A test to determine whether, in an unfamiliar environment where one is not already known (such as a shopping centre), when one asks to be directed to the toilet, one would be directed to the toilet appropriate for the birth sex or the sex in which one claims now to be living.

Patients with appropriate medical help may sometimes be ineligible for treatment with sex steroids because the risks outweigh the benefits. Such circumstances would include smoking, a clotting diathesis and history of thromboembolic disease.

Rarely, there are psychiatric reasons precluding treatment with sex steroids. One such was a female patient displaying a sexual attraction to peripubertal males (experienced as homosexual paedophilia). It was felt too risky to augment this patient's libido with androgen treatment. The patient had polycystic ovary syndrome that was sufficiently severe to androgenise her to some extent.

No male patient should undergo gender reassignment surgery without first experiencing a total lack of androgens, because this is exactly what they will experience after such surgery. If this has not been attained with female sex steroid therapy alone, it could be achieved with gonadotrophin-releasing hormone analogue treatment.

It is probably not a good idea to achieve a low-androgen state by means of orchidectomy because this would represent an irreversible step and thus prejudge the result of what is being tested. For this reason, it is debarred by the Harry Benjamin Gender Dysphoria Association guidelines. In addition, it may render subsequent gender reassignment surgery more difficult (*see* 'Orchidectomy in a female role', p. 90).

Reversion to former gender role during real life experience but before gender reassignment surgery

In the context of a real life experience, reversions to former gender role comprise brief episodes of reversion for 'special' or other occasions, sustained periods of reversion, and permanent reversion. Each has a different cause and prognostic implication.

It is essential that both patient and clinician grasp that a change of role is not always easily reversible. Reversion to the original gender role might be simple early in a real life experience, but after hormone treatment (especially for female patients) it will be very much less so.

Gender reassignment surgery makes no difference to how easily social gender role may be reverted, but makes psychological adjustment to reversion more difficult and sexual adjustment very difficult indeed. Patient and clinician need to be acceptably sure that reversion is not likely before hormone treatment is commenced (especially for female patients) and wholly sure it is not going to happen before the patients are referred for gender reassignment surgery.

Brief reversions may occur to meet the perceived needs of 'special occasions' such as weddings, funerals, court appearances and so forth. Oddly, brief reversions can also occur because there is nothing at all special about the day, and the patient could not be bothered to go to the effort of changing role. Of these two, the latter has the worse implication, since such days are common in anyone's life. Both sorts of brief reversion carry with them both the implication that the patient views a change of role as something that can easily be reversed, and that the patient has a low threshold for such reversion. This is not compatible with the decreasingly reversible nature of what is being embarked upon. It needs to be addressed before any step that is at all hard to reverse is undertaken.

Lengthier reversions to a former role may occur in the context of relationships. They may imply that the drive to change role may not have been quite as strong as was suggested or might have had different motivations from those first suspected.

Case report: reversion in the context of a relationship

PQ presented with a vague history of dual-role transvestism, seemingly without a preceding fetishistic transvestite phase. His sexual interests and activities had always been with women.

PQ changed social gender role, but reported feeling very self-conscious in a female role. He hoped that this would diminish with time. He changed his name to a female one that was a homophone for his former name. PQ had previously always been employed, and for the first time experienced difficulty getting a job.

While in a nominally female role, PQ met a woman whom he described as androgynous but attractive. They formed a relationship, and as part of this PQ ceased his female hormone treatment to allow him to improve his sexual performance. He quickly reverted to a male role, with the partner's support.

At review, PQ remained in a male role, but remained gender dysphoric. He saw the relationship as more important than whether he was male or female, and did not want to do anything drastic and irreversible while the relationship remained incompletely explored.

Case report: reversion to a male role

DB presented in his mid-40s, with a stated desire to change gender role. He was sexually attracted to women, and had a history of initially fetishistic and later dual-role transvestism.

DB changed social gender role with moderate ease, but experienced difficulty gaining an occupation. It seemed that there was a lacklustre performance at job interviews, of which there were said to have been many.

As time passed, DB gained occupation in a voluntary capacity with a tolerant organisation, despite having formal qualifications that should have made a much higher level of occupational functioning possible.

DB reported that time in a female role proved more of a strain than had been expected, and that at times returning home and divesting himself of his female clothing came as a great relief. No very great time later, he reverted to a male role, and wanted no further contact with the gender identity clinic.

In due course DB again contacted the gender identity clinic, saying that the earlier reversion to a male role had been regretted fairly soon after the last appointment. The regret was said to have grown with time rather than to have diminished. He once again adopted a female role, and gained a slightly better level of occupational functioning than before, although still far below that which would have been expected given the level of training and qualifications he had.

Thereafter his pattern of attendance at the gender identity clinic became erratic, with many appointments cancelled on the grounds of minor physical ill-health. The level of attendance and reasons for non-attendance were such that it was not possible for DB formally to be discharged, but neither was it possible for treatment greatly to progress.

Reversions to a male role may come late in a real life experience, as the following illustrate.

Case report: late reversion to a male role (1)

DY presented at a gender identity clinic aged 48. He had a history of service as a police officer, and of relationships with both men and women. DY had been married, and had three children.

DY consulted a psychiatrist, who advised him that he was transsexual. Estrogen therapy was started despite DY's male social gender role. DY's children objected to his breast growth, and his relationship with them deteriorated.

DY changed gender role while remaining in his work as a housing officer. He underwent facial feminising surgery, but nonetheless reverted to a male role after 7 months, losing his job in the process.

DY again attempted to live in a female role, and estrogen therapy was restarted. After 14 months this role was again abandoned. DY described having lost any drive to live in a female role, and reported having found his unusually great height as a woman rather uncomfortable.

Case report: late reversion to a male role (2)

MR presented to a gender identity clinic at the age of 30, requesting gender reassignment surgery. He was male, and seemed to have a very passive personality. There was a history of relationships with men, libido being low and accompanied by vague sadomasochistic fantasies. He also had odd ideas about extraterrestrial influences, none of which seemed frankly delusional.

MR attended the gender identity clinic for many years, consistently requesting gender reassignment surgery. Continued failure to obtain occupation was seen as a problem by the clinic. Insistence on this was seen as unnecessarily obstructive by MR.

MR's passivity led her complainingly to endure suboptimal social circumstances, always bitterly protesting that it was someone's job to help her and provide her with therapy of some sort. A referral to psychotherapeutic services was made. Psychotherapists felt that her continued use of cannabis precluded much useful work being done.

After 6 years in a female role, MR dropped out of the gender identity clinic follow-up. Two years later she re-presented at her own request. She had reverted to a clearly male role and was asking whether estrogen-induced breast growth would spontaneously reverse or whether surgery would be needed. She said that she could no longer be bothered with the effort of maintaining a female role. She had not troubled to change her name to a clearly male form, and still used a female name. It seemed that her social circumstances remained unchanged and that any drive to improve them remained absent.

It is much less common for patients to revert to a female role than to a male. Two such are described below.

Case report: reversion to a female role (1)

CR had a childhood history of tomboy behaviour, and an earlier social identification as lesbian. He changed role to male in his early 20s, being particularly glad that hormone treatment would induce menopause. He changed his name to a clearly male choice, and started to live in a male role.

A year later CR had reverted to an androgynous role and stopped treatment with androgens, accepting that menstruation (still greatly disliked) would inevitably return.

Over the year, CR had made a casual relationship with a straight man that was described as having felt to CR like a gay relationship, but to the man concerned like a straight one. In the same period, there had been a similarly unserious relationship with a lesbian woman. This was said to have felt straight to CR but lesbian to the woman. It did not seem to trouble CR that partners had a different perception of the nature of the relationship.

CR accepted that she had earlier felt distress at being taken to be female most of the time, and had wanted an exclusively male social role. She now thought that having returned to an ambiguous role was all right. She felt that an unmistakably male role was a stage she had to go through. At review, CR was being taken as male most of the time, but occasionally was viewed as a masculine female, which she did not mind.

Lesbians seemed to feel CR came across as mainly lesbian, straight males felt CR seemed to be mostly like a straight man. It was postulated that CR might somehow accept the projection of whoever was encountered, and the sexual identity preferred by the partner of that moment.

Case report: reversion to a female role (2)

JR reverted to female role after 18 months living as a man. The initial change of social gender role to male was at the time seen as very certainly the right thing to do, even though treatment with androgens was withheld until official documentation had been changed.

JR reported an initial state of mild euphoria, feeling as if something that had been a preoccupation since childhood had at last been turned into action. JR had talked of a change of gender role to her whole social circle, which had consisted mainly of lesbians of varying degrees of politicisation. They were said to have offered their principled support, but seemed to have been persuaded rather than convinced.

Following a change of social gender role to male, JR experienced a loss of her lesbian social circle's emotional if not principled support, along with the loss of her relationship. This proved to be more to bear than she had expected.

A new relationship followed, with a female partner who was careful never to express any view about the wisdom of the change of gender role. JR became increasingly unhappy in a male role, and after 18 months reverted to a masculine lesbian identity, feeling that she ought instead to work through her personal issues around social androgyny. She was very glad that she had not been treated with androgens, as had she been so treated she would have had the additional problems of facial hair, cliteromegaly and a deep voice.

Patients who never quite change gender role

Patients seem sometimes to spend long periods maintaining that they are about to change social gender role, or claiming that they have done so, when by any objective measure they have not. This can be so despite the diagnosis being one of transsexualism, differential diagnoses having been excluded.

These patients easily divide into those who acknowledge that they have not changed role and those who maintain that they have. Whether this distinction is useful is unclear.

In the following case, the patient seemed to have acted out ambivalence in an impulsive act that served substantially to postpone any possibility of a permanent change of gender role. Interestingly, the impulsive act followed a brief episode of successfully passing in the other gender role.

Case report: acting out ambivalence

HP, aged 47 years, presented later in life with a history of initially fetishistic cross-dressing and later dual-role transvestism. His sexual drive had been moderate and towards women, but had diminished as the cross-dressing had increased. HP maintained that he wished to change his social gender role, and was held back only by the risk of losing his job. He had been buying expensive but pharmacologically inactive 'hormone precursors', having electrolysis and had grown his hair to shoulder length. HP was advised that active hormone treatment from a gender identity clinic would depend upon a change of role. He accepted this without protest.

When next seen, HP had, as advised, investigated the risk to his employment. He had discovered that this was minimal. His employer was said to have acknowledged that there was a legal obligation to support him and to have added that such support would be very willingly given. Despite this, HP had not changed role. He had undergone further electrolysis, arguing that he could not be expected to change role unless he was entirely without facial hair.

At the next appointment, HP had exceedingly short hair. It seemed that he had been in a large shopping complex, dressed in androgynous winter garments. He had been taken as female in a number of stores, despite not attempting to present himself as a woman. After this experience, which he described as 'uplifting', HP developed an intense feeling of low mood that lasted a week. During the course of it, he went to the barber and demanded that all his hair be cut off. He was said to have cried bitterly as he walked home.

Later, HP could find no reason for his request for a drastic haircut. He willingly accepted a suggestion that it might have reflected some sort of ambivalence. HP felt that it would take him about a year to grow his hair back and planned to have further electrolysis, despite having passed as female literally effortlessly with the electrolysis he had already undergone.

Sometimes the patient seems more easily to accept that the drive to change role is low, fluctuating or diminishing, as the following illustrates.

Case report: dwindling drive to change gender role (1)

SE presented in his early 20s, as a male university student. He had no history of childhood femininity, but did present with an adolescence characterised by bookish unmasculinity. This had served to gain him a place at university. His sexual drive was good, and directed towards women.

SE initially presented with the clear aim of changing gender role. He readily accepted it would be necessary for him to do so before he could be treated with hormones. He went on to inform the university authorities of his intention, and gained their unqualified support. He described himself as 'about to make a move'.

When next seen, SE had made a relationship with a fellow student. She had been attracted to him, it seemed, as much because of his gender confusion as anything else. The relationship proved stormy but provided intense emotional and sexual release for SE. He had postponed any change of gender role while in this relationship, but still described himself as 'about to make a move'.

When next seen, the woman concerned had rejected SE. His gender role had not changed, though, because his degree project had proved to be of commercial interest. Most of his spare time was taken up developing a university project into a saleable product. SE was excited by this unexpected development. He described himself as 'still ready to make a move'

Almost a year later SE had left university. His project had proved of only modest commercial value, but had been useful in opening doors to other, more lucrative, work. He was intrigued to learn that others could see uses for the things he developed which had not occurred to him, and was greatly enjoying his occupational life. His comments about his gender role had an increasingly abstracted quality, and he freely admitted that any change of role seemed to get ever more distant as time passed.

A similar story is seen in the following case.

Case report: dwindling drive to change gender role (2)

NP also presented while at university, partway through a degree in architecture. Born female, NP had a history of childhood tomboyishness. Her fellow students had initially assumed her to be a lesbian. NP was in fact attracted to men. This attraction was experienced as being of a gay male nature.

NP had extensive contact with the university counselling service, and performed very well on her course. She made many social friendships, often through sport, but did not make a relationship at university.

NP was described by the counselling service as being on the brink of informing the university authorities of her intention to change gender role. She never did so. Qualifying at the end of the long course, she decided to hold off on changing her gender role until she had completed an architectural internship. It seemed that internships were scarce, essential for career development, and likely to be jeopardised by any unusual personal circumstances.

NP prospered as an intern, and described the pressure to change social gender role as having become, at that time at least, secondary to the pleasures and pressures of work.

The above patients accepted that they seemed never to get round to changing their social gender role, but such a failure to change may not be acknowledged by the patient, as the following illustrates.

Case report: suggestions of a change of role that has not in fact occurred

LP was a middle-aged woman with a very limited and largely religiously based social circle. She had a lifelong romantic attraction to women. The first had inhibited any expression of the second. LP articulated lifelong feelings of masculinity, and requested bilateral mastectomy and treatment with androgens. She presented in an androgynous, decidedly unsexual way.

LP found it hard to accept any suggestion that she might formally change her social gender role. She at first maintained that she was already treated as if she was a man, but withdrew from this when it was suggested that this would make an official change of role little more than an effortless formality.

LP's religious and social circle would have been best described as a collection of associates rather than as friends, and she felt that her feelings were not their concern. It had not occurred to her that others would notice that she had lost her breasts. When asked what they would think of this development she weakly suggested that they might assume that she had undergone cancer treatment. She confessed to being unable honestly to say that she could bring herself to lie about this. LP wanted treatment with androgens, and was unable to think how she would explain gross virilisation to her associates.

LP ruefully accepted that a change of role seemed to be necessary, and returned claiming that this had occurred. She had changed her name, but to one that was a male homophone of her original name. On closer enquiry, it seemed that when people expressed surprise about the masculine spelling of her name she would retort 'many women now spell it that way'. She had not changed in appearance, and still had her androgynous hairstyle prepared by her usual ladies' hairdresser. It seemed that any 'change of role' had certainly been nothing more than a paper exercise.

A small proportion of patients, usually with a background of dual-role transvestism with moderate dysphoria, seem never to change social gender role. They may cite the pressures of work or domestic life as their main obstacle to so doing, at the same time as admitting that these obstacles might fairly easily be overcome. These patients may attend a gender identity clinic for very many years, always saying that the time is not yet right. For many, it seems, the time will never be right.

It is understandable that some might regard the many appointments attended by patients such as these as in some sense 'wasted'. This may well not be the case. The patients describe the appointments as 'a lifeline' and 'a safe place to discuss things'. Patients in this position may remain stable and high functioning for very many years, at the small expense of infrequent appointments. Their discharge, they often say, would lead to psychological instability and a sharp reduction in their functioning and quality of life.

Patients who hesitate at the brink of gender reassignment surgery

Patients may complete a real life experience, sometimes with ease, and hesitate to commit themselves to gender reassignment surgery. Others decline surgery at the last minute, or fail to attend for their pre-operative work-up.

There is sometimes a marked discrepancy between the patient's actions and their dogged insistence that gender reassignment surgery is deeply desired. In such circumstances, it seems that actions speak louder than words. Sometimes it is possible to discern a probable reason for the failure to enact a stated aim.

Case report: failure to show up for gender reassignment surgery

BJ presented to a gender identity clinic in his early 60s, with a long history of cross-dressing, initially and briefly fetishistic and subsequently lengthily dual role. A change of role to that of a late middle-aged woman proved untroubling. BJ worked full time, even after reaching 65 years of age, in a stereotypically female unskilled occupation.

At presentation, BJ had a relationship with a woman that had endured for a number of years, and which survived BJ's change of role. It seemed that BJ's partner was not happy with the prospect of genital surgery, though, despite there having been no sexual relations between them for a number of years. Over time, BJ reported that this unhappiness had diminished slightly, but remained unsure whether the relationship would survive if the gender reassignment surgery occurred. BJ claimed to want gender reassignment surgery whatever the consequences for the relationship.

BJ attended a pre-surgical assessment but failed to arrive for gender reassignment surgery itself, leaving an operating theatre standing idle. Her absence was attributed to minor transportation difficulties combined with a claimed belief that it would be easy to find another patient to fill her place. She offered apologies and assurances that this would not be repeated

A second pre-operative assessment was uneventfully attended, BJ again being given a detailed information sheet and a consent form to fill out. BJ arrived for admission having left her consent form at home, and claimed to be too upset by its absence to be able to fill out another. She was sent home.

BJ's apologies and assurances were intensified at the outpatient appointment prior to her next and final admission for surgery – which she failed to attend. She made no further contact. It was assumed that BJ had found herself unable to act as if her relationship had as little value as she claimed.

Patients who hesitate on the brink of gender reassignment surgery need not be doing so because of fundamental doubts about the wisdom of the gender reassignment surgery itself, but rather may do so because of independent personality factors, as the following illustrates.

Case report: hesitating on the brink of gender reassignment surgery because of personality factors

CW came from an upper-middle class background, and achieved well at an academic Catholic secondary school. She entered an accountancy firm and worked her way up to a position of some seniority. CW changed gender role from male to female with some success. The change of role was timed to coincide with a civilian post in the police service, working in a major fraud investigation unit. The unit had known of the change of role and had proved wholly supportive, as did her family. She was described as having been too busy to make a relationship, but had a history of half-hearted relationships with women.

CW was anankastic in both her employment and leisure roles, having a keen interest in sustainable transport and organic catering. She prospered in a female role, passing so well that many suspected nothing. A candidate for gender reassignment surgery after 2 years, aged 28, at just the time when she would have been eligible she began to be plagued with increasing obssesionality and doubts, once in the form of what seemed to be a particularly significant dream. Her doubts were intense, but occurred only about 2 days in a typical week. CW reported having been bothered by the morality of gender reassignment surgery after reading criticism in a newspaper, but was unable particularly to enlarge on this. Her Catholic schooling was said to have left her not a believer, but nonetheless very conservative in her social behaviour. She reported she could not rid herself of a fundamentalist Christian viewpoint, although she felt no emotional resonance with it, and could not see a return to a male role being possible. CW was feeling stuck at work as well, saying that it would be hard for her to find a job outside the police, and that her change of gender role probably precluded employment in the private sector.

CW had received workplace romantic advances from both men and women, but reported that some men were put off by her pre-surgical status and felt it might be easier for them to cope if she was a post-operative patient. CW rejected those men who were not so troubled.

It was felt that CW's perpetual ambivalence reflected an excessive superego more than any fundamental problem with her female gender identity. She herself had earlier remarked that she expected to be 40 before she 'knew where she was going in life'.

A refusal to go through with gender reassignment surgery may sometimes be presented as a fear of surgical procedures in themselves. Fear of surgery can be reasonable in someone who has never undergone a surgical procedure or a general anaesthetic as an adult, but can usually be allayed by a pre-operative tour round a surgical ward and a conversation with a specialist nurse. 'Surgical fears' in someone who has earlier undergone surgery with no difficulties should raise suspicions. Similarly, concerns over safety or hygiene that are said to be so great as to preclude going through with surgery raise worries about one fear hiding behind another.

Case report: one fear hiding behind another

TF changed role from male to female with some difficulty and limited social and family support. After an uncertain start her progress became steady if not spectacular, and she was eventually referred for gender reassignment surgery.

TF twice left the surgical ward the night before the gender reassignment surgery was due to occur. On each occasion, concerns about the professionalism of the nursing staff were cited as the reason for her departure. It was suggested that she might have other fears about gender reassignment surgery, which she was not expressing. TF indignantly refuted this suggestion, saying that if she was not to be provided with gender reassignment surgery under the auspices of the NHS, she would castrate herself and thus force the issue. She could not explain having both this stated determination to castrate herself and her refusal to endure a far safer setting for full gender reassignment surgery.

Patients who choose not to have gender reassignment surgery

Some patients complete a real life experience, but choose not to have gender reassignment surgery. Their reasons are various, but their choice does seem to be a very active one. This seems clearly to distinguish them from patients who seem to hesitate on the brink of gender reassignment surgery. Kockott and Fahrner found that those with an unaltered wish for surgery, but who had not had gender reassignment surgery, did not differ substantially from transsexuals who had had surgery.[9] By contrast, the 'hesitating' patients were noticeably older, more often married and more often had children of their own; their partnerships were of long duration, and exclusively with partners of the opposite biological sex. These characteristics had been seen when the diagnosis was first made and were thought to be prognostic for this subgroup. Transsexual people who relinquished their wish for surgery did not differ substantially from transsexuals with an unaltered wish for surgery. Their reasons for relinquishing the wish for surgery could not clearly be established. It was concluded that it was hesitating patients who required particular scrutiny.

These patients seem sometimes to have a clear identity as 'a transsexual', and to be content forever to so distinguish themselves from born men or women.

Case report: patient actively choosing not to have gender reassignment surgery

SC presented to the gender identity clinic in her early 40s, having already changed gender role from male. Tall and statuesque, she had always been narcissistic. She reported a lifelong romantic and sexual interest in men. Her increasing sense of femininity had led her to make a change from a beautiful gay man to a striking, slightly androgynous, female form.

SC had a very successful career revolving around her ability to present herself well. This continued, seemingly unaffected by a change of gender role, although she was said to find it increasingly boring and superficial.

As time passed, SC's appearance became ever less androgynous. Augmentation mammoplasty combined with skilled dress sense to produce an appearance consistent with modelling.

SC was referred for gender reassignment surgery, at her request, but subsequently declined as the surgery date approached, with generous notice. She described herself as very happy as she was, and said that she had become unenthusiastic about any form of surgery, feeling that she had essentially changed her gender role and was too successful to consider messing things up at that stage. She viewed herself as 'transsexual'. While not opposed to the right for herself and others like her to change their birth certificate, she said that she did not want to do so, feeling that the past was something that could not be changed, and had rather to be embraced.

Other patients actively refuse gender reassignment surgery but do not discount the possibility of wanting the surgery at an unspecified later date. Again, their refusal seems a distinct and very active choice, even though it is stated to not necessarily be an enduring one.

Case report: gender reassignment surgery actively postponed

NM presented to the gender identity clinic in his late 20s, giving an account of lifelong feminine homosexuality that had gradually changed into distinct feelings of femininity, associated with a decrease in libido. The change had not distressed him, and both he and his circle of friends expected a change of gender role to female to go smoothly.

These expectations were realised. NM prospered in a female role, and held a series of temporary clerical posts that had been obtained through an employment agency. She reported little trouble from others, and suspected that only a minority of those with whom she worked suspected she was genetically male, and that those whom she thought had noticed seemed unconcerned.

NM had never been in single-minded pursuit of gender reassignment surgery, but was nevertheless pleased to be referred after 2 years. She went on to postpone the surgery on two occasions 'because work commitments did not easily accommodate it'. These postponements were backed with valid evidence to support them. NM's career prospered and work became ever more demanding, as well as more rewarding. She asked to be removed from the surgical waiting list because she could not easily see when she was going to be able to have enough free time to have gender reassignment surgery. She pointed out that her life was working out well anyway, and that she might later want the gender reassignment surgery. The department of surgery was happy to accede to her request because her postponements had made the mean waiting time seem longer than it would otherwise have done.

Sometimes patients decline gender reassignment surgery and one never knows why. They may sever contact with the gender identity clinic and the surgical waiting list by means of a postcard from Turkmenistan declaring a desire to travel, but failing to explain why they are happy to abandon the gender reassignment surgery they had so stridently demanded.

References

1 Hepp U, Milos G and Braun-Scharm H. Gender identity disorder and anorexia nervosa in male monozygotic twins. *International Journal of Eating Disorders* 2004; **35**: 239–43.

2 Marks IM and Mataix-Cols D. Four-year remission of transsexualism after comorbid obsessive-compulsive disorder improved with self-exposure therapy. *British Journal of Psychiatry* 1988; **172**: 452–4.

3 American Psychiatric Association. *Diagnostic and Statistical Manual of Mental Disorder* (4e) (DSM-IV). Washington DC: APA; 1994.

4 Kielhofner G. *Model Of Human Occupation Theory and Application* (3e). Baltimore: Lippincott Williams and Wilkins; 2002.

5 Department of Health. *Valuing People*. London: Department of Health; 2001.
6 Department of Health. *Seeking Consent: working with people with learning disabilities*. London: Department of Health; 2001.
7 Cambridge P and McCarthy M. Developing and implementing sexual policy for learning disability provider service. *Health and Social Care in the Community*. 1997; **5**: 227–36.
8 Kraemer B, Delsignore A, Gundelfinger R, Schnyder U and Hepp U. Comorbidity of Asperger syndrome and gender identity disorder. *European Child and Adolescent Psychiatry* 2005; **14**: 292–6.
9 Kockott G and Fahrner EM. Transsexuals who have not undergone surgery: a follow-up study. *Archives of Sexual Behavior* 1987; **16**: 511–22.

Part 3

Non-surgical treatments

Non-capital treatments

11

The role of the speech and language therapist

Christella Antoni

Speech and language therapists (SLTs) working in the field of gender dysphoria work in a highly specialist, challenging and relatively small field within the remit of speech and language therapy as a whole. The specialism falls under the larger specialist field of voice.

In the UK, with the exception of the speech and language therapy post at Charing Cross Hospital, SLTs treat gender-dysphoric individuals as part of their general voice caseload. A voice therapist's caseload, excluding head and neck cancer patients, comprises clients diagnosed with a wide range of vocal difficulties. These range from the hyperfunctional voice associated with excessive muscular tension in the larynx, to those many laryngeal pathologies and structural anomalies that result in a variety of voice disorders. In addition, a voice therapist treats psychogenic voice disorders such as those relating to chronic anxiety state, personality disorder, and conversion aphonia.

Rising referral rates have led to an increasing number of voice therapists who work with transsexual patients. However, not all voice therapists have experience with this client group, either by choice or by circumstance. Very often, therapists feel that due to lack of experience working with transsexuals lies outside the level of their clinical competency. There are a few well-established services nationally, and more therapists nowadays willing to treat individuals within this client group. More often than not, patients have difficulty accessing services in their local areas and may find themselves travelling to Charing Cross Hospital for treatment, the only tertiary referral centre within the UK. As a leading centre for the treatment of transsexual clients, the gender identity clinic at Charing Cross Hospital will be used as a model for discussion within this chapter.

Within the gender identity clinic at Charing Cross Hospital, the SLT forms part of the multidisciplinary team (MDT). In addition to an understanding of the transsexual condition, the SLT needs to be conversant with the medical model of treatment for transgender clients, for both male and female individuals.

Psychiatric and medical elements (hormonal and surgical treatment) and various non-medical-associated aspects of transition (hair removal, legal change of name), are likely to be current issues in a patient's life at the time of SLT intervention. As well as these medical and practical aspects of gender transition, awareness is required of the psychological and emotional aspects that frequently feature in transsexualism.

There is a far greater number of male-to-female patients referred to speech and language therapy than female-to-male patients. This corresponds to the greater incidence of male-to-female transsexualism within the general population. In addition, estrogen hormone treatment given to male-to-female patients has no effect on the cartilaginous framework of the larynx or the vocal cords.[1] Thus estrogen has no effect on the pitch (fundamental frequency) of the voice. Consequently, male-to-female patients need to learn to produce a higher-pitched voice and a more characteristically female voice, despite the constraints of a biological male larynx, vocal folds (vocal cords), and vocal tract, the latter of which is both longer and wider than a natal female larynx.

In the female-to-male client group, androgen treatment leads to an increase in the mass of the vocal folds. The thickened vocal folds result in a lower-pitched voice. Although female transsexuals are therefore at a distinct advantage in acquiring their desired voice, some speech and language therapy intervention may still be indicated. A Swedish study by Scheidt *et al* concluded 'that voice therapy seems to be advisable for female-to-male transgenders'.[2] The authors cite studies made of biological females who had received testosterone hormone treatment for gynaecological reasons. Deleterious effects on female voice may occur in the aspects of 'vocal stability, singing voice, vocal power, quality and pitch'.[2] Some female-to-male patients therefore may remain dissatisfied with their male voice, despite testosterone treatment and seek the services of a SLT. Furthermore, female transsexuals who are professional voice users or who have high vocal demands may require voice therapy as well as counselling regarding some of the possible vocal restrictions outlined above.

The bulk of the voice therapist's involvement with transgender clients nevertheless falls within the male caseload. Certainly, the therapy intervention with the latter client group is longer in duration and generally covers a far wider number of speech and vocal aspects, as well as related issues such as general female presentation. This chapter will therefore seek to provide an overview of the SLT's involvement with male clients from the point of referral to the stage of discharge. The chapter will include assessment, treatment and management approaches as well as describing the SLT's role with ear, nose and throat (ENT) vocal surgery interventions.

The overall aim of treatment is to aid the client to produce a convincing-sounding female voice. Aspects of female voicing and communication are first taught to the client, along with general aspects of voice production and voice care. The therapy room provides a safe environment for the client to experiment with her voice and to try out the exercises with the SLT, prior to practising the exercises at home and in public. An additional goal is the client developing a confident manner in speech and voicing. Inherent in these goals are emotional and psychological aspects of voicing. These require the therapist to work beyond the remit of perceptual voice. Counselling therefore often forms a large part of the voice therapy, and will be addressed later in the chapter.

Referral

Acceptance to a speech and language therapy programme requires a medical referral. Within the gender identity clinic at Charing Cross Hospital, and similarly for the smaller established gender identity units nationally, the majority of referrals come from the allied consultant psychiatrists. Occasionally, a general practioner (GP) may refer a patient or a patient self-refers directly, but prior to acceptance to the service a patient's confirmed psychiatric diagnosis of gender dysphoria must be established. At Charing Cross Hospital, all patients referred to speech and language therapy must be registered patients of the gender identity clinic. SLTs not allied to specific gender identity units, servicing local communities, receive referrals from both GPs (based on the above criteria) and consultant psychiatrists.

Increasingly, referrals to speech and language therapy are being made by ENT consultants for opinion, assessment and treatment both before and after vocal cord surgery. Voice surgery intervention is offered in only a few centres nationally, but the referral rates for vocal surgery are increasing. At Charing Cross Hospital, where the majority of UK vocal surgery is carried out, the ENT consultant forms a part of the gender identity clinic service. Close liaison between ENT and speech and language therapy is therefore a strong feature of MDT working.

The timing of referral to speech and language therapy for male clients can vary widely and may range from referral while an individual is still living in a male role to a referral only when the patient has undergone vocal pitch-raising surgery. However, the majority of referrals are for patients with no previous experience of speech and language therapy and in most cases, clients will have commenced their real life experience, or will be close to it.

Although it is felt that current best practice is to offer vocal surgery only after a course of voice therapy has been completed, and when a patient is well established on their real life experience, some patients access voice surgery (in most cases privately) without having any previous speech and language therapy.

While formal data regarding outcomes in these cases is lacking, clinical experience suggests that surgery without any speech and language therapy generally leads to less effective outcomes post-surgically, and increased incidences of dysphonia.

Patients already embarked on their real life experience tend to progress more quickly in speech and language therapy. The speech and voice work becomes more relevant for them and forms part of their endeavour to present as female. Generally speaking, speech and language therapy is not strongly recommended with clients who are not yet living fully in a female role, but it may be considered with some individuals who are highly motivated and close to embarking on their real life experience. Suitability for treatment, following referral, is determined by the SLT's initial consultation with the client.

Initial assessment

As with any voice client, a thorough initial assessment is crucial to the planning of treatment and therefore requires a substantial time allocation. Approximately 75–90 minutes is recommended.

This may be the longest appointment time a client has experienced with a professional, and clients are often nervous and unsure of what to expect. It is worthwhile outlining the session briefly to the client to help dispel anxieties. As Chaloner wrote, 'The speech and language therapy consultation provides some transsexuals with the first safe, accepting and relaxed setting to "be themselves"'.[3] As well as a detailed case history, the aim is to impart the necessary information regarding what can be offered by speech and language therapy, and to obtain recordings of the patient's voice if possible.

Standard voice history forms are designed to capture information regarding vocal disorders or difficulties, including details concerning onset of vocal symptoms, the type of voicing difficulty and influencing factors. With gender-dysphoric clients, the voicing difficulties do not fit specifically into the category of a disorder. After all, in the vast majority of patients, the voice is physically healthy and intact. The issue for the client is that their voice requires modification and does not fit with their perception of self. They have 'a strong wish to make the voice more congruent with their psychological gender identity'.[4] There are several similarities between a standard voice case history form and an initial assessment form used with a transsexual client, in that each will include sections on the client's vocal habits and level of voice use. In addition, however, an initial assessment form for a gender-dysphoric client should include sections that pertain specifically to gender reassignment. A speech and language therapy department offering a service to gender-dysphoric clients will probably adapt their standard voice assessment form. At Charing Cross Hospital, an initial assessment form has been devised and includes the headings:

- *Summary of status in gender reassignment programme,* including medical information, e.g. whether a client is receiving hormone treatment, and details regarding a client's real life experience
- *Medical history*: this includes physical and mental health status or factors
- *Social history,* including employment, marital status and current level of support from family and friends and other social networks
- *The presentation of the client*: this includes an outline of the patient's physical presentation made by the SLT as well as the client's perception of self and concerns regarding the overall presentation. Observations should also be made with respect to the client's 'social skills and competence as a communicator'[5]
- *Voice history,* including vocal abuse and misuse – factors such as smoking, previous voice difficulty, level of voice use and whether there are any laryngeal symptoms
- *Voice presentation*: a listener judgement should be made by the SLT, and the client's own perception of voice should be noted. It is useful for the therapist to ask the client how their voice serves them both in face-to-face contact with others in everyday life, and when visual cues are absent, most commonly when using the telephone.
- *Perceptual assessment,* including vocal characteristics and any dysphonia. The latter is graded according to the GRBAS* perceptual assessment.[6] An audio recording should, if possible, be made of a client reading a standard voice text, such as *The Rainbow Passage,*[7] as well as a sample of free speech, such as 'what I did at the weekend'

---

* GRBAS – G = Grade (the dysphonia is graded from 0–3, with 0 meaning no dysphonia and 3 meaning severe dysphonia; R = Roughness (in the voice) graded 0–3, as are the following: A = Breathiness; A = Aesthenia; S = Strain.

- *Objective assessment*, using instrumentation such as Visipitch or the electro-laryngograph to obtain a reading of the client's habitual vocal pitch
- *ENT history*: this includes whether the patient is considering a thyroid chondroplasty, pitch-raising surgery or both
- *Indications/suitability for treatment*, particularly the client's level of motivation, degree of voice concern and ability to commit to therapy, as well as the client's expectations of treatment and any factors that may impede or aid progress
- *SLT management*: following assessment there may be many indications, including delaying treatment until a more appropriate time or referral to an alternative service local to the patient. In most cases a full treatment block is offered, which may at some point lead to a referral for ENT surgery. All patients at Charing Cross Hospital gender identity clinic undergo individual therapy sessions with SLT. In addition, some may be invited to attend a voice practice or communication skills group.

In addition to the above the SLT outlines the expectations of the client, which will include regular attendance at sessions and a commitment to practising communication and voice exercises. There is a mutual decision about whether a client should begin treatment.

Occasionally, a client attends the speech and language therapy assessment simply out of curiosity and has no overt concerns regarding voice. Although the SLT may feel a patient's voice is not convincingly feminine, it is unwise to treat clients who are not highly motivated, as this usually wastes scarce treatment sessions.

Voice therapy covers many aspects and can be a long and difficult journey. Some individuals present at initial assessment with a good female voice and overall presentation. In these cases, the client is usually merely seeking confirmation of this by 'an expert', or is seeking some additional tips to ensure they are using best voice possible. Others present with a perceptually close to feminine-sounding voice or with an easily adaptable voice, and will therefore require a short speech and language therapy intervention. The majority of clients present with unmistakably masculine voices. For these individuals, a full course of speech and language therapy intervention is required.

Speech and language therapy treatment

At the early stage of voice work, there may be an overlap between standard voice clients and clients with gender dysphoria. Almost all voice therapy begins with a treatment session that will include advice and information regarding vocal hygiene, voice care, voice production and voice education. The last is a logical starting point with gender-dysphoric individuals, but the information needs to be expanded to include issues related to the differences between male and female voices. Aspects of treatment, both direct and indirect will be listed and outlined below.

Indirect treatment and therapy centres around increasing a client's awareness of all aspects of female presentation and on providing background information to speech and voice in general, rather than direct therapy exercises. The following are included.

Voice education

This may include information about how voice is produced, and voice care advice, also, the different ways male and female vocal tracts shape sound and how pitch and resonance are produced

Physical presentation

Although physical presentation is crucial the NHS rarely provides help with a client's general female presentation. It generally falls to clients themselves to work on their 'total look'. Clients are advantaged or disadvantaged in this respect by their build, their perception and their social circumstances. Thus, while many clients have an excellent presentation, others struggle to look convincing or even appropriate in the female role, particularly those who are socially isolated or who have limited financial means. It may thus form part of the SLT's role to offer advice and suggestions in areas that are not directly related to speech and voice but are directly related to the client's success in presenting as female. This supports the voice therapy and should, if possible, be client led. It is useful for the SLT to have a list of resources to offer the client if they seeking services regarding their physical presentation.

Aspects in this area include hair removal, which nearly all male clients require. Both electrolysis and laser removal are costly, lengthy, and often painful. Clients undergo treatment not only for removal of facial hair, but also to eliminate body hair and sometimes genital hair prior to gender reassignment surgery (if advised by the surgeon). It is common for clients to attend voice sessions with blotchy red faces, or expressing physical discomfort relating to hair removal. The SLT merely needs to be aware of this lengthy commitment for the client and the practical implications. Often clients have voice therapy and electrolysis on the same day to minimise time off work.

Although an SLT is unlikely to be an expert in hairdressing, clothes, make-up and accessories, he or she can still offer guidance in the form of practical advice and basic suggestions in these areas. (Note there are far fewer male SLTs than female. A small percentage, however, do work with transgender individuals.) Many clients hold stereotypical views of female presentation and therefore, regardless of their age and shape, tend to strong make-up, short skirts, high heels and long wigs. Conversely, a number of clients present very androgynously, either because they are happier this way (not all clients feel they have to present as stereotypically female), because they are fearful of discrimination or abuse, or are simply lacking in confidence. The therapy sessions can be a useful and safe situation for a client to experiment in these matters.

Communication and social skills

Work in this area is another departure from the traditional form of voice therapy (although not for many other areas of speech and language therapy as a whole). While it will certainly not be an area of focus for many patients, for approximately half the clients referred to the service at Charing Cross Hospital gender identity clinic, attention to these areas occurs throughout the SLT intervention.

The aim is to aid the individual to 'have a convincing image within the frame-work of the client's personality and ability'.[8]

Socially challenged or isolated individuals or those who have concomitant mental health issues will generally benefit from assistance in this area, provid-ing that they are cognitively intact. Perhaps through a longstanding sense of 'being different', or because of others' negative reactions or lack of social contacts, gender-dysphoric clients may lack general communication, interpersonal and social skills and come across as being particularly self-referential. According to Cavalli and Chaloner,'The transsexual can be a very self-absorbed and egocentric individual who makes little effort to relate in any but the most superficial way to other people, and has failed to develop many social conversational skills'.[8] Clients may conversely present as being so lacking in confidence and experience with others that they find it very difficult to talk about themselves. Often there is a marked paucity of personal interests or employment, and therefore the range of conversational subjects is limited.

It is also not unusual for clients to perseverate on certain topics, frequently about their physical presentation, viewing this as the major obstacle to their successful life as a woman.

Once a rapport has been established with an individual and some basic voice skills acquired, the majority of clients are willing to attend a voice and com-munication skills group which allows for practice in all the above areas based on specific tasks such as role-play, turn-taking in conversation, giving biographical details and asking questions about others.

As well as general communication skills, specific communication features pertaining more specifically to women may need addressing, including posture, the increased use of gesture, eye contact and facial expression. Dr Lillian Glass identifies 105 'sex talk differences' in her book *He Says, She Says*.[9] Referring to body language differences, she lists that women provide more listener feedback through their body language than men, and that men 'are not as sensitive to the communication cues of others'. In her examples of facial language differences between the sexes, she writes, that women 'provide more facial expressions in feedback and more reactions'.[9]

Again, there is a variety of presentations among this client population, with some individuals' body language and non-verbal communication presenting them very naturally as women. Others have overt masculine presentations, sometimes compounded by a large stature and strong masculine physical char-acteristics. The majority of patients referred to speech and language therapy will wish to present as successfully as possible and tend to welcome suggestions in this area. It is worthwhile noting how a client walks down a corridor or sits in a chair for example. Legs kept wide apart (sometimes despite the wearing of tights and a knee-length skirt), and a masculine gait is frequently one of the most telling aspects of presentation – one that the client is often unaware of, especially if in other ways, there is a reasonable female presentation.

Direct therapy with male clients centres on the speech and voice parameters of pitch, resonance, intonation, articulation, prosody, intensity, language use, communicative style and manner of voicing. The aim is to modify the client's voice so that it presents as female. At best, this means that listeners will identify the voice as female, both in face-to-face exchanges and exchanges where visual cues are absent, usually a telephone conversation. This last is the decisive test.

Although formal data are lacking, there is more success achieving an adequate voice for face-to- face situations and general voicing. This is because visual cues aid listener perceptions. A client who presents convincingly as female, perhaps due to small stature, attention to grooming and confident social and speaking manner, will be accepted as female despite a rather idiosyncratic voice or lower pitch. Feminising a voice is difficult. It is easier for a client to feminise some aspects of voicing, rather than all. To put it simply, every little bit helps the overall perception. A unisex-type voice can often be achieved, which may not be distinctly female but nevertheless serves the individual well.

As Soderpalm *et al* wrote 'astonishingly little has been published on voice therapy and specifically the efficacy of vocal intervention'.[4] Chaloner points out that 'The speech gender indicators are at present ill-defined' and that 'Speech and Language Therapy intervention is still largely driven by empirical observations and subjective criteria'.[3]

The three most salient aspects that are most likely to distinguish male and female voices however are pitch, intonation and resonance.[10]

Pitch is the most researched aspect of male transsexual voice. Pitch is the perceptual correlate of frequency and is measured in hertz (Hz). As air passes through the glottis, the vocal folds vibrate. 'The rate of the vibration of the vocal folds is dependent on vocal fold length, tension, elasticity and mass, and resistance to subglottic air pressure. As the vocal folds increase in length and the vocalis muscles thin and stiffen them, frequency increases'.[11]

Many studies have sought to determine the speaking fundamental frequency (SFF), that separates male and female voices. The dividing line is around a fundamental frequency of 155–160 Hz.[10,12] Greene and Mathieson recorded the average speaking fundamental frequency to be 128 Hz in males, and 225 Hz in females.[11] Pitch varies according to the individual and the circumstances. Emotional status influences pitch as does the age of the speaker. Mild increases in pitch are associated with older males as the vocal folds decrease in mass with age. The opposite is true for females where the vocal cords tend to thicken slightly with ageing. Oates and Dacakis found that 'the range for males and females overlaps considerably'.[13] For males between 20 and 29 years of age, the mean of fundamental frequency is noted as being 138 Hz, with a range of 60–260 Hz. For females of the same age group, the mean is 227 Hz with a frequency range of 128–520 Hz. In the study of Wolfe *et al*, the mean fundamental frequency of their transsexual subjects ranged from 93 Hz to 202 Hz, clearly overlapping the range of male and female speakers.[10]

It is useful to experiment with the client's pitch early on in therapy to gain a sense of the client's natural vocal ability in this area. Much of the client's success will be determined by whether they have an 'ear' for pitch. Without it, altering pitch will prove very difficult. The main aim of therapy is to encourage a slightly higher pitch to begin with, which is easily achievable for the client. A further increase in pitch may be possible over time with increased experimentation and confidence. Clients who attempt to self-modify their voices generally aim too high regarding pitch, and present with a hyperfunctional voice that may be characterised by strain, breathiness, roughness or hoarseness. At worse, they will habitually employ a falsetto voice quality (also known as loft register), which will result in an unnatural-sounding voice akin to that of a pantomime dame.

While many clients will be focused on their pitch as the essential marker for vocal femininity, in reality, 'high pitch is not necessarily the result of high frequency but may be caused by the acoustic characteristics imparted to the voice by the supraglottic vocal tract'.[11] Longer, wider vocal tracts are likely to impede the production of higher pitch in transsexuals. Spencer's study found that transsexuals who were perceived as female were of small build (170 cm or below). '[Since] shorter individuals are likely to have shorter vocal tracts, small stature is likely to be an advantage for transsexual voice when combined with high fundamental frequency'.[12]

An essential part of speech and language therapy therefore often lies in teaching the client ways of gaining differentiated control of varying parts of the vocal tract, such as altering tongue and lip positions, and raising the larynx. This type of work lends itself better to professional voice users, actors or performers rather than to the lay public who, in the main part, have a low insight and limited experience regarding the workings and potential of the human voice. Modelling sounds and vocal tract positions helps the patient fully to grasp what is intended by the exercises. Alteration of vocal tract parameters allows for alterations in intonation, resonance and formant frequencies of vowels all of which play an important role in the feminisation of a male voice. Regarding the latter for example, 'Lowering the larynx would tend to lower the formant values while raising the larynx would tend to raise them'.[14]

Voice quality can be altered in a variety of ways. Raising the back of the tongue raises the larynx. This, in turn, shortens the length of the vocal tract, which can help a client develop or sustain higher pitch. In addition, developing the ability to use thinner vocal folds will also lead to a higher-pitched voice. The voice quality 'twang',[15] lends itself very well to voice feminisation. The quality can be adapted successfully to use with transgender clients to develop higher-pitched, brighter voices.[16] Apart from a larynx free from constriction, its main features are a high larynx setting, a high- and forward-placed tongue and aryepiglottic sphincter narrowing. Twang also allows for safe voice projection, if taught correctly, another reason why it is especially useful for working with transgender voice, as one of the key worries of clients is that they are unable to use raised volume in their 'female' voice. This is especially true if they have favoured the use of a breathy voice quality.

Experience with a large volume of patients has led me to believe that work on the overall tone and tonal range of a patient's voice can prove to be the single most discerning factor regarding female identification by a listener. The overall tone usually needs to be less forceful and more expressive. This again is a challenging aspect for the majority of patients to develop skill in and alter sufficiently. Practising different tones of voice to convey different emotions is one way of developing this skill. Above all, the voice must be as far away from a monotone as possible, and display a variety of intonation shifts, even with relatively short-length speech utterances, as the latter is more characteristic of female speech. Gelfer and Schofield defined an intonation shift as 'A change in frequency, with or without interruption of phonation, of at least two semitones'.[17] Further, the male-to-female transsexuals in their study who were perceived as female used a greater number of upward intonation shifts and a greater range (in semitones) of downward intonation shifts.[17]

Regional accents can sometimes be a useful feature of a client's voice and can be built on. The natural lilt and peaking of a Welsh accent lends itself very well to uprising tone and tonal shifts. Conversely, some London accents, especially when coupled with a low pitch, can prove very resistant to increases in tone variation.

It is vital for patients to grasp that reduced chest resonance is a characteristic of female voice quality. Chest and oral resonance can easily be contrasted, and the patient is encouraged to feel vibrations both on the upper part of the chest and on the face, to gain an understanding of how sound is altered in the various resonance chambers of the body. The resonating system of the voice is made up of the structures and air-filled cavities above and below the larynx, such as the nasal, oral and oro-pharyngeal spaces, which can be manipulated to produce specific harmonics. Indeed, 'the laryngeal note is insignificant without its system of resonators'.[11]

Carew and coworkers have investigated the effectiveness of oral resonance therapy on the perception of femininity in voice in a group of 10 male-to-female subjects.[18] This type of therapy targets increased lip spreading and forward tongue carriage. Their preliminary findings suggest that this type of therapy 'may be effective in increasing the VFF and mean fundamental frequency of male-to-female transsexual clients. This may in turn result in an increased perception of femininity in male-to-female transsexuals'.[18] No correlations were conducted on the data due to poor inter-rater agreement; therefore further research is clearly warranted. Interestingly, all ten subjects rated themselves as sounding more feminine following therapy; listeners however, judged only seven subjects out of ten as sounding more feminine.

The overall aim of treatment in this area is for the client to develop skill in using oral, oro-pharangeal and facial resonance when voicing, aiming for a physically higher 'placement' of speech, which usually involves increased focus on articulation also. In the majority of cases, patients are helped by learning to soften the contacts with the articulators for consonant sounds and by using more precise diction. The latter has been identified as being a more common feature of female speech rather than male speech.[9] In addition, increased or altered oral shaping for vowels can be a crucial element of successful female voice.

The resonant pitches of vowels are known as formants and can be identified spectographically as F1, F2, etc. In studies by Gunzburger, F3 increased in frequency in male-to-female transsexuals using their female voice.[19,20] A previous study indicates that F3 appears to be an important element of influencing listener judgements of gender.[21] Gelfer and Schofield, found that female perceived subjects had consistently '... higher vowel formant frequencies for isolated productions of /i/ and /a/'.[17]

Additional aspects of voice and communication that may be worked on in varying degrees, depending on the presentation of the patient, are intensity (volume), language use and prosody. The usual focus in therapy for the parameter of intensity is for the client to aim for a slightly quieter volume in speaking, as male voices tend to be louder. However, with some patients, the opposite focus is required. It is not uncommon, for example, for patients who have attempted to self-modify their voices to overcompensate and present with a very quiet or overly breathy voice. This kind of voice attracts untoward attention and challenges the listener not only in the way of gender recognition but more importantly because it is difficult to hear!

Language use and choice of conversational topic frequently gains attention in the literature, especially articles or advice sheets written by transsexuals themselves. It is one example of how clients may conform to stereotypical views of female communication. From my own experience, this area tends not to feature strongly in therapy sessions. As boundaries between male and female language use have blurred since the feminist movement, working on this aspect seems less relevant.[22,23]

Regarding choice of conversational topic for example, clients for the most part continue to have the same interests and hobbies in their life as a female as they did in their male existence; therefore they are likely to be interested in talking about similar things. A client who devoted hours of attention to his train set as a man is likely to devote further hours of attention to it during and post-transition. Feeling under pressure to develop interests in new activities that are more 'feminine' can contribute to a client feeling as if she is putting on an act rather than being herself. As a client's transition progresses, they may indeed begin to have different perspectives on life, new interests or altered feelings but this is by no means guaranteed and devoting therapy time to these aspects may therefore prove unwise.

The debate around sex talk differences is vast and ongoing. 'Few feminists would dispute that discourse in often gendered'.[24] However, within the feminist movement itself there are different theories relating to the ways males and females communicate. Socio-linguistic elements of language, both form and function, are complex, and while language can reflect inherent sexism or pejorative notions against women, gender transition can act as a bridging factor between the embedded sexual politics of language. Clients changing gender inevitably take with them, to varying degrees, the speech, language and communication patterns according of the gender they have been socialised in. These patterns may feature strongly in terms of presenting as overtly male or female, but the majority of speech and language therapy intervention focuses on acquiring a perceptually acceptable voice rather than encouraging the client to adopt a 'female style' of communication.

It is, however, well worth drawing the client's attention to some of the general differences suggested for the ways men and women communicate, such as the female conversational tendencies to use more descriptors, more facial animation and to give more listener feedback than do males. Working on these aspects as well as the sound of an individual's voice could help overall presentation. In some clients, this type of work will be strongly indicated; with others it may never feature as an aspect that requires addressing.

Many clients comment that they fear sounding unnatural. Reassurance should be given that the aim is to modify their voice and speech, not to adopt a totally alien sound. The goal is for the voice to be acceptable and believable. Some patients have sought the services of a voice coach or teacher. Working with transsexuals is one potential area where the boundaries of a voice therapist and a voice/drama coach may merge. While some highly stable individuals, coping well with all aspects of transition, may benefit from this approach, Chaloner states that transsexuals 'are not professional actors but troubled individuals who need the help of someone who is used to dealing with people under stress, and where there is medical back-up available'.[3]

There are indeed challenges in working with this client group; challenges which on a daily basis often exceed the challenges of working with a standard voice client group. The complexities involved in gender dysphoria require awareness not only of the condition itself but of the whole process of transition with its incumbent psychiatric, endocrinological, psychosocial and surgical aspects. The progress for clients is very rarely linear, and high levels of stress, anxiety and frustration are common.

Counselling

Counselling commonly forms a part of all forms of voice therapy treatment. Because of the psychological and emotional considerations outlined above, it is not surprising that this role forms a significant part of the SLT's involvement with transgender patients. In a standard voice caseload, counselling skills are employed as part of the patient's vocal rehabilitation, perhaps in identifying personality and emotional factors that negatively influence voice production. These factors may lead to vocal pathology such as vocal fold nodules. In transgender voice, emotional issues are rarely related to vocal misuse or abuse, but may prevent the patient's progress. Very often the latter is linked to an overall lack of progress in the individual's gender transition. It is not unusual for emotional issues to dominate some treatment sessions, but when this tendency frequently overrides the voice and communication work, a referral to a counselling or psychotherapeutic service is indicated and should be sought where possible.

The above area is a potentially tricky one for SLTs. While there is access to psychiatry for these patients, accessing counselling services can prove to be difficult. The most obvious route is a referral to local services via the GP but sessions, if available, are generally limited and therefore do not offer the kind of long-term support that is indicated for many patients. In addition, a referral to a generalist counsellor can prove to be an ineffective intervention. There is a marked scarcity of counsellors and psychotherapists who specialise in gender issues, and those who do remain largely in the private sector.

A further psychosocial consideration is the patient's need emotionally to adjust to the modified voice. This aspect is rarely given attention in the literature or by clinicians or patients themselves. Very often, patients wish to move quickly with their voice and speech feminisation, but cease to make progress or plateau early on in treatment because of reluctance, conscious or unconscious, to adopt the 'new' voice. They fear sounding unnatural, or 'too high', and experience embarrassment, especially when trying to use a more feminine voice in front of family members, friends or work colleagues. A common finding is that patients have more success using their feminised voice with strangers than with people who are well known to them. Family members in particular can have difficulty accepting any or every level of a relative's gender transition, including voice. Patients who have supportive families and friends, or who are determined and confident in nature, tend to progress more successfully and adopt the changes more permanently than those who struggle with their own resistance to transition, or the resistance of others. It is worth pointing out to clients that it takes time to learn new voice skills and time to adapt to having, and using, a different voice.

Surgical voice modification: the role of the speech and language therapist

It is not within the remit of this chapter to discuss specific surgical interventions and techniques regarding phonosurgery. However, SLTs working in this field need to have an understanding of the pitch-raising surgeries offered most commonly the crico-thyroid approximation surgery (CTAS). In addition, therapists should be very familiar with the chondroplasty procedure carried out for reducing the thyroid cartilage. A prominent Adam's apple is frequently cited by patients as being of great concern to them. Even patients who present with a relatively small laryngeal prominence may show concern that it is a tell-tale sign of masculinity.

Increasingly, patients have an awareness regarding the above and an interest in learning about the procedures and how to access them. Correspondingly, and because the above procedures are now more routine than they used to be, an increasing amount of pitch-raising vocal surgeries are carried out. Current criteria for referral to ENT at Charing Cross Hospital include the patient having received a course of speech and language therapy treatment. The individual must also be well embarked on their real life experience. In addition to this, the patient should have a voice that is free from any dysphonia and possess a moderate to high level of voice use and/or voice concern. The referral is made after both the SLT and a member of the psychiatric team have evaluated the patient's suitability regarding the above surgery.

Limited data exist regarding the formal outcomes of vocal surgery with transsexuals. However, empirical observation suggests that patients who successfully modify parameters of voice and speech other than pitch, for example, prosody, intonation, manner of voicing etc, tend to have a more successful surgical voice outcome than those patients who seek surgery without previous speech and language therapy. This is a logical conclusion, as the surgery only addresses the aspect of pitch. Post-surgically, a patient may still sound male, albeit high pitched, without attention to other speech and voice features. In the Spencer study, the transsexuals related that they 'alter more than pitch', citing in particular more precise consonant production and the use of a 'softer tone'.[12]

Pitch surgery can therefore support and extend the progress made in speech and language therapy, but is rarely a total substitute for it, much to the disappointment of many patients who are hoping for a quicker 'fix' to the problem of their voice. This should be made clear to patients. Of course, some patients, (with or without speech and language therapy), manage to make reasonable modifications to their voices and communicative style, but find sustaining pitch consistently the single most problematic factor regarding feminising their voice adequately. For these individuals phonosurgery can yield a satisfactory to excellent outcome. Psychologically, too, there may be a boost for patients who often report that they experience less fear post-surgically that their voice will 'suddenly drop' when they are in mid-conversation. Activities such as coughing or laughing, or emotional states such as anger or sadness are also potential trouble areas for sustaining pitch consistently. Vocal surgery may also increase emotional security concerning these areas, which in turn, can lead to a more confident communicator overall.

Matai et al conducted a survey on patients who had received CTAS, and/or chondroplasty.[25] Of the 42 completed questionnaires, 33 patients had the CTAS procedure, 79% of whom indicated an improvement in their voice. Comments by patients included: 'It has given me the confidence to face the world', and 'It's the best thing I've ever had done!'. Nine patients, (21%) indicated that they 'were not pleased with surgery'.[25]

Pre- and post-surgery intervention

In most cases the patient is known to the SLT and therefore baseline measurements of the individual's voice will already exist. Pre-surgically, an audio recording and a pitch measurement should be made, if possible. The therapist should also provide post-surgical voice care advice, which includes limiting all voice use for the first 72 hours after surgery, and conservative voice use for approximately 2 weeks following surgery.

Post-surgically, the patient should be followed up with a view to assessing the outcome of surgery and to help the patient in establishing a comfortable voicing manner if there are signs of vocal strain. Audio and objective recordings should be taken if possible for comparison with pre-surgical voice. Follow-up speech and language therapy may also be required to address any dysphonia that may result from the surgery. Kanagalingam et al carried out an evaluation of medium-term outcome for 21 transsexuals who had a crico-thyroid and subluxation procedure.[26] They concluded that 'Cricothyroid approximation effectively raised pitch in male-to-female transsexuals. There was a concomitant rise in voice irregularities which is effectively addressed by speech therapy'.[26]

It is likely that a lack of sufficient speech and language therapy intervention prior to surgery will yield less successful vocal outcomes for the patient and possibly an increase in dysphonia. The bulk of the SLT's involvement with the transsexual patient should therefore occur prior to surgery rather than following it. In my experience, this approach tends to minimise post-surgical dysphonia which, if present, tends to resolve in 23 weeks, as the patient adapts to the altered laryngeal dynamics.

A full evaluation of the published data regarding these patients is difficult, as the speech and language therapy input they received had been variable. Matai et al agree too that 'it is difficult to judge the relative contribution of the two methods: probably both surgery and speech therapy work in conjunction and increase the likelihood of a good result'.[24]

Length of intervention

Length of intervention varies greatly with the transsexual client group due not least to the individual nature of voices in general and the unique presentation of each client. An average course of speech and language therapy intervention with standard voice patients in the UK tends to be around six sessions, and in many centres in the UK this applies to the transsexual patients too. Unless a patient has made significant voice modifications prior to the onset of speech and language therapy treatment, a treatment block of at least around 10 to 12 sessions is recommended for the majority of patients, with a review of progress around the sixth session. Further treatment sessions may be planned if indicated and/or a referral to ENT based on each individual's circumstances and abilities. It is recommended that up to four sessions of treatment should be allocated for follow-up prior to discharge for both surgical and non-surgical patients, as this kind of support tends to minimise re-referrals to the service.

The study by Soderpalm *et al* suggests that the patients who had received more than 14 sessions of therapy achieved higher fundamental frequency than those patients who received fewer than 14 sessions.[4] Although the finding did not reach statistical significance. Their study did show that at follow-up sessions both groups continued to increase the fundamental frequency of their voices to a small degree. The mean value for the group that received longer therapy intervention was 165 Hz; above the pitch threshold for female perception. The fact that fundamental frequency may continue to increase after therapy is an important observation, as techniques may have been adopted and vocal modification will continue.[4]

Discharge criteria

Discharge criteria with all voice patients centre on the patient achieving the maximum gains possible. This does not necessarily mean that the patient will be totally satisfied with their voice. Therein lies an issue that frequently requires addressing during the course of treatment. Many patients assume that if they continue attending therapy sessions, their voice will continue to improve. This can be especially true of gender-dysphoric patients. In reality, however, as with all courses of speech and language therapy, to successfully generalise the 'new' voice into everyday life the onus of responsibility lies with the patient. Therapy requires active client participation; once the voice skills and techniques have been taught to the patient and practised with the therapist the goal is to make the 'new' voice the patient's habitual voice. This requires dedication on the part of the therapist, but more on the part of the patient who needs to keep practising and applying the work. The ultimate goal is that the feminised voice will become second nature. While some patients achieve this fairly easily, many others do not. Generally, some change and improvement is possible with almost all motivated patients, but it is not uncommon for patients to feel that their voice is not 'feminine' enough, despite a long course of treatment.

Summary and conclusion

Each patient responds differently to therapy and has variable natural ability regarding manipulating and altering voice production. The skill of the voice specialist, as with all voice patients, is in finding which exercises and techniques work best with which patient, and in breaking those tasks down in order that the patient can master them.

So much of an SLT's work revolves around restoring or improving function, and working with impaired systems. In working with transsexual individuals, however, the work centres on the teaching of new skills or in modifying fully functioning systems to work, or to present, in a different way. Within the speech and language therapy intervention, many aspects may be covered, both direct and indirect.

Speech and language therapy is just one aspect of a myriad of issues that the patient may be trying to modify or adapt to including hair removal, transitioning at work, adapting to the female self generally, and gender reassignment surgery. It is not unusual therefore for the therapy to be interrupted or delayed.

An SLT's involvement with transsexuals tends to be longer than with standard voice patients. Indeed, a patient may in total spend more time with an SLT than with other members of the MDT professionals allied to the gender identity unit. The intervention tends to be lengthy, not least because, for non-voice professionals, the learning of new voice skills is challenging. Very often, the bulk of the therapist's intervention centres around helping the client to generalise the acquired voice and communication skills into everyday life.

Phonosurgery with this client group may also be an aspect of the SLT's role, and further increase the therapy intervention period. Surgical intervention, usually combined with speech and language therapy, has proved successful for many patients. However, the outcomes of surgery remain highly variable, and further research is warranted in this area.[27]

As well as a respect for human diversity, the unique and often highly complex presentations by the patients require the therapist to be flexible, adaptable and skilled in both treatment and management approaches. Strong interpersonal skills are vital to build an effective rapport with each individual client. Working within this field allows for creativity and innovation regarding therapy techniques and the speech and language therapy intervention as a whole. It also provides a unique opportunity of working within a large team of highly specialist health professionals including psychiatrists, counselling psychologists, otolaryngologists, endocrinologists and plastic surgeons.

Many transsexual individuals are uncomfortable with the pathologising of gender dysphoria that is inherent in the medical model of treatment. As the provider of the least medical form of gender reassignment intervention, the SLT lies further outside this model than the other members of the MDT. On the whole a good rapport can be established with the patients, the majority of whom are motivated towards speech and language therapy treatment. Even those with limited natural vocal ability manage some successful voice modifications if they have a generally positive attitude.

The teaching of voice, communication and social skills by the SLT can be as challenging as the learning by the patient. This can make the speech and language therapy involvement highly interesting and rewarding. There are also rewards in assisting an individual to achieve their goals not only regarding speech and language therapy, but also regarding their life as a whole, by helping them to transition as effectively as they wish or are able to.

Voice and speech patterns are complex and crucial aspects of every individual's personal identity. Many clients report that modifying their voice successfully is one of the most essential aspects of transition. The role of the SLT is therefore a necessary and often vital component in the holistic treatment of transsexuals, and one that is generally highly valued by the patients themselves.

References

1   Money J and Walker P. Counselling the transsexual. In: Money M (ed). *Handbook of Sexology*. Amsterdam: Elsevier; 1977, pp. 1289–1301.
2   Scheidt D, Kob M, Willmes-von Hinckeldy K and Neuschaefer-Rube C. *Do we Need Voice Therapy for Female-to-male Transgenders?* Proceedings of the IALP Congress, Brisbane, Australia, 2004.
3   Chaloner J. The voice of the transsexual. In: Fawcus M (ed). *Voice Disorders and their Management*. London: Chapman and Hall; 2000, pp. 245–67.
4   Soderpalm E, Larsson A and Almquist S. Evaluation of a consecutive group of transsexual individuals referred for vocal intervention in the west of Sweden. *Logopedics Phoniatrics Vocology* 2004; **29**: 18–30.
5   Elias A. *Does the Speech Therapist have a Role in the Assessment and Treatment of the Male Transsexual?* (Abstract) International Conference on Gender Identity, London, 1986.
6   Hirano M. *Clinical Examination of Voice*. Heidelberg: Springer Verlag; 1981.
7   Fairbanks G. *The Rainbow Passage. Voice and Articulation Drillbook* (2e). New York: Harper; 1960.
8   Cavalli L and Chaloner J. Gender identity disorders. In: France J and Kramer S (eds). *Communication and Mental Illness – theoretical and practical approaches*. London: Jessica Kingsley; 2001, pp. 269–81.
9   Glass L. *He Says, She Says*. London: Judy Piatkus Ltd; 1992.
10 Wolfe V, Ratusnik D, Smith F and Northrop G. Intonation and fundamental frequency in male-female transsexuals. *Journal of Speech and Hearing Disorders*. 1990; **55**: 43–50.
11 Greene M and Mathieson L. *The Voice and its Disorders* (6e). London: Whurr; 2001.
12 Spencer LE. Speech characteristics of male-to-female transsexuals: a perceptual and acoustic study. *Folia Phoniatrica* 1988; **40**: 31–42.
13 Oates J and Dackakis G. Speech pathology considerations in the management of transesualism – a review. *British Journal of Disorders of Communication* 1983; **18**: 139–51.
14 Estill J. *The Control of Voice Quality*. Eleventh Symposium: Care of the Professional Voice, 1982, New York
15 Colton RH and Estill J. Elements of voice quality: perceptual, acoustic, and physiologic aspects. In: Lass NJ (ed). *Speech and Language: advances in basic research and practice* Vol V. New York: Academic Press; 1981.
16 Bagnall A. *Voicecraft for Transsexuals. 1st National Gender Dysphoria Course For Speech and Language Therapists, Charing Cross Hospital, London*. London: Charing Cross Hospital; 2002.
17 Gelfer MP and Schofield KJ. Comparison of acoustic and perceptual measures of voice in male-to female transsexuals perceived as female vesus those perceived as male. *Journal of Voice* 2000; **14**: 22–33.
18 Carew L, Dacakis G and Oates J. The effectiveness of oral resonance therapy on the perception of femininity of voice in male-to-female transsexuals. *Journal of Voice* 2006; 3 July epub ahead of print.
19 Gunzburger D. An acoustic analysis and some perceptual data concerning voice change in male-to-female transsexuals. *European Journal of Disorders of Communication* 1993; **28**: 13–21

20 Gunzburger D. Voice adaptations by transsexuals. *Clinical Linguistics and Phonetics* 1989; **3**: 163–72.

21 Gunzburger D and De Vries M (1989). How do minor acoustical cues affect male and female voice quality? *Proceedings of the European Conference on Speech Communication and Technology.* 1989; **2**: 143–5. Edinburgh: CEP Consultants.

22 Hass A. Male and female spoken language differences: stereotypes and evidence. *American Psychological Bulletin*: 1979; **86**: 616–26.

23 de Klerk V. *How Taboo are Taboo Words for Girls? Language Soc.* Cambridge: Cambridge University Press; 1992; **21**: 277–89.

24 Speer SA. *Gender Talk. Feminism, discourse and conversation analysis.* London: Routledge; 2005.

25 Matai V, Cheesman AD and Clarke PM. Cricothyroid approximation and thyroid chondroplasty: a patient survey. *Otolaryngology Head and Neck Surgery* 2003: **128**: 841–17.

26 Kanagalingham J, Georgalas C, Wood GR *et al.* Cricothyroid approximation and subluxation in 21 male-to-female transsexuals. *Laryngoscope* 2005; **115**: 611–18.

27 Brown M, Perry A, Cheesman AD and Pring T. Pitch change in male-to female transsexuals: has phonosurgery a role to play? *International Journal of Language and Communication Disorders* 2000; **35**: 129–36.

12

The practical management of hormonal treatment in adults with gender dysphoria

Leighton J Seal

Introduction

Gender identity disorder occurs in 1:11 900 to 1:37 000 males and 1:30 400 to 1:107 000 females. As we have seen previously, it is defined by the *Diagnostic and Statistical Manual for Mental Disorders IV* (DSM-IV)

> A strong and persistent cross-gender identification and a persistent discomfort with their sex or a sense of inappropriateness in the gender role of that sex[1]

and by the *International Classification of Diseases* version 10 (ICD-10) as:

> The desire to live and be accepted as a member of the opposite sex usually accompanied by the wish to make his or her body as congruent as possible with the preferred sex through surgery and hormone treatment.[2]

This latter definition implies that hormonal manipulation of the individual to achieve the secondary sexual characteristics of their desired gender is intrinsic to the diagnosis in the majority of cases.

The endocrinologist has two main roles in the treatment and evaluation of individuals with gender identity disorder: firstly the diagnosis and management of organic disorders that may present with gender confusion, and secondly the supervision of the hormonal treatment of individuals diagnosed as having a gender identity disorder. The aim of treatment is to provide a smooth successful gender transition while minimising the side-effects of treatment, by using the minimal effective amount of hormone and screening for adverse effects.

Disorders that may present with gender confusion

There are many conditions that can present with intersex states, and some but not all of these can be associated with gender confusion. Future gender orientation and the possibility of developing gender dysphoria if the incorrect sex of rearing is chosen in these conditions is now a major consideration in the management of intersex conditions. All of these conditions are rare, but gender role reversal has been described in 3β-hydroxysteroid dehydrogenase deficiency, 17-hydroxysteroid dehydrogenase deficiency and most notably in 5α-reductase deficiency.

To understand how endocrine diseases can result in gender confusion it is important to examine the normal development of gender identity and from this we can postulate how disruption of this process can result in gender confusion.[3] The development of gender orientation has been the subject of intense research; the study of intersex conditions and of gender-specific behaviours in animal models have provided invaluable insight into the development of gender. Current models of gender development are centred on the masculinisation of the central nervous system and behavioural patterns *in utero* and how, in the absence of these masculinising signals, female differentiation of the brain, with female patterning of hormonal responses and behaviours, results.[3]

Models of gender identity

In animal models such as the development of birdsong in finches, exposing chicks to androgen or aromatisable estrogens during critical windows of development permanently masculinises the female brain so that later exposure of the female to androgens will result in the development of birdsong. In females not so exposed to androgen, the administration of androgen as an adult cannot induce birdsong. The later exposure to androgen does however affect aggressive and mating behaviour. A similar situation occurs in rodents where the application of androgens to XX animals can masculinise elements of reproductive behaviour in later life and castration or the application of anti-androgens to male animals can feminise them. These hormonal manipulations can only alter behaviour during certain temporal windows in development. Outside these critical periods hormonal exposure has no effect on future behavioural patterns. This has led to a model where neuronal structure and synaptic patterning are set as critical phases of development, and this nascent patterning can be activated later by an appropriate hormonal *milieu.*

With this model in mind, in a genetic XY individual failure of testosterone action or production during the critical periods for masculinisation of the brain would lead to feminine neural development. Conversely exposure to high testosterone levels in an XX individual could result in masculinisation of a female fetus brain.

The conditions that result in a decrease in androgen action or synthesis are outlined in Table 12.1. The biochemical features that form the diagnostic criteria for these conditions are also described. As they are so rare, many of these have not been reported in the transsexual population, but as they alter testosterone action and this is believed to be critical to the gender-appropriate development of the central nervous system, they could in theory alter gender-specific development and thus gender identity. I will now discuss the more common conditions that present with gender identity disorder.

Androgen-insensitivity syndrome

The androgen receptor is encoded on X1q11–12, there have been more than 250 mutations described that effect androgen receptor function but in more than

Table 12.1 Conditions that result in a decrease in androgen action or synthesis and can produce intersex states.

	Chromosome	Inheritance	Clinical features	Biochemistry
Male pseudohermaphroditism				
17β-HSD deficiency	9q22	Recessive	Female phenotype, testis in inguinal canal, virilisation at puberty, well-developed Wolffian structures	High Androstenedione low testosterone
Congenital lipoid adrenal hyperplasia	8p11.2	Recessive	Severe salt wasting, female phenotype or ambiguous genitalia	Low androgens cortisol aldosterone
17α-hydroxylase deficiency	10q24–25	Recessive	Hypertension, ambiguous genitalia	High progesterone, low 17-OH-progesterone, low Androstenedione
5α-reductase deficiency	2p23	Recessive	Pseudovagina, urogenital sinus to hypospadius testis in inguinal canal, virilisation at puberty	High testosterone low Dihydrotestosterone
3β-hydroxysteroid dehydrogenase (II) deficiency	1p13.1–2	Recessive	Salt wasting, penoscrotal hypospadius, normal Wolffian structures,	Increased Δ5/Δ4-steroids, low aldosterone, low cortisol, high Dehydroepiandrosterone pregnenolone and **high** 17-OH pregnenolone
LH receptor defects (Leydig cell hypoplasia)	2p21	Recessive	Female phenotype, no pubic hair, no breast development, penoscrotal hypospadius	Low androgens
Female pseudohermaphroditism				
21 hydroxylase deficiency	6p21.3	Recessive	Excess sex steroids cause virilisation, hirsutism, premature adrenarche, infertility salt-losing crisis	Low cortisol, low aldosterone, excess androgens, high 17-hydroxyprogesterone
11β-hydroxylase deficiency	8q	Recessive	Excess sex steroids cause virilisation, hirsutism, premature adrenarche, infertility, hypertension	Low cortisol, low aldosterone, excess androgens, high 17-hydroxyprogesterone, high deoxycorticosterone
Aromatase deficiency	15q21.1	Recessive	Virilisation of female fetus, virilisation of mother during pregnancy	high Dehydroepiandrosterone sulphate, testosterone, Androstenedione

80–90% of familial cases the mutation is known.[4] The condition is divided into two grades: complete androgen insensitivity and partial androgen insensitivity, where there is mutation in the androgen receptor gene resulting in a partial or complete loss of androgen receptor function. Although the individual has abnormally high plasma testosterone levels they are not responsive to them and so androgen action is absent.

Complete androgen insensitivity is also known as testicular feminisation syndrome. The affected individual has a female habitus with normal external genitalia. There are no internal genitalia present and the vagina is a shortened blind-ending pouch.[4] Despite this, the majority of subjects report satisfactory sexual functioning. Axillary and pubic hair are absent as there is no testosterone action. The subject may present in childhood with a groin swelling (inguinal or labial testis), or at puberty with primary amenorrhoea. If the testes have not been removed prior to puberty then breast development is normal due to the aromatisation of testosterone to estradiol. Their psychometric profiles are un-equivocally female in gender identity and sexual orientation.[5]

Partial androgen insensitivity has had several other names such as partial complete androgen insensitivity, Refenstein's syndrome and Aiman's syndrome, depending on the degree of genital abnormality.[4] We now know that all these are caused by a spectrum of androgen receptor mutations that result in varying amount of functional loss of the receptor action and therefore androgen effect. The phenotype of these individuals can vary from normal female genitalia but the absence of sexual hair, to an intersex state, to minor genital abnormality with retained fertility depending on the degree of residual androgen receptor function. These patients can present with gender dysphoria especially when the sex of rearing has been assigned to female and corrective genital surgery has been performed to facilitate this.

The diagnosis is based on biochemical markers. If the testes are in place then post-puberty the patients have a normal or high testosterone with high luteinising hormone (LH) levels. Estradiol is high, but does not reach that seen in females.

Pre-puberty plasma testosterone levels are normal. Human chorionic gonado-trophin (hCG) stimulation (7×1500 iu/l intramuscular (i.m.)) can be used, and there is an exaggerated testosterone response to hCG stimulation in androgen insensitivity syndrome with plasma levels above 35 nmol/l (normal response is >10 nmol/l).[4]

After orchidectomy the biochemical diagnosis of androgen insensitivity is extremely difficult, however the response of plasma sex hormone-binding globulin levels to stanozolol stimulation can be measured. In complete androgen insensitivity there is no decrease in plasma sex-hormone binding globulin (SHBG) following stanozolol suppression. In partial insensitivity there was a fall in plasma SHBG by <40% of the baseline value whereas in normal individuals the fall is to 50% of the baseline value.[6]

The gold standard, however, is the analysis of androgen receptor function from genital skin fibroblasts supplemented with genetic screening of the individual for molecular defects in the androgen receptor gene.

The management of these patients is gonadectomy to prevent the occurrence of testicular cancer (extremely high as the testes are intra-abdominal). Female hormone replacement can then be instituted at puberty following standard hormone replacement protocols with either topical or oral agents.[4] The vagina is often adequate for intercourse, but occasionally augmentation of the vagina or dilation with acrylic moulds is required to allow the vagina to be functional.

If the chosen gender of these patients is female, then the management of such individuals in the gender identity clinic is the same as a post operative transexual patient as they have reduced sensitivity to testosterone and often achieve excellent feminisation. Biochemically, testosterone levels fall rapidly with estrogen treatment as the pituitary gland decreases gonadotrophin release and so testicular function is suppressed.

If the patients request gender assignment to male, then higher than normal doses of testosterone are required. Doses of up to 500 mg/week have been administered for 1–3 years in partial androgen insensitivity syndrome, and in these cases useful penile growth can occur but is often limited.[7,8] The best predictor of response as an adult is the response to testosterone in childhood. The degree of response appears to depend on the severity of receptor dysfunction.

5α-reductase deficiency

Testosterone can be converted to the more potent androgen dihydrotestosterone (DHT) by the enzyme 5α-reductase. There are two isozymes present: the type I enzyme is present in the scalp and peripheral tissues, and the type II enzyme is found in the male reproductive tract. The type II enzyme is coded on chromosome 2p23. Mutations in this gene can lead to a loss of function in the type II enzyme; this was first reported in a Dominican kindred in the 1970s[9]. The clinical phenotype is an individual with normal male internal genitalia, but feminised external genitalia. The scrotum is bifid with severe penoscrotal hypospadius and a short blind-ending vagina. The phallus is small and held in chordee, resembling a clitoris.[9] The testes are usually palpable in the inguinal canal. Prostate formation is rudimentary and so these patients are infertile. These individuals have normal action of the type I enzyme, but this enzyme is not normally expressed until puberty. At puberty there is testicular descent and enlargement of the genitalia, although not normally sufficient for sexual activity.[9] Despite this, there have been reports of normal sperm production in the testes, providing they descend, and there are even cases where individuals have fathered children.[10] There is an increase in muscle mass and erectile activity commences, but facial and body hair is reduced. Male pattern baldness has never been described in this condition.[9] Gender identity usually changes from female to male with the surge of testosterone at puberty, despite the individuals being raised as female. This is an interesting phenomenon because gender identity is believed by some to be fixed by the age of 5 years, and yet even thought their socio-cultural rearing is as female, these individuals respond to their biological sex and become male.[11] These individuals progress to function psychosexually as male.

Biochemically they present with high plasma testosterone but reduced testosterone to DHT ratio. In infancy HCG stimulation testing with measurement of urinary steroid profile may be required to demonstrate this.

As many of these subjects developed a definite male gender identity, the management of their genital abnormalities is complicated; gender assignment to female with feminising surgery can be associated with gender dysphoria later, especially if the testes are not removed until late childhood.[11] Thus there needs to be prolonged evaluation of the child before decisions about gender assignment are made, even if it is felt that the genitalia may be inadequate for sexual function in the male role, to prevent the problems of gender dysphoria later. Even though these patients are not transsexual, they may well present to gender identity clinics as the surgical reconstructions are generally performed by surgeons with an interest in this field. Indeed, only 7% of cases had a female gender identity past puberty in one reported series.[12] If the final gender is female, hormone replacement in these subjects can follow standard protocols. If the patients are male, then a trial of DHT cream applied to the genitalia is often trialled in infancy, in an attempt to improve penile growth. This may produce a doubling in penile size but will not correct other genital abnormalities. If the testes are present and descended then hormonal supplementation may not be necessary, but supplementation of DHT may be appropriate if there is under-virilisation. High-dose testosterone therapy as sustenon 500 mg/week has been shown to provide a good clinical response in 5α-reductase deficiency.[7] The aim is to bring the plasma DHT into the normal male range. This virilisation can then be maintained using oral testosterone undecanoate, as 5α-reductase 1, present in the lacteals of the gut, can convert the testosterone to DHT.

Congenital adrenal hyperplasia

Steroid hormones are synthesised from cholesterol by a common pathway in the adrenal glands and gonads. The expression of the enzyme systems for the production of cortisol and aldosterone is, however, limited to the adrenal cortex. An outline of this pathway is given in Figure 12.1. Defects in the enzymes in this pathway can lead to congenital adrenal hyperplasia (CAH).

These are autosomal recessive conditions causing defects in the P_{450} enzyme systems involved in the production of cortisol and aldosterone. The enzyme defects lead to an accumulation of the intermediary steroid 17-hydroxyprogesterone, which is then diverted into androgen production for disposal. The commonest defect is a deficiency in the action of 21-hydroxysteroid hydroxylase.[13]

CAH is classified into classical and non-classical forms. Classical CAH presents with severe loss of function of the cytochrome P450 dependant 21-hydroxylase enzyme, and presents in infancy or early childhood. It is rare, with an incidence of 1:10000 live births. In an XX individual, this exposure to excess androgen *in utero* can lead to virilisation and abnormalities of the genitalia, resulting in an intersex state. In both sexes, due to a lack of both aldosterone and cortisol production, a salt-losing crisis where sodium loss from the kidney due to a lack of aldosterone action causes circulatory collapse. Here, the condition is detected in infancy.[13]

In non-classical CAH the clinical presentation may be later as there is partial functioning of the 21-hydroxylase enzyme; XX individuals present with varying degrees of virilisation and menstrual disturbance.[14] XY individuals, although usually asymptomatic, may present with premature puberty or testicular tumours.[14] These tumours are usually benign and arise from adrenal rest cells that are found in the testis, as both glands are derived from a common lineage in embryogenesis.[15]

Less common is a reduction in the action of 11β-hydroxysteroid hydroxylase. This accounts for approximately 5% of cases of CAH. Here there is a lack of

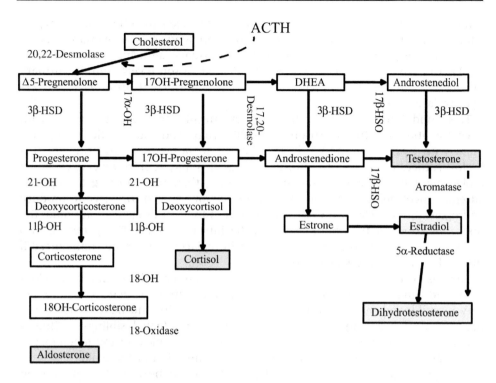

Figure 12.1 The steroid hormone synthesis pathway. Key: ACTH, adrenocorticotrophic hormone; 20,22-desmolase, side chain cleavage enzyme; 3β-HSD, 3β-hydroxysteroid dehydrogenase; 21-OH, 21-hydroxysteroid hydroxylase; 11β-OH, 11β-hydroxysteroid hydroxylase; 18-OH, 18-hydroxysteroid hydroxylase; 18 Oxidase, 18-oxidase aldosterone synthetase; 17α-OH, 17α-hydroxysteroid hydroxylase; 17,20, desmolase; 17β-HSO, 17β hydroxysteroid oxidase; aromatase.

aldosterone and cortisol production but the intermediate steroid deoxycorticosterone (DOC) is increased as well as 17-hydroxyprogesterone. DOC has partial activity at the mineralocorticoid receptor, and so salt wasting does not occur.[16] These patients may present in childhood with hypertension. There is excess androgen production, and in XX subjects virilisation of the external genitalia. Some individuals can be completely masculinised and they present as undescended testis or premature puberty in a male. As the condition is not usually detected in infancy, individuals may be untreated for a prolonged period, and the androgen excess can lead to premature fusion of the epiphyses resulting in short stature.

Biochemical diagnosis relies on the demonstration of excess 17-hydroxyprogesterone in the plasma, with a level of >6 mmol/l highly suggestive of the diagnosis. To confirm the diagnosis Synacthen testing is used with 250 µg synacthen injected at time 0, and blood samples taken at 0, 30 and 60 minutes post-injection. Plasma 17-hydroxyprogesterone rises to >30 nmol/l, whilst plasma cortisol levels fail to rise above 550 nmol/l with synacthen stimulation.[14] Other changes on baseline testing include raised plasma testosterone and dehydroepiandrosterone sulphate, but these often overlap with the range seen in other female hyper-androgenic conditions such as polycystic ovarian syndrome or ovarian tumour, and are not diagnostic. There is an increase in urinary $\Delta4$ urinary metabolites.[14] In 11β-hydroxylase deficiency, plasma deoxycortisol levels and its urinary metabolites are markedly raised, which distinguishes it from classical 21-hydroxylase deficiency.[16]

This condition is managed by replacement of the missing steroids with a combination of fludrocortisone 50–200 μg/day and glucocorticoid replacement with hydrocortisone or dexamethasone at doses that can bring the 17-hydroxyprogesterone into the normal range. This may require reverse circadian replacement with higher doses in the evening than the morning to suppress adrenocorticotrophic hormone (ACTH) production, and so the drive to produce androgens. In non-classical CAH where signs of hyperandrogenism are mild, the only indication for treatment may be if fertility is affected. The patient is also advised to carry a steroid card so that steroid replacement can be commenced if they suffer major illness or injury.[9,14]

There is evidence that this androgen exposure can masculinise neural development and behaviour too. Girls with CAH display more male gender-appropriate play in childhood, have a deceased desire for maternity and have an increased occurrence of bisexuality compared with their unaffected siblings.[17] Thus a patient with congenital hyperplasia is treated with steroids during pregnancy if she is carrying a female fetus, to prevent masculinisation of the child.

CAH provides us with a source of information on hormonal influences on human gender identity formation, where XX individuals are exposed to unusually high levels of testosterone *in utero*. A few cases have been reported where girls with CAH have developed male gender identity.[3] However, a significant number of studies have found that CAH patients who are assigned and consistently raised as girls do not develop a gender identity disorder. However, during childhood, a number of these girls show increased masculine play behaviour.[17,18]

Polycystic ovarian syndrome

The polycystic ovarian syndrome (PCOS) is extremely common. It is estimated to affect up to 20% of the female population. It has a familial component and the phenotype in males appears to be premature balding before the age of 30 years.[19] It is characterised by oligomenorrhoea, hyperandrogenism and a metabolic syndrome that includes insulin resistance, dyslipidaemia and premature ischaemic heart disease.

PCOS is characterised by a failure of ovulation, which leads to oligomenorrhoea. There is also increased androgen production from both the ovaries and the adrenals. The increase in plasma testosterone decreases hepatic SHBG production, and this further increases free androgen levels, causing hyperandrogenism. Clinically this presents as hirsuitism, acne and, rarely, mild cliteromegally.

PCOS is also associated with obesity and the development of insulin resistance. The insulin resistance can progress to glucose intolerance and frank diabetes mellitus. Clinically this is marked by pigmentation and a thickening in the skin termed acanthosis nigricans. Along with this, dyslipidaemia consisting of low plasma high-density lipoprotein (HDL), and raised total cholesterol and low-density lipoprotein (LDL) cholesterol, can occur. This combination of cardio-vascular risk factors can lead to premature vascular disease and is termed the metabolic syndrome. One of the commonest presentations, however, is that of subfertility, and it is the commonest endocrine disease in women seen at fertility clinics.

Women with PCOS fall into two categories: ovulatory and anovulatory. Those who maintain a normal body mass index are generally ovulatory with regular menses. These women do not display the metabolic syndrome, although they may have mildly raised fasting insulin. Weight gain can lead to anovulation and the expression of the metabolic syndrome, which suggests that obesity and the concomitant increase in insulin resistance may be the key factor in the pathogenesis of this syndrome.

The management of PCOS depends on the patient's presenting complaint. In all cases, however, weight reduction can lead to a significant improvement in the clinical condition of the patient, with a decrease in androgen production and a return of ovulation. The insulin resistance is treated with the biguanide drug metformin. This increases the peripheral tissue sensitivity to insulin, and also decreases appetite leading to weight reduction. Doses of 500 mg once daily up to 850 mg three times daily are used. Even in patients who are not diabetic, hypoglycaemia does not occur. The major side-effect of the medication is gastro-intestinal upset, which can limit its effectiveness. The hepatic lipase inhibitor orlistat is also effective in PCOS, producing its effects by weight loss. On treat-ment with metformin 89% have a return of ovulation.[20]

Hirsuitism and menstrual irregularity can be controlled using the oral con-traceptive pill. These medication induce SHBG production whilst suppressing ovarian androgen production and effectively reducing hirsuitism. Dianette is especially effective as it contains a combination of the ethinylestradiol with the anti-androgenic progestin cyproterone acetate, which helps to control the effects of androgens on the hair follicle. An alternative approach is to use a topical preparation eflornithine (Vaniqa 11.5%), which inhibits the enzyme ornithine decarboxylase in the hair follicle and so reduces hair growth. Local measures such as waxing, sugaring, laser and electrolysis are also extremely effective in controlling excess body hair.

If the features of the metabolic syndrome are present then intervention in lifestyle, with advice on weight loss, smoking cessation, healthy eating and exer-cise are important. If dyslipidaemia is present and these measures fail to correct the disturbance, treatment with lipid-lowering agents such as statins is necessary.

As these women are oligomenorrhoeic and obese there is a risk of endometrial hyperplasia, and so ultrasound scanning is important. If the endometrium is thickened endometrial biopsy may be necessary. Other tumours linked to excess estrogen exposure in obese PCOS patients include breast cancer and ovarian cancer. Reassuringly, recent analysis of the data suggest that this association is limited to endometrial carcinoma.[21]

Subfertilty is linked to anovulation. Metformin and weight reduction are both effective means of increasing ovulation. When these simple measures fail, referral to an assisted fertility clinic is appropriate. These patients respond well to clomifene, but are at risk of experiencing excess follicle formation and so require ovarian tracking by ultrasound during treatment. If this fails then *in vitro* fertilisation (IVF) may be effective.

There has been an association between PCOS and transexualism in genetic females. In one report, PCOS was present in 58% of their population.[22] It is attractive to postulate that excess androgen production in these women has masculinised their gender identity, but we must remember that PCOS is very common and with such a small cohort it is difficult to make any firm conclusions. Another biological factor is that androgen production does not become excessive until after puberty, long after gender identity is determined. The excess androgens may, however, be important in the expression of these subjects' male gender identity. In patients with PCOS it is important to screen for the elements of the metabolic syndrome, as testosterone therapy will exacerbate them. The patients should have a formal fasting blood glucose and a full lipid profile to define their metabolic status. They should be given appropriate lifestyle advice on diet, exercise and smoking cessation. Screening for endometrial hypertrophy is important if the subject has been oligomenorrhoeic prior to testosterone therapy. This is important, as testosterone can be aromatised to estradiol, which is mitogenic for the endometrium and can increase the risk of endometrial malignancy.

Initiation of hormone therapy

The principle of treatment is triadic therapy, which consists of three critical elements; real life experience, hormonal therapy of the desired gender and finally sex reassignment surgery. The reason for adopting this strategy is that the patient advances through a sequence of therapy with progressively more irreversible effects on their body, and therefore avoiding more significant physical alterations should they choose to revert to their birth gender. It is therefore important that hormonal therapy is undertaken in close collaboration with a mental health professional who is experienced in the assessment of these patients, and who ideally has a close working relationship with the endocrinologist.

Hormonal therapy can be recommended by one mental health practitioner (MHP) following a period of assessment by them. The World Professional Association for Transgender Health, Inc. (formerly Harry Benjamin) guidelines state that the client should have either a documented real life experience living in their new gender role of 3 months, or 3 months of psychotherapy by the referring MHP prior to the initiation of hormone therapy. Commencement of hormonal therapy should generally be deferred until the client has demonstrated consolidation of their gender identity during real life experience, and they have made progress in mastering the problems their new social role has brought. Ideally the client should also be in a state of stable or improving mental health. It is also important that the MHP felt that the client is likely to take hormones in a reliable manner before hormone treatment is commenced. If this last criterion is not fulfilled then hormonal manipulation must be cautious and involve a clear therapeutic contract between the patient and doctor administering the hormones, allowing a clear understanding by the client that the physician involved in their hormonal care cannot take clinical responsibility for their use of any non-endorsed products and that the use of these products may be detrimental to their health. In certain circumstances the use of non-endorsed products may reasonably lead to termination of the therapeutic relationship between the hormonal prescriber and the client. In general, clients are not treated until they reach 18 years of age. In paediatric practice puberty may be arrested using gonadotrophin-releasing hormone (GnRH) agonists before this age to facilitate gender transition later. This will be dealt with later in this chapter.

Under certain circumstances the normal triadic pattern of therapy may not be appropriate, but in these circumstances the use of hormones must be recommended by the MHP involved in the patient care. If, following assessment, it is felt that the withdrawal of illicitly used black market hormones would be detrimental to the individual's mental health, approval may be given by the MHP for the initiation of hormonal therapy prior to a change in gender role. This approach can occasionally lead to problems in the patient–doctor relationship later, and it is therefore much preferable to have a real life experience first. The other situation where hormonal therapy is used without a change in gender role is to provide symptomatic relief of gender dysphoria when, following diagnosis and psychotherapy, the client does not wish to proceed to gender role change.

Prior to the initiation of hormonal therapy, the patient should be counselled about the risks and benefits of the hormonal therapy they are about to undertake, and this counselling should be performed by a health professional experienced in the use of these agents.

Hormonal regimens in common use

Male-to-female transsexuals

The use of hormonal manipulation in the treatment of transsexual individuals is hampered by a lack of any randomised controlled trials to assist in our therapeutic decisions. There has, however, been a significant amount of experience in the treatment of this condition over the last 30 years, using several well-established hormonal protocols. These are summarised in Table 12.2.

Treatment protocols

The longest experience is with the use of ethinylestradiol; this estrogen is synthetic and has some affinity for the androgen receptor. The major disadvantage is that it negatively affects the elements of the clotting cascade making it procoagulant. The reason for its popularity is that it is effective and indeed has been shown to be more effective than conjugated estrogens in one study[23] but this was not reproduced in the same group's later work.[24]

Ethinylestradiol doses of at least 100 μg/day are needed to suppress testosterone production in pre-operative patients, and in a significant proportion plasma testosterone is still not suppressed. This requires either escalating doses of estrogen with the attendant risk of DVT, or the use of adjuvant therapy. In light of the Toorians et al paper[25] we now administer estrogen valerate as our primary estrogen of choice.

Estrogen valerate 2 mg/day is approximately equivalent to ethinylestradiol 50 μg/day, and doses of 2–6 mg/day have been used, resulting in good feminisation. Unlike ethinylestradiol, estrogen valerate can be measured using standard estrogen radioimmunoassays, allowing the dose to be accurately titrated with the aim of achieving a plasma estrogen level in the mid- to upper-part of the normal

Table 12.2 A list outlining the published treatment protocols for the feminisation of Male to Female transsexuals.

Clinic	Feminising hormone regimens		Masculinising hormone regimens	n
	Estrogen	Adjuncts		
Academic Hospital Vrije Universeit Amsterdam	Ethinylestradiol 100 μg/day or transdermal 17β-estradiol 100 mg × 2/week	Cyproterone acetate 100 mg/day	Testosterone esters 250 mg/2 week or testosterone undecanoate 160 mg/day	816 MtF, 293 FtM
Psycholneurology Unit Liège, Liège	Ethinylestradiol 50–100 μg/day or Conjugated Equine Estrogens 1.25–2.5 mg/day or estrogen benzoate 25 mg/week	Optional: spironolactone 100–200mg/day or cyproterone acetate 100 mg/day	Testosterone 240 mg/day or testosterone esters 250 mg/2–4 week	
Mount Sinai School of Medicine New York	Ethinylestradiol 100 μg/day or Conjugated Equine Estrogens 1.25–2.5 mg/day or estrogen benzoate 25 mg/week	Medroxyprogesterone acetate 510 mg/day for 10 days/month for the first 6 months Optional: spironolactone 100–200 mg/day or cyproterone acetate 100 mg/day	Testosterone esters 250–400 mg/2–3 week	93 FtM
Department of Endocrinology, University of British Colombia, Vancouver	Conjugated Equine Estrogens 0.625 mg increasing to 5 mg/day for 3 weeks per month	Spironolactone 100–200 mg/day; medroxyprogesterone acetate 10 mg/day for 14 days/month or continuously	Unreported	50 MtF
Max-Planck Institute Endocrinological Unit Munich	Estradiol 80–100 mg i.m. 2 weekly for 1 year; 17β-estradiol 2–8 mg/day to continue	Cyproterone Acetate 100 mg/day for 6–12 months	Testosterone Esters 250 mg/2 week for 9–12 months, then testosterone esters 250 mg/2–4 week Optional: progesterone 500 mg i.m. × 2 3–4 days apart between testosterone doses	129 total

Clinic	Oestrogen regimen	GnRH analogue	Testosterone regimen	Numbers
Gender Clinic University of Texas Medical Branch Galverston	Ethinylestradiol 50–100 µg/day or Conjugated Equine Estrogens 7.5–10 mg/day	Unreported	Testosterone cyprionate 200 mg/2 week i.m.	60 MtF, 30FtM
Department of Obstetrics and Gynaecology National University of Singapore, Singapore	Unreported		Testosterone esters 250 mg/2–4 week or testosterone Cyclopentylpropionate 100 mg/week i.m.	70 FtM
Gender Identity Clinic Charing Cross Hospital London	Estrogen valerate 2–6 mg/day or ethinylestradiol 50–150 µg/day or Conjugated Equine Estrogens 2.5–7.5 mg/day or transdermal 17β-estradiol 50–100 mg 2/week	Goserelin 3.6 mg/4 week or 10.8 mg/12 week or leuporelin 3.75 mg/4 week or 11.25 mg/12 week	Testosterone esters 250 mg/2–4 week *Post-operative*: testosterone esters 250 mg/3–5 week or transdermal testosterone 50–100 mg/day or buccal testosterone 30 mg twice daily or testosterone undecanoate 1000 mg/3 months i.m. or testosterone implant 300–600 mg/6 months	

FtM, female-to-male; MtF, female-to-male.

range for a woman in the follicular phase of the menstrual cycle. At our centre there has been a move away from using high doses of estrogen to suppress testosterone production pre-operatively; these, historically, have been administered in doses up to 250 μg/day, but adjuvant therapy use is now more common. The use of anti-androgen therapy in the form of cyproterone acetate or finasteride has been associated with abnormalities of liver function and also depression, which can be particularly marked in this patient group. To minimise the doses of estrogen required for feminisation, we have moved to using primary chemical castration with GnRH analogues and immediate administration of estrogen valerate. They are well tolerated, and with the co-administration of estrogen relatively side-effect free, as sex steroid replacement prevents the most severe side-effects such as vasomotor flushing and tiredness associated with these compounds. The only disadvantage of this approach is that for the first 2 weeks after the first administration, gonadotrophin levels increase with an increase in plasma testosterone levels, increased feelings of masculinity and increased frequency of erection. If this is likely to be psychologically detrimental for the patient, then cyproterone acetate 100 mg/day can be administered for these 2 weeks. Subsequent injections will not induce this flare phenomenon, as the hypothalamo-pituitary-gondal axis is thereafter suppressed. Using this approach, much lower doses of estrogen can be used and this should result in a reduction in the rate of thromboembolic events.

In some patients this regimen is not well tolerated. The major objection from some patients is the need for regular injections, hair loss, which although rare can occur, and in patients who have had ethinylestradiol previously a feeling of being less feminine during estrogen valerate therapy. In these cases either high-dose estrogen valerate or ethinylestradiol can be used.

Parentral adminsitratiaon of estrogen benzotate has been advocated by some centres. This preparation has the advantage of only requiring administration 2–4 weekly and results in good feminisation. The disadvantage of this preparation is that it is open to abuse with some patients using topical or oral supplementation of estrogen obtained illicitly in addition to the estrogen injection. There has been a case of a prolactinoma developing in a patient who used estrogen benzoate in combination with illicit ethinyl estradiol.

Post-operative management

If the patient was on suppressive doses of oestrogen pre-orchidectomy, the dose of estrogen can be significantly reduced. Typically, the patient can be maintained on long-term treatment with estrogen valerate 2 mg/day, ethinylestradiol 50 μg/day or transdermal 17β-estradiol 100 mg $\times$ 2/week.

If the patient was being treated with a GnRH analogue pre-operatively then the pre-operative estrogen dose is continued after the gender reassignment surgery.

The aim of therapy is to maintain good bone health, general well-being and cardiovascular health. Standard hormone replacement doses can be used although in many case higher levels, such as twice the normal amount, are administered. This reflects the generally larger body habitus of the transsexual woman. The replacement is monitored on clinical parameters and estrogen monitoring.

Charing Cross Clinic regimen

The standard hormonal regimen used at our clinic is the initiation of estrogen valerate 2 mg increasing to a maximum of 6 mg/day (*see* Box 12.1). This is titrated to give a plasma estradiol level of 400–600 pmol/l. Dose increases are made after 3 months of therapy. Goserelin 10.8 mg/3 months is added to suppress testosterone production. To cover the flare in testosterone levels for the first 2 weeks, cyproterone acetate 100 mg once daily is added. The anti-androgen is only required for the first injection. The aim is to achieve a plasma testosterone in the normal female range (<3 nmol/l). If testosterone is not controlled with 3-monthly injection, then this can be increased to 11 or 10-weekly. As an alternative goserelin 3 mg every 4 weeks can be used.

In older patients, estrogen monotherapy may be adequate to achieve testosterone suppression. In those aged over 45 years, estrogen valerate 2 mg is commenced and titrated 3 monthly. If plasma testosterone is not suppressed on 4 mg once daily then goserelin may be added.

Box 12.1   Standard pre-operative treatment protocol at Charing Cross Hospital Gender Identity Clinic

- Estrogen valerate 2–4 mg/day
- Goserelin 10.8 mg/12 week

Optional:
- Cyproterone acetate 100 mg/day for 2 weeks

or
- Estrogen valerate 4–6 mg/day

or
- Ethinylestradiol 50–150 µg/day

In patients that cannot tolerate estrogen valerate therapy, ethinylestradiol 50–150 µg/day or conjugated equine estrogens 2.3–7.5 mg/day are alternative treatments. The usual reasons for discontinuation of estrogen valerate are nausea, headache or a lack of breast development although, in our experience, breast development does not appear to be any better with ethinylestradiol.

Six weeks prior to gender reassignment surgery, estrogen therapy is discontinued to reduce the incidence of peri-operative deep vein thrombosis (DVT). It is recommenced 1 week post-operatively. Post-gender reassignment surgery the estrogen valerate dose is reduced to a maintenance level of 2 mg once daily.

Alternative therapies include transdermal estrogen with 50 or 100 µg twice per week, ethinylestradiol 50 µg daily, or conjugated equine estrogens 2.5 mg once daily. These doses tend to be at the upper end of those used in standard hormone replacement therapy (HRT) regimens, and are frequently necessary as the transsexual female is often of a larger frame that a genetic female. Estrogen valerate has the advantage of allowing plasma estradiol levels to guide therapy, aiming for a plasma estradiol of 400–600 pmol/l. Goserelin is stopped post-operatively.

Effects of hormone replacement

Estrogens

The cornerstone of hormone treatment of the male-to-female transsexual is the use of estrogen. Many preparations have been used and these are listed in Table 12.2. Typically, doses of estrogen that are 2–3 times that used for HRT are used in the treatment of transsexual individuals. The route of administration is usually oral, but some centres recommend the use of transdermal preparations, especially over the age of 45 years.

Facial hair

The beneficial effects of estrogen in the transsexual are induction of female characteristics. In the skin the texture of the facial skin becomes finer, and there is a reduction in the growth of facial hair. Both facial and truncal hair shaft diameters decrease and this effect is maximal after 4 months of treatment. There is not an ongoing improvement after this.[26]

Although slowed, estrogen therapy itself seldom reduces facial hair growth adequately to provide a female facial appearance once a male has adult beard development. Local measures such as electrolysis, waxing, shaving, sugaring or laser therapy are needed to reduce the appearance of facial hair and facilitate female presentation.

The topical ornithine decarboxylase inhibitor eflornithine has been used to treat hirsuitism in genetic females. It takes 6–8 weeks to have any effect and 24 weeks to reach its maximum action.[27] The drug is applied twice daily as a 15% cream to the hirsute areas. Side-effects include redness and itching. In transsexuals there are no published data, but it may be of benefit once plasma testosterone levels are in the normal female range. Male pattern baldness also slows and may arrest as plasma testosterone levels fall in response to estrogen treatment; however regrowth of hair, once it is lost, does not occur.

Breast growth

Breast development, which for the transsexual patient is often the most important alteration they wish to achieve, occurs with estrogen treatment. During normal puberty breast growth is estrogen dependent. The stages of breast development can be characterised using the system of Tanner and described in five stages from prepubertal to adult breast development:

- *stage 1*: prepubertal with no elevation of the breast bud
- *stage 2*: elevation of the breast bud with enlargement of the areola
- *stage 3*: further elevation of the breast with no separation of their contours
- *stage 4*: projection of the areola and papilla to form a secondary mound above the level of the breast
- *stage 5*: mature breast with projection of the papilla only, due to recession of the areola to the general contour of the breast.[28]

Breast development during normal puberty occurs over 18 months to 2 years once telearche has been attained. Estrogen therapy in transsexual individuals mimics this process. Breast development begins about 2–3 months after the initiation of treatment and the maximum effect of estrogen on breast development is not seen until 2 years of estrogen therapy. Doses of estrogen in the order of 100 μg ethinylestradiol are adequate for this to occur. Using higher doses of estrogen does not appear to have additional benefit in inducing breast development; a dose of 500 μg/day ethinylestradiol resulted in breast development identical to that seen when premarin is used in doses of 2.5 to 5 mg/day.[24]

The average breast development was to 14.5 ± 1.2 cm, which was not statistically different from the baseline characteristics of the female-to-male transsexual population studied (14.5 ± 0.9 cm).[24] This equates to a B cup size. In general the maximum breast development a patient can expect to achieve is a cup size less than their mother, as the first-degree female relatives are the best guides to the genetic programming for breast development that the patient carries.

However, the majority of transsexual individuals do not reach their desired breast size and may develop pointed or conical breasts. This phenomenon has been seen in the past in genetic females undergoing induction of puberty. In these cases, the use of large doses of estrogen early leads to growth of the breast but premature termination of ductal branching, resulting in small conical breast formation. The need to suppress androgen production has necessitated the use of high-dose estrogens at an early stage in the past, but now with the availability of gonadotrophin-releasing hormone (GnRH) analogues, testosterone suppression can be achieved independently of feminisation, and initiation of estrogen therapy at lower doses may result in better breast development. This approach has not yet been tested to see if it results in improved breast development.

Breast development is dependent on the deposition of fat into the breast, and encouraging underweight patients to gain some weight can result in enhanced breast growth.

Despite hormonal manipulation 60% of transsexual subjects progress to breast augmentation surgery.[29] The major reason for this is the poor response of patients to estrogen therapy but there are also differences in anatomy between the male and female thorax. In genetic females the thorax is shorter and more conical and there is a greater layer of subcutaneous fat over the thoracic wall, which obscures the muscle bulk of the chest. And so, even with a response to hormonal therapy, some patients still require augmentation so that the breast contour appears proportionate for their larger body frame.

Body fat distribution

Estrogen therapy results in changes in the distribution of body fat. There is an increase in subcutaneous fat especially around the hips and buttocks to give a more rounded form to the body. There is an average 3.8 kg weight gain, with a 38% increase in subcutaneous fat deposits.

This is accompanied by a decrease in muscle bulk and upper body muscle strength. The increase in subcutaneous fat also decreases muscle definition, promoting a more female body outline.

Genital effects

Estrogen therapy in males reduces libido and erectile function. Due to gonado-trophin suppression there is a decrease in testicular volume. Spermatogenesis is also decreased, and before commencing estrogen therapy patients should be counselled about their loss of fertility, and offered sperm storage if future fertility may be required.

Cognition

In peri- and postmenopausal women, estrogen therapy has mood-modulating effects. It increases feelings of well-being and decreases depression scores.[30,31] Estrogen therapy in transsexuals is reported to have a calming effect and to promote euthymia. Anecdotally many patients report an increased feeling of femininity on estrogen therapy and a calmer mood in reaction to a reduction in their feelings of being male.

Hormonal adjuncts

Some centres use either anti-androgens such as cyproterone acetate or progestin to augment the action of estrogens.

Cyproterone acetate is a potent androgen receptor-blocking drug. It is derived from progesterone and is metabolised in the liver. Its use is associated with hepatic dysfunction, and although this rarely leads to discontinuation of the drug it does require regular monitoring of liver function.[32,34] More importantly there is a significant incidence of depression associated with the use of cyproterone in up to 30% of users.[32] In this patient population depression is a significant problem, and cyproterone acetate can often exacerbate these symptoms. The same problems occur with the use of finasteride; both depression and liver function disturbance have been described with the use of this drug.[35-37] Anti-androgens have been necessary in the past, as many patients fail to suppress their production of testosterone with estrogen therapy. Now we have the availability of GnRH analogues. These drugs work by over-stimulating the LH receptors on the gonadotrophin cells of the pituitary, which become downregulated decreas-ing LH release which leads to reduced testosterone production. There has been extensive experience in using these drugs both in the treatment of prostate cancer and infertility, and they have an excellent side-effect profile.

Progesterone is used by some centres and is widely purported by trans-sexual websites to improve breast development. In the only study published comparing estrogen with estrogen and progesterone there was no additional benefit of progesterone on breast growth over estrogen alone. More worryingly, we know that in trials of hormone replacement in women there is an increased incidence of cardiovascular events and a trend towards increasing levels of breast cancer. These risks were not seen in the estrogen-only arm of these trials, suggesting that progesterone is detrimental for both cardiovascular and breast health.[38,39]

Negative effects of estrogen therapy

Estrogen therapy is safe and effective, but several side-effects of this treatment have been described in the transsexual population. The most important of these are thromboembolic complications, breast cancer risk, hyperprolactinaemia and liver function abnormalities.[40]

Thromboembolic disease

The incidence of deep venous thrombosis (DVT) in transsexual patients is approximately 2.6%; however in this young population this represents a risk that is 20 times that of the untreated population. The majority of these incidents occur during the first 2 years of treatment. There is however an ongoing risk of 0.4% per year which continues.[41]

The risk of DVT is affected by several factors. The type of estrogen may be important. It has been demonstrated that ethinylestradiol alters the levels of plasma protein S, C and prothombin, which results in a procoagulant haemostatic profile in transsexual subjects.[25] These changes were not observed when either transdermal estrogen or oral estrogen valerate were used.[25] There were no thromboembolic events seen in either group, but this was a short-term study. Due to the high incidence of thromboembolic (TE) disease, the Liège clinic in Belgium began a policy of using transdermal estrogen after the age of 45 years, and they have noticed a decrease in incidence of DVT in their clinic population from a 40-fold to a 20-fold increased risk.[42] In our own clinic we have moved away from using ethinylestradiol to estrogen valerate, however we have not yet demonstrated any change in the incidence of DVT in our population.

Smoking in women taking the oral contraceptive pill increases the risk of stroke and DVT.[43] The incidence appears to be dose related, with the higher dose pill (80 μg estrogen) having a higher incidence of DVT. The doses of estrogen used in the contraceptive pill are approximately half those used for feminisation in the transsexual population, and so it is strongly recommended that patients stop smoking prior to commencing on estrogen therapy to minimise the risk of DVT. Subsequent studies on the contraceptive pill have failed to demonstrate this association, but these have examined pills with lower estrogen doses.[43–45]

Breast cancer

The incidence of breast cancer with standard HRT in genetic females is estimated at an excess of 3.2/1000 aged 50–59 years and 4/1000 aged 60–69.[46] This is based on large population-based studies. We know from both the Heart and Estrogen/Progestin Replacement Study (HERS)[39] and Women's Health Initiative trial[38] that the inclusion of progesterone in the HRT regimen increases this risk. There are no similar studies available in the transsexual population. There have only been four case reports of breast tumours occurring in treated transsexual patients, suggesting that the risk of breast cancer secondary to feminising hormone therapy is very low. Some units do use progestins routinely as part of their hormonal regimen and have not reported excess breast cancer incidence in comparison with other transsexual populations.

In view of the fact that progestins are not involved in normal pubertal breast development, are of no proven benefit in breast development induction in trans-sexuals, and that there is evidence they may increase breast cancer risk, their use for the feminisation of transsexual women has to be seriously questioned.

Hyperprolactinaemia

The lactotroph is sensitive to the ambient estrogen levels in the serum. Estrogen not only causes increased prolactin release from these cells, but also causes proliferation of them, which can result in hyperprolactinaemia and pituitary hypertrophy. The incidence of significant hyperprolactinaemia has been reported to be up to 15%.[40] There have only been two case reports of prolactinomas in transsexual subjects and none have needed withdrawal of estrogen treatment.[47,48] The incidence of hyperprolactinaemia appears to be related to the dose of estrogen used and if plasma prolactin becomes elevated then reduction of the estrogen dose and the use of GnRH analogues or anti-androgens can be useful. Indeed, one of the patients who developed a prolactinoma had self-administered i.m. estrogen benzoate in addition to her prescribed estrogen therapy.[47]

Abnormal liver function

Abnormalities of liver function are, rarely, associated with the use of estrogen therapy. Estrogen use can be associated with obstructive jaundice.[49,50] This is particularly seen in orally administered estrogens. If the liver function disturbance is mild, with enzyme changes of less than three times the upper limit of normal, then this condition can often be successfully managed by either dose reduction or changing the patient to a transdermal estrogen preparation. Other risks of estrogen therapy are Budd–Chiari syndrome, which has a relative risk of 2.37 times in oral contraceptive users.[36] Estrogen use also increases the prevalence of hepatic adenomas as a function of duration of treatment. While hepatocellular carcinoma is very rare, its risk is increased by a factor of 7–20 in women using oral contraceptives for 8 years or more,[51] although there are no cases reported in transsexual individuals. Use of combined oral contraceptives appears to speed development of cholelithiasis in predisposed women and this risk of cholelithiasis is linked to the dose of estrogen administered in women aged under 30 years.[52] Several cases of acute pancreatitis in the first 3 months of treatment have been reported in women with pre-existing lipid metabolic abnormalities.[52] For this reason, monitoring of the liver function 3-monthly is needed in the first year of treatment; this can then be reduced to 6–12-monthly thereafter.

The risk of abnormal liver function tests is approximately 3% in male-to-female transsexuals.[40,41] In half of these, the abnormalities persist for more than 3 months. However the increases are mild and only rarely require discontinuation of treatment.

Prostate cancer

Prostate cancer has only been reported in two transsexual women in the world literature.[53,54] As this is such a common malignancy in the male population with an incidence of up to 50% by the eighth decade, it is difficult to attribute these cases to hormonal therapy.[55] Indeed, in one series the use of long-term estrogen in men there was no evidence on biopsy of either hypertrophy or dysplasia.[56]

Fertility

Estrogen therapy leads to a suppression of gonadotrophin production and subsequent reduction in spermatogenesis. Patients should be counselled that treatment will reduce their fertility, and offered the chance of sperm storage if desired.

Other side-effects

Estrogen therapy is associated with other minor side-effects that appear in the literature as isolated case reports. These are often minor and include dry hair and brittle nails that maybe due to a decrease in sebum production following estrogen treatment. Other skin changes include the development of cholasma and abdominal striae. There is also the risk of the development of periondontal disease in susceptible individuals, although there have been no reports of this in male to female transsexuals as yet.

Safety monitoring

The safety monitoring for this ongoing treatment is outlined in Table 12.3. This monitoring is designed to detect the major side-effects of hormonal therapy as we have outlined above. The risks of estrogen exposure appear to be related to the duration of estrogen treatment in genetic females. For this reason, the long-term monitoring of transsexual individuals includes health screening for breast cancer and monitoring of bone health in any individuals who have had a significant break from sex steroid treatment (>6 months).

To attempt to minimise the cumulative exposure to estrogen it is advisable to use the lowest estrogen dose tolerated by the patient, and when a preparation that can be monitored is used, to use plasma levels of estrogen to guide replacement therapy. Gonadotrophin level measurements are unhelpful. When the patient reaches 40 years of age, consideration of transdermal estrogen preparation has been recommended by one group;[42] in our practice however there does not appear to be an increased risk of thromboembolic events after this age , possibly reflecting the fact that we insist on patients stopping smoking which was not the case in their series. When the individual reaches 55 years, then the discontinuation of HRT should be discussed. It is known that prolonged HRT use beyond 7 years after the menopause is associated with an increased risk of breast cancer. These data apply to genetic females, and although this is the best evidence available on the long-term effects of estrogen therapy, we do know that the standardised mortality ratio for transsexual people is normal suggesting that in this patient group longer-term estrogen therapy is not detrimental. With this in mind discussion around stopping HRT should include this information, and if the patient decides to continue estrogen therapy for life there are no data available to suggest that this is harmful.

Table 12.3 Safety montoring for ongoing hormonal treatment of transsexual patients

	Male to female	Female to male
Initial visit	LH FSH Testosterone Estradiol SHBG Prolactin Dihydrotestosterone PSA Weight Blood pressure Lipid profile Glucose	LH FSH Testosterone Estradiol SHBG Prolactin Dihydrotestosterone Weight Blood pressure Lipid profile Glucose
Every 3–6 months	Testosterone levels until stable Estradiol blood level (if on estrogen valerate) LFTs Breast examination Blood pressure Weight	Testosterone levels LFTs FBC (polycythaemia) Blood pressure Weight
Every 6–12 months pre-operatively	Serum prolactin *Over 50 years*: PSA	Lipids Cervical smear (every 3 years) Endometrial ultrasound (every 2 years)
Every 12 months post-operatively	Decrease estrogens to high HRT dose Serum prolactin LFTs Blood pressure Weight *Over 40 years*: Consider transdermal estrogen *Over 50 years*: Discuss stopping HRT Mammography every 5 years PSA	Decrease testosterone to standard HRT dose Lipid profile LFTs Blood pressure Weight Testosterone levels FBC (polycythaemia) (DEXA scan)

FBC, full blood count; FSH, follicle-stimulating hormone; HRT, hormone-replacement therapy; LFT, liver function test; LH, luteinising hormone; PSA, prostate-specific antigen; SHBG, sex hormone-binding globulin.

Management of therapy complications

Although the use of hormonal manipulation is very safe, complications from therapy can occur. These can be managed effectively, and in the vast majority of cases, estrogen therapy can be continued.

Thromboembolic effects

In the acute situation, the estrogen therapy should be stopped. The patient is formally anticogulated to treat the embolic event. It should be borne in mind that as the estrogen wears off the patient will become progressively more warfarin sensitive, due to a decrease in liver warfarin metabolism, and so the patient requires close monitoring of the international normalised ratio (INR). It is advisable to manage such cases in conjunction with a haematologist, but if the patient wishes to continue with estrogen therapy it is our practice to recommend lifelong anticoagulation, as the incidence of recurrent thromboembolism is extremely high. The estrogen dose chosen should be minimal and the least procoagulant. If the patient is pre-operative, then goserelin implants can be commenced once the INR is stable, and used in conjunction with estrogen valerate 2–4 mg/day or transdermal estradiol patches 50–100 mg 2/week. Post-operatively, the same estrogen dose can be used without GnRH analogue treatment.

Breast cancer

This is a hormonally sensitive tumour. The use of ongoing estrogen therapy is not safe and so it should be discontinued. If the patient is post-operative then clonidine hydrochloride 50–100 μg three times daily can be helpful in controlling the vasomotor flushing. Bone health must be monitored and osteoporosis managed with bisphosphonate therapy, Selective Estrogen Receptor Modulators (SERMs) or stronitium ranelate. Cardiovascular risk factors should be monitored and addressed as appropriate to minimise the adverse effect on the cardiovascular system that is associated with hypogonadism.

Hyperprolactinaemia and galactorrhoea

Minor hyperprolactinaemia is relatively common. With plasma prolactin level below 1000 mu/l there is a negligible chance of there being any significant pituitary enlargement. The patient should have an assessment of the visual fields by confrontation and measurement of thyroid function, insulin-like growth factor (IGF-1) and 9 am cortisol to assess the other pituitary axes. If these are normal, then the prolactin level should be repeated in 3 months' time. If it is stable, then 6-monthly monitoring should be undertaken. Hyperprolactinaemia secondary to estrogen therapy is often transient and may spontaneously resolve.

Prolactin levels above 1000 mu/l should be assessed further, in conjunction with an endocrinologist. Formal perimetometry should be performed and magnetic resonance imaging (MRI) scanning of the pituitary gland is often undertaken. In these cases, minimising the estrogen dose by combining GnRH therapy with estrogen treatment, or changing from ethinylestradiol to transdermal or oral estrogen valerate usually leads to resolution of the hyperprolactinaemia. If the patient is taking spironolactone or cyproterone acetate, these too should be withdrawn as they can induce hyperprolactinaemia.

Abnormal liver function

Minor derangement of liver function with increases in liver enzyme levels to less than twice the upper limit of normal do not require withdrawal of estrogen therapy. Screening for other causes of hepatic dysfunction should be performed (*see* Box 12.2), as well as ultrasound scanning of the liver to exclude any hepatic lesion or the presence of gallstones. If there is minor derangement then transferring the patient to a topical estrogen preparation decreases the estrogen dose delivered to the liver and may improve liver function. It is known that the natural estrogens have less effect on liver function than synthetic estrogens.[57] In a patient taking ethinylestradiol, liver dysfunction may resolve if the patient is changed to oral estrogen valerate or i.m. estrogen benzoate if they find topical estrogen ineffective. Severe cholestatic jaundice has been reported; if this occurs, estrogen therapy is contraindicated and measures to treat hypogonadism and sex steroid deficiency should be initiated as we have discussed in the section on breast cancer (*see* p. 179).

Box 12.2   Screening tests for liver disease

Autoimmune screen
- Anti-nuclear antibody (ANA)
- Anti-mitochondrial antibody
- Anti-smooth muscle antibody

Viral titres
- Hepatitis A
- Hepatitis B
- Hepatitis C
- Epstein–Barr virus

Metabolic disease
- Ferritin
- mean corpuscular volume (MCV)

Treatment of capital hair loss

Male pattern baldness is distressing for transsexual clients. Hormonal manipulation has been used in both males and females with hair loss; however it is of limited benefit. The best treatment to stabilise hair loss is suppression of androgen production. As plasma testosterone levels fall, there is a slowing of the hair cycle and a reduction in the loss of androgen-sensitive hair. Once the plasma testosterone is in the normal female range, the addition of either an anti-androgen such as cyproterone acetate 100 mg/day, or spironolactone 100–200 mg/day, or a 5α-reductase inhibitor such as finasteride 2–5 mg/day may provide some additional benefit to the patient. These are standard treatments that are used in genetic females with male pattern alopecia. The effects are slow and take 6–12 months to reach their maximum, which is likely to be a stabilisation of hair loss but no significant regrowth of hair.

Minoxidil 2–4% topical solution doses result in clinically significant hair regrowth. This preparation in the UK is not available on NHS prescription. The major side-effects of it are dermatitis and headache. The hair regrowth is only maintained while the solution is used, and the hair will be lost when the solution is discontinued.

As hormonal manipulation is poorly effective in treating male pattern hair loss, it is often advisable for the patient to use local measure such as a wig to facilitate passing in the female role.

Female-to-male patients

Virilisation of female-to-male transsexuals is achieved by the administration of testosterone. Traditionally this has been in the form of testosterone enanthate esters given as Sustanon injections 2–4-weekly. At this dose, testosterone suppresses ovarian function even in pre-operative patients, obviating the need for other endocrine manipulation. Menses normally suppress within one or two injections of testosterone, but the process of virilisation is slow and takes between 2 and 4 years to complete.

Charing Cross regimen

Testosterone treatment is commenced at 250 mg testosterone enthatnate esters (Sustanon) 4-weekly. Doses of 250 mg every 2–4 weeks are usually adequate to suppress menstruation, and the aim of therapy is to achieve testosterone levels in the high normal male range (25–30 nmol/l) 1 week after the injection, and to have a trough level at the bottom of the normal male range (8–12 nmol/l) on the day the injection is due before the injection is administered. Monitoring should be performed in the steady state, i.e. following at least three injections. Titration of the peak value is achieved by varying the dose administered with each injection, while the trough level is controlled by changing the length of time between the injection. If the levels are too high, it is best to adjust the dosing frequency first and then the dose. Alterations are generally made by weekly intervals, i.e. the dose is administered 2–6-weekly and the doses altered by 50 mg at a time, which is an alteration of 0.2 ml of a 250 mg dose vial.

Non-injectable preparations are monitored by plasma testosterone level. The level should be measured at least 4 h after the administration, and the aim is to get the plasma testosterone level into the normal male range (10–28 nmol/l).

Oral testosterone undecanoate is directly converted to dihydrotestosterone by 5α-reductase 1 in the lacteals of the gut. Plasma testosterone levels are usually undectable if measured. Treatment is monitored by measuring plasma dihydrotestosterone levels 4 h after a dose; it should be in the normal male range of 1–3 nmol/l.

Cessation of menses

Menstruation is distressing for female-to-male transsexuals. The suppression of menses is often found to be the most psychological beneficial effect of hormonal therapy. It is usual for menses to cease within 2–3 injections of Sustanon, as gonadotrophin and therefore ovarian function is suppressed by the high levels testosterone.

The use of oral testosterone supplements results in lower androgen levels than with injectable testosterone, which may fail to suppress menses without the addition of a progestin. In this situation, medroxyprogesterone acetate 10 mg three times daily or norethisterone 15–25 mg/day can be used to suppress menstruation.

Facial effects

Testosterone therapy results in the development of facial hair growth in the beard area and a coarsening of the facial features, resulting in a more masculine facial appearance. This is the most important effect for the patient and the most noticeable change in outward appearance for the patients. There is an increase in body hair and a change of the sexual hair to a masculine pattern, with hair growth on the face, chest, abdomen, sacrum and inner thighs. The eschuteon takes a concave contour. In susceptible individuals, there is a loss of capital hair in a male pattern baldness distribution, with temporal thinning and crown hair loss.

Somatic changes

Testosterone therapy results in an increase in lean body mass and upper body strength; there is a concurrent decrease in body fat, resulting in a more masculine body shape with increased muscle definition and a decrease in hip to waist ratio. There is an increase in body hair development with increased hair on the chest, legs, sacrum and abdomen, with the pubic hair taking a convex upper border.

Genital changes

There is an increase in clitoral size; usually reaching 4–5 cm in length over 1 year, however this growth is never of a degree that will allow penetrative intercourse. There is an increase in ovarian stromal tissue and cyst formation identical to the changes seen in polycystic ovarian syndrome.[58] These changes occur after 6 months of therapy; their significance is unclear.

Cognition

Testosterone therapy increases aggression and general drive when used in hypogonadal men. Female-to-male transsexuals report that they have more energy, aggression and there is an increase in libido.[59] Psychologically, patients feel more masculine and generally more settled in their new gender role once testosterone therapy has commenced. There is also an improvement in visuospatial ability in these patients.[60]

Voice changes

Testosterone promotes growth in the laryngeal cartilage and vocal cords. With the elongation of the vocal cord, the fundamental frequency of the voice drops. The fundamental frequency of speech in females is 200 Hz (160–500 Hz), while that in males is 120 Hz (60–260 Hz) and takes a more masculine timbre. The vocal cords also thicken, further decreasing the pitch. The changes in laryngeal anatomy through normal puberty are complete within 6 months in the majority of cases, but the process can take up to 3 years. These laryngeal changes are usually accompanied by increased growth of the facial sinuses, increased lung capacity and chest wall strength in genetic males none of which can occur after bony growth is complete. The lack of growth of accessory structure can therefore affect the final timbre of the voice.

Side-effects

Polycythaemia

Testosterone induces the production of erythropoietin and so increases the production of red blood cells. Testosterone replacement can be associated with polycythaemia and this increase in blood viscosity can lead to an increased incidence of stroke in those who have a haematocrit above 48%.[61] This can occur even in young subjects as both stroke and myocardial infarction have been reported in athletes who abuse testosterone.[62]

Polycythaemia is seen more frequently when injectable testosterone is used, and appears to be proportional to the amount of supraphysiological testosterone that is administered. For this reason the aim of treatment is to keep the peak testosterone within the upper normal male range, i.e. 25–30 nmol/l, while keeping the trough level at the bottom of the normal male range (8–12 nmol/l). Polycythaemia is seen much less frequently with other formulations.

Polycythaemia usually responds to a decrease in the dose of testosterone, especially if this is changed to a non-injectable formulation. When this is inadequate, regular venesection to bring the haematocrit down into the normal range can be instituted, and this allows the testosterone therapy to be continued. The frequency of the venesection is variable, but in this situation it often needs to be performed 4–6-weekly to control the haematocrit.

Liver dysfunction

The incidence of hepatic dysfunction with alkylated steroid preparations such as methyl testosterone is high. There have been reported cases of fulminant hepatic failure.[63] These preparations have been used as drugs of abuse by body builders and athletes, which means that some transsexual individuals can get supplies of these medications illicitly. These anabolic steroids are no longer used in routine testosterone replacement, and so the incidence of hepatic dysfunction associated with testosterones use is less. In one series, however, transient increases in liver function enzymes were seen in 4.4% of female-to-male transsexuals and this was prolonged (>6 months) in 6.8%.[41] It is unclear from this study if this required cessation of the testosterone treatment; however, as the liver function was demonstrated to be abnormal for >6 months, we can infer that the disturbance was not great enough to merit cessation of therapy. Routine monitoring of the liver function in patients on testosterone replacement is recommended.

There has been one report of a hepatic tumour in a female-to-male patient[64] who had been treated with methyl testosterone. As stated earlier, this drug is no longer used for testosterone replacement. There have been no reports of liver tumours with testosterone esters.

Metabolic derangement

Lipid profile

There is a large difference in the plasma lipid parameters between males and females. Males have higher total cholesterol, LDL cholesterol and triglyceride, with lower plasma HDL cholesterol. The fear is that in female-to-male trans-sexuals testosterone administration would result in an adverse lipid profile and lead to premature heart disease. The administration of testosterone in female-to-male transsexuals is associated with a deterioration of lipid parameters such that they are more atherogenic; however not all lipid parameters change. There is an increase in triglyceride and a decrease in plasma HDL levels, both of which are proatherogenic. However total cholesterol and LDL cholesterol remain unchanged.[65] It is interesting that these changes in lipid profile do not appear to translate into an alteration in cardiovascular risk, as there is no increase in cardio-vascular mortality in treated female-to-male transsexuals; indeed the myocardial infarction rate is approximately half that expected.

Insulin resistance

Testosterone replacement in hypogonadal men is known to decrease insulin resistance. If used in excess amounts however, such as steroid abuse in athletes, insulin resistance increases. It has been assumed that the high doses used in masculinisation of female-to-male transsexuals would lead to an increase in insulin resistance. This does not appear to happen; in the only published study on this topic insulin resistance did not change following 1 year of testosterone treatment.[65]

Gynaecological malignancy

Testosterone can be aromatised to the estrogen estradiol. This is especially likely to occur when supraphysiological testosterone replacement is used. This is often the case in female-to-male transsexual subjects. When it is unopposed by the action of cyclical progesterone, estrogen is mitogenic for the endometrium, and therefore is a risk for the development of endometrial cancer in the long term. The reported risk of endometrial hyperplasia is 15% in male-to-female transsexual.[40] Monitoring of the endometrial thickness by ultrasound scanning biannually is recommended. It is our usual practice to recommend hyster-ectomy after 2 years of testosterone therapy, and several other groups also take this approach.

If irregular vaginal bleeding occurs then the patient should undergo ultrasound scanning and endometrial biopsy to rule out any neoplastic alteration in the endometrial epithelium.

Ovarian cancer risk appears to be very low; there have been only two cases reported following testosterone therapy for a prolonged period.[66] Exogenous testosterone treatment cannot be ruled out as a precipitating factor, and so it is recommended that bilateral salpingo-opherectomy is carried out at the time of hysterectomy after 2 years' real life experience.

Osteoporosis

In male-to-female subjects, estrogen therapy appears to maintain bone mineralisation despite testosterone withdrawal. The same may not be true of testosterone treatment in female-to-male transsexuals. In one study testosterone did not prevent the loss of bone mineral density that occurs post-ovariectomy.[41] These results however were not confirmed in another study in transsexual subjects.[67] In the large outcome trial of van Kesteren et al mortality rates did not differ between transsexuals and the general population, suggesting that any osteoporosis risk is not translated into an increase in hip fracture mortality.[41]

Obstructive sleep apnoea

Obstructive sleep apnoea is a common condition in which there is nocturnal hypoventilation or apnoea either due to airway obstruction or a decrease in central ventilatory drive. The condition is characterised by excess somnolence, snoring and carbon dioxide retention that results in morning headache. The apnoea occurs during rapid eye movement (REM) sleep, and so poor-quality sleep results in increasing somnolence. It is associated with obesity and a crowded pharynx. Obstructive sleep apnoea has serious health implications as the condition is associated with cardiac arrhythmia, and these patients are at increased risk of sudden death.

Testosterone therapy exacerbates the symptoms of obstructive sleep apnoea and, more worryingly, increases the occurrence of cardiac arrhythmia in this condition. In a female-to-male transsexual who has symptoms of obstructive sleep apnoea, symptom scores should be assessed and referral made to a specialist in sleep disorders for treatment if the patient displays any deterioration in their condition.

Summary

Hormonal treatment is intrinsic to the management of gender dysphoria. It should be undertaken only in the context of an active multidisciplinary approach involving both the mental health professional and the endocrinologist. The principles of treatment follow the World Professional Association for Transgender Health, Inc. (formerly Harry Benjamin Society) guidelines and should not be initiated without approval from a mental health practioner with a special interest in gender dysphoria.

For male-to-female patients the hormone regimen consists of estrogen, usually as estrogen valerate, in combination with testosterone suppression, usually as goserelin. This combination allows measurement of plasma sex steroid levels to guide therapy. Alternative approaches include the use of the synthetic estrogen ethinylestradiol, and anti-androgens such as cyproterone acetate, spironolactone and finasteride.

The major side-effect of estrogen therapy is the development of thromboem-bolism, usually as deep venous thrombosis with a rate of 2–3%. Other important risks are breast cancer, liver enzyme derangement and hyperprolactinaemia.

Treatment is very successful, with good feminisation in the majority of cases. Many patients, however, do require breast augmentation. Breast development occurs over 2 years of hormone therapy, and treatment beyond this will not produce further breast development. High dose estrogen therapy does not increase breast size and may adversely affect the final breast outcome.

There is no evidence that progestins improve breast development in male-to-female transsexuals. They may be proatherogenic and promote breast cancer development. For these reasons their use is difficult to justify.

Following gender reassignment surgery, estrogen doses can be reduced to levels used for high-dose standard HRT. If estrogen valerate is used, plasma monitoring can be used to get the estradiol level to the upper follicular range.

In female-to-male transsexuals, testosterone administered as an i.m. injection 2–4-weekly results in masculinisation over 2–4 years. Male sexual characteristics such as beard growth, deepened voice and increased musculature are pronounced. Clitoral growth does occur, but is not usually adequate for sexual function. Menstruation usually stops rapidly following testosterone administration, as the doses used effectively suppress ovarian function. The aim of treatment is to get the testosterone levels into the normal male range.

The major side-effects of testosterone treatment are polycythaemia, and the development of endometrial hyperplasia due to aromatisation of testosterone to estradiol. Polycythaemia can be treated with dose reduction or venesection. Endometrial hyperplasia can be screened for with serial ultrasound scanning, but it is usually recommended that the patient undergoes hysterectomy after 2 years of testosterone treatment, to prevent the development of endometrial neoplasia. Other more minor side-effects of treatment include increased triglyceride level, abnormal liver function tests and possible osteoporosis.

Hormonal manipulation of patients with gender dysphoria does not alter their standard mortality ratio, confirming that these treatments are safe as well as effective. They also do not increase the incidence of any conditions that one might predict would be more common in hormonally treated patients, such as breast cancer in male-to-female patients and myocardial infarction in female-to-male patients, with the exception of thromboembolism in estrogen-treated patients.

References

1   American Psychiatric Association Work Groupon DSM-IV-PC. *Diagnostic and Statistical Manual for Mental Disorders IV*. 1995.
2   World Health Organization. *International Classification of Diseases*. Geneva: World Health Organization; 2004.
3   Meyer-Bahlburg HF. Hormones and Psychosexual Differentiation: Implications for the Management of Intersexuality, Homosexuality and Transsexuality. *Clin Endocrinol Metab* 1982; **11**(3): 681–701.
4   Sultan C, Lobaccaro JM, Belon C, Terraza A, Lumbroso S. Molecular Biology of Disorders of Sex Differentiation. *Horm Res* 1992; **38**(3–4): 105–13.

5   Wisniewski AB, Migeon CJ, Meyer-Bahlburg HF, Gearhart JP, Berkovitz GD, Brown TR, Money J. Complete Androgen Insensitivity Syndrome: Long-Term Medical, Surgical, and Psychosexual Outcome. *J Clin Endocrinol Metab* 2000; **85**(8): 2664–9.

6   Sinnecker GH, Hiort O, Nitsche EM, Holterhus PM, Kruse K. Functional Assessment and Clinical Classification of Androgen Sensitivity in Patients With Mutations of the Androgen Receptor Gene. German Collaborative Intersex Study Group. *Eur J Pediatr* 1997; **156**(1): 7–14.

7   Price P, Wass JA, Griffin JE, Leshin M, Savage MO, Large DM, Bu'lock DE, Anderson DC, Wilson JD, Besser GM. High Dose Androgen Therapy in Male Pseudohermaphroditism Due to 5 Alpha-Reductase Deficiency and Disorders of the Androgen Receptor. *J Clin Invest* 1984; **74**(4): 1496–508.

8   Mendonca BB, Inacio M, Costa EM, Arnhold IJ, Silva FA, Nicolau W, Bloise W, Russel DW, Wilson JD. Male Pseudohermaphroditism Due to Steroid 5alpha-Reductase 2 Deficiency. Diagnosis, Psychological Evaluation, and Management. *Medicine (Baltimore)* 1996; **75**(2): 64–76.

9   Imperato-McGinley J, Guerrero L, Gautier T, German JL, Peterson RE. Steroid 5alpha-Reductase Deficiency in Man. An Inherited Form of Male Pseudohermaphroditism. *Birth Defects Orig Artic Ser* 1975; **11**(4): 91–103.

10 Ivarsson SA. 5-Alpha Reductase Deficient Men Are Fertile. *Eur J Pediatr* 1996; **155**(5): 425.

11 Imperato-McGinley J, Zhu YS. Androgens and Male Physiology the Syndrome of 5alpha-Reductase-2 Deficiency. *Mol Cell Endocrinol* 2002; **198**(1–2): 51–9.

12 Peterson RE, Imperato-McGinley J, Gautier T, Sturla E. Male Pseudohermaphroditism Due to Steroid 5-Alpha-Reductase Deficiency. *Am J Med* 1977; **62**(2): 170–91.

13 Hughes IA. Congenital Adrenal Hyperplasia: 21-Hydroxylase Deficiency in the Newborn and During Infancy. *Semin Reprod Med* 2002; **20**(3): 229–42.

14 Dewailly D. Nonclassic 21-Hydroxylase Deficiency. *Semin Reprod Med* 2002; **20**(3): 243–8.

15 Kirkland RT, Kirkland JL, Keenan BS, Bongiovanni AM, Rosenberg HS, Clayton GW. Bilateral Testicular Tumors in Congenital Adrenal Hyperplasia. *J Clin Endocrinol Metab* 1977; **44**(2): 369–78.

16 Peter M. Congenital Adrenal Hyperplasia: 11beta-Hydroxylase Deficiency. *Semin Reprod Med* 2002; **20**(3): 249–54.

17 Dittmann RW, Kappes MH, Kappes ME, Borger D, Stegner H, Willig RH, Wallis H. Congenital Adrenal Hyperplasia. I: Gender-Related Behavior and Attitudes in Female Patients and Sisters. *Psychoneuroendocrinology* 1990; **15**(5–6): 401–20.

18 Dittmann RW, Kappes MH, Kappes ME, Borger D, Meyer-Bahlburg HF, Stegner H, Willig RH, Wallis H. Congenital Adrenal Hyperplasia. II: Gender-Related Behavior and Attitudes in Female Salt-Wasting and Simple-Virilizing Patients. *Psychoneuroendocrinology* 1990; **15**(5–6): 421–34.

19 Ferriman D, Purdie AW. The Inheritance of Polycystic Ovarian Disease and a Possible Relationship to Premature Balding. *Clin Endocrinol (Oxf)* 1979; **11**(3): 291–300.

20 Nestler JE, Jakubowicz DJ, Evans WS, Pasquali R. Effects of Metformin on Spontaneous and Clomiphene-Induced Ovulation in the Polycystic Ovary Syndrome. *N Engl J Med* 1998; **338**(26): 1876–80.

21 Gadducci A, Gargini A, Palla E, Fanucchi A, Genazzani AR. Polycystic Ovary Syndrome and Gynecological Cancers: Is There a Link? *Gynecol Endocrinol* 2005; **20**(4): 200–8.

22 Baba T, Endo T, Honnma H, Kitajima Y, Hayashi T, Ikeda H, Masumori N, Kamiya H, Moriwaka O, Saito T. Association Between Polycystic Ovary Syndrome and Female-to-Male Transsexuality. *Hum Reprod* 2006.

23 Meyer WJ, III, Finkelstein JW, Stuart CA, Webb A, Smith ER, Payer AF, Walker PA. Physical and Hormonal Evaluation of Transsexual Patients During Hormonal Therapy. *Arch Sex Behav* 1981; **10**(4): 347–56.

24 Meyer WJ, III, Webb A, Stuart CA, Finkelstein JW, Lawrence B, Walker PA. Physical and Hormonal Evaluation of Transsexual Patients: a Longitudinal Study. *Arch Sex Behav* 1986; **15**(2): 121–38.

25 Toorians AW, Thomassen MC, Zweegman S, Magdeleyns EJ, Tans G, Gooren LJ, Rosing J. Venous Thrombosis and Changes of Hemostatic Variables During Cross-Sex Hormone Treatment in Transsexual People. *J Clin Endocrinol Metab* 2003; **88**(12): 5723–9.

26 Giltay EJ, Gooren LJ. Effects of Sex Steroid Deprivation/Administration on Hair Growth and Skin Sebum Production in Transsexual Males and Females. *J Clin Endocrinol Metab* 2000; **85**(8): 2913–21.

27 Balfour JA, McClellan K. Topical Eflornithine. *Am J Clin Dermatol* 2001; **2**(3): 197–201.

28 Marshall WA, Tanner JM. Variations in Pattern of Pubertal Changes in Girls. *Arch Dis Child* 1969; **44**(235): 291–303.

29 Kanhai RC, Hage JJ, Asscheman H, Mulder JW. Augmentation Mammaplasty in Male-to-Female Transsexuals. *Plast Reconstr Surg* 1999; **104**(2): 542–9.

30 Onalan G, Onalan R, Selam B, Akar M, Gunenc Z, Topcuoglu A. Mood Scores in Relation to Hormone Replacement Therapies During Menopause: a Prospective Randomized Trial. *Tohoku J Exp Med* 2005; **207**(3): 223–31.

31 Morgan ML, Cook IA, Rapkin AJ, Leuchter AF. Estrogen Augmentation of Antidepressants in Perimenopausal Depression: a Pilot Study. *J Clin Psychiatry* 2005; **66**(6): 774–80.

32 Frey H, Aakvaag A. The Treatment of Essential Hirsutism in Women With Cyproterone Acetate and Ethinyl Estradiol. Clinical and Endocrine Effects in 10 Cases. *Acta Obstet Gynecol Scand* 1981; **60**(3): 295–300.

33 Willemse PH, Dikkeschei LD, Mulder NH, van der PE, Sleijfer DT, de Vries EG. Clinical and Endocrine Effects of Cyproterone Acetate in Postmenopausal Patients With Advanced Breast Cancer. *Eur J Cancer Clin Oncol* 1988; **24**(3): 417–21.

34 Ylostalo P, Laakso L, Viinikka L, Ylikorkala O, Vihko R. Cyproterone Acetate in the Treatment of Hirsutism. *Acta Obstet Gynecol Scand* 1981; **60**(4): 399–401.

35 Pope JE, Makela EH. Response to Article "Depression Circumstantially Related to the Administration of Finasteride for Androgenetic Alopecia" (J Dermatol, 29, 665–669, 2002). *J Dermatol* 2003; **30**(11): 837–9.

36 Altomare G, Capella GL. Depression Circumstantially Related to the Administration of Finasteride for Androgenetic Alopecia. *J Dermatol* 2002; **29**(10): 665–9.

37 Ciotta L, Cianci A, Calogero AE, Palumbo MA, Marletta E, Sciuto A, Palumbo G. Clinical and Endocrine Effects of Finasteride, a 5 Alpha-Reductase Inhibitor, in Women With Idiopathic Hirsutism. *Fertil Steril* 1995; **64**(2): 299–306.

38 Rossouw JE, Anderson GL, Prentice RL, LaCroix AZ, Kooperberg C, Stefanick ML, Jackson RD, Beresford SA, Howard BV, Johnson KC, Kotchen JM, Ockene J. Risks and Benefits of Estrogen Plus Progestin in Healthy Postmenopausal Women: Principal Results From the Women's Health Initiative Randomized Controlled Trial. *JAMA* 2002; **288**(3): 321–33.

39 Hulley S, Grady D, Bush T, Furberg C, Herrington D, Riggs B, Vittinghoff E. Randomized Trial of Estrogen Plus Progestin for Secondary Prevention of Coronary Heart Disease in Postmenopausal Women. Heart and Estrogen/Progestin Replacement Study (HERS) Research Group. *JAMA* 1998; **280**(7): 605–13.

40 Futterweit W. Endocrine Therapy of Transsexualism and Potential Complications of Long-Term Treatment. *Arch Sex Behav* 1998; **27**(2): 209–26.

41 van Kesteren PJ, Asscheman H, Megens JA, Gooren LJ. Mortality and Morbidity in Transsexual Subjects Treated With Cross-Sex Hormones. *Clin Endocrinol (Oxf)* 1997; **47**(3): 337–42.

42 Michel A, Mormont C, Legros JJ. A Psycho-Endocrinological Overview of Transsexualism. *Eur J Endocrinol* 2001; **145**(4): 365–76.

43 Burkman RT. Oral Contraceptives: an Update. *Drugs Today (Barc)* 1999; **35**(11): 857–66.

44 Mishell DR, Jr. Oral Contraception: Past, Present, and Future Perspectives. *Int J Fertil* 1991; **36** Suppl 1: 7–18.

45 Zeitoun K, Carr BR. Is There an Increased Risk of Stroke Associated With Oral Contraceptives? *Drug Saf* 1999; **20**(6): 467–73.

46 Beral V, Banks E, Reeves G. Evidence From Randomised Trials on the Long-Term Effects of Hormone Replacement Therapy. *Lancet* 2002; **360**(9337): 942–4.

47 Gooren LJ, Assies J, Asscheman H, de SR, van KH. Estrogen-Induced Prolactinoma in a Man. *J Clin Endocrinol Metab* 1988; **66**(2): 444–6.

48 Serri O, Noiseux D, Robert F, Hardy J. Lactotroph Hyperplasia in an Estrogen Treated Male-to-Female Transsexual Patient. *J Clin Endocrinol Metab* 1996; **81**(9): 3177–9.

49 Adlercreutz H. Cholestatic Jaundice Caused by Contraceptive Steroids and Its Relation to Intrahepatic Cholestatic Jaundice of Pregnancy. *Res Steroids (Amst)* 1966; **2**: 521–3.

50 Card IR, Sneddon IB, Talbot CH. Oral Contraceptives and Jaundice. *Br Med J* 1966; **1**(5489): 739–40.

51 Grimaud JC, Bourliere M. [Contraception and Hepatogastroenterology]. *Fertil Contracep Sex* 1989; **17**(5): 407–13.

52 Lindberg MC. Hepatobiliary Complications of Oral Contraceptives. *J Gen Intern Med* 1992; **7**(2): 199–209.

53 Thurston AV. Carcinoma of the Prostate in a Transsexual. *Br J Urol* 1994; **73**(2): 217.

54 Goodwin WE, Cummings RH. Squamous Metaplasia of the Verumontanum With Obstruction Due to Hypertrophy: Long-Term Effects of Estrogen on the Prostate in an Aging Male-to-Female Transsexual. *J Urol* 1984; **131**(3): 553–4.

55 Sanchez-Chapado M, Olmedilla G, Cabeza M, Donat E, Ruiz A. Prevalence of Prostate Cancer and Prostatic Intraepithelial Neoplasia in Caucasian Mediterranean Males: an Autopsy Study. *Prostate* 2003; **54**(3): 238–47.

56 van KP, Meinhardt W, van d, V, Geldof A, Megens J, Gooren L. Effects of Estrogens Only on the Prostates of Aging Men. *J Urol* 1996; **156**(4): 1349–53.

57 Astedt B, Jeppsson S, Liedholm P, Rannevik G, Svanberg L. Clinical Trial of a New Oral Contraceptive Pill Containing the Natural Oestrogen 17 Beta-Oestradiol. *Br J Obstet Gynaecol* 1979; **86**(9): 732–6.

58 Spinder T, Spijkstra JJ, van den Tweel JG, Burger CW, van KH, Hompes PG, Gooren LJ. The Effects of Long Term Testosterone Administration on Pulsatile Luteinizing Hormone Secretion and on Ovarian Histology in Eugonadal Female to Male Transsexual Subjects. *J Clin Endocrinol Metab* 1989; **69**(1): 151–7.

59 Van Goozen SH, Cohen-Kettenis PT, Gooren LJ, Frijda NH, Van de Poll NE. Gender Differences in Behaviour: Activating Effects of Cross-Sex Hormones. *Psychoneuroendocrinology* 1995; **20**(4): 343–63.

60 Slabbekoorn D, Van Goozen SH, Megens J, Gooren LJ, Cohen-Kettenis PT. Activating Effects of Cross-Sex Hormones on Cognitive Functioning: a Study of Short-Term and Long-Term Hormone Effects in Transsexuals. *Psychoneuroendocrinology* 1999; **24**(4): 423–47.

61 Krauss DJ, Taub HA, Lantinga LJ, Dunsky MH, Kelly CM. Risks of Blood Volume Changes in Hypogonadal Men Treated With Testosterone Enanthate for Erectile Impotence. *J Urol* 1991; **146**(6): 1566–70.

62 Ferenchick GS. Anabolic/Androgenic Steroid Abuse and Thrombosis: Is There a Connection? *Med Hypotheses* 1991; **35**(1): 27–31.

63 Wilder EM. Death Due to Liver Failure Following the Use of Methandrostenolone. *Can Med Assoc J* 1962; **87**: 768–9.

64 Coombes GB, Reiser J, Paradinas FJ, Burn I. An Androgen-Associated Hepatic Adenoma in a Trans-Sexual. *Br J Surg* 1978; **65**(12): 869–70.

65 Elbers JM, Giltay EJ, Teerlink T, Scheffer PG, Asscheman H, Seidell JC, Gooren LJ. Effects of Sex Steroids on Components of the Insulin Resistance Syndrome in Transsexual Subjects. *Clin Endocrinol (Oxf)* 2003; **58**(5): 562–71.

66 Hage JJ, Dekker JJ, Karim RB, Verheijen RH, Bloemena E. Ovarian Cancer in Female-to-Male Transsexuals: Report of Two Cases. *Gynecol Oncol* 2000; **76**(3): 413–5.

67 Schlatterer K, Auer DP, Yassouridis A, von WK, Stalla GK. Transsexualism and Osteoporosis. *Exp Clin Endocrinol Diabetes* 1998; **106**(4): 365–8.

13

Feminisation of the larynx and voice

Guri Sandhu

Introduction

The larynx is a complex structure, and its principal function is to protect the airway during swallowing. In humans the larynx is uniquely designed also to play a pivotal role in communication through speech. To serve these functions the larynx possesses some of the fastest muscles in the body, and is richly supplied with both sensory and motor nerves.

Laryngeal anatomy

The skeleton of the larynx consists of a series of single and paired cartilages united by ligaments and membranes (*see* Figure 13.1). The larger single cartilages are the

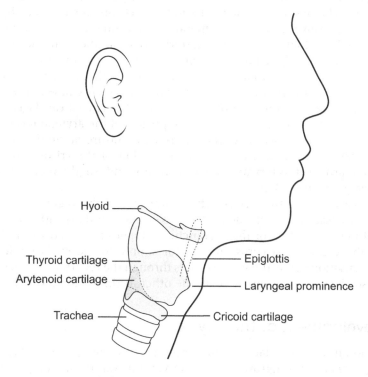

Figure 13.1 Anatomy of the larynx in the neck.

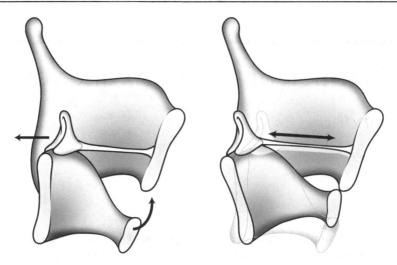

Figure 13.2 Section of larynx to show how the action of the cricothyroid muscle leads to tensioning and lengthening of the vocal cords.

thyroid and cricoid. The principal paired cartilages are the arytenoids which lie on the superior edge of the lamina of the cricoid cartilage. The epiglottis consists of a thin sheet of elastic cartilage lined on all surfaces with mucous membrane. During swallowing, the epiglottis flops down and back over the laryngeal inlet and protects the airway. This protection is reinforced by the closure of the true and false vocal cords and by the tongue base pushing back during swallowing. The hyoid bone supports the larynx in the neck, and is suspended by muscles and ligaments from the skull base, mandible and tongue. The thyroid cartilage has two laminae that are fused anteriorly to form the anterior commisure. The posterior border of each thyroid lamina has a superior and inferior horn. The inferior horns of the thyroid cartilage articulate with the cricoid cartilage at the cricothyroid joint. There is a synovial joint between the base of the arytenoid cartilages and the superior edge of the lamina of the cricoid cartilage. The vocal fold and vocal ligament attach to the vocal process of the arytenoid cartilage and insert into the posterior aspect of the anterior commisure of the thyoid cartilage, approximately halfway down. Through the action of the cricothyroid muscle, the thyroid cartilage tilts forwards and downwards and lengthens and tensions the vocal folds (*see* Figure 13.2).

The nerve supply to the larynx is from branches of the vagus nerve. The two vagus nerves descend either side of the neck in the carotid sheaths. The superior laryngeal nerve, the first of these branches, supplies sensation to the laryngeal mucosa above the vocal cords, and motor supply to the cricothyroid muscle. Larngeal sensation below the vocal cords is through the recurrent laryngeal nerve, which also gives a motor supply to all the other intrinsic muscles of the larynx.

The development of the larynx

The primordium of the larynx and respiratory system (trachea, bronchi and lungs) appears as an outgrowth from the ventral wall of the foregut when the embryo is 4 weeks old. Growth and maturation continue until birth. The infant

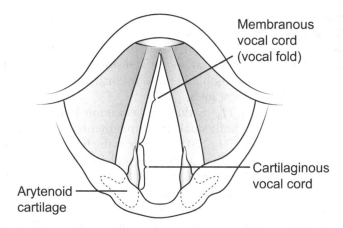

Figure 13.3 View of the glottis showing the structure of the vocal cords.

larynx differs markedly from the adult larynx. It is smaller in absolute and relative terms and lies higher in the neck. During the first 3 years of life, the child's larynx descends to an adult position, lower in the neck. Until puberty the larynx grows proportionately to crown–heel length. At puberty the female larynx grows slightly, whereas the male larynx enlarges in all directions. The effects of androgens are irreversible and lead to vocal cord lengthening, increased muscle bulk and the production of more viscous mucous. This leads to 'breaking' of the voice and lowered vocal pitch. The estrogen surge at female puberty also causes thickening of mucus but there is no effect on muscle bulk, and laryngeal growth is so slight that the breaking of the voice is much less marked.

There is a process of calcification of the laryngeal cartilages that begins in the third decade of life and starts in the thyroid cartilage. Calcification is more marked in men, and by the fifth decade of life the thyroid cartilage consists largely of bone and may even possess a bone marrow.

The angle between the two laminae of the thyroid cartilage is 90° in men and 120° in women. This sharper angle in men and the relatively greater anterior to posterior dimension leads to the more obvious laryngeal prominence ('Adam's apple').

The vocal cord (*see* Figure 13.3) comprises the vocal process of the arytenoid (cartilaginous vocal cord) and the vocal fold (membranous vocal cord). It is only the vocal fold that vibrates during speech. The length of the vocal fold is the same in both males and females until the age of 10 years (6–8 mm). After puberty the male vocal fold has doubled in length (16–18 mm), whereas the female vocal fold has increased by one-third (8.5–12 mm).[1]

Voice production

The requirements for voice include an air source (lungs), vibrating organ (larynx), articulators (lips, teeth and tongue) and resonators (pharynx, nose and sinuses, and oral cavity).

The epithelium of the vocal folds vibrates to produce a sound of varying pitch (frequency) that is then modified by the articulators and resonators. Although one may consider the vibration of the vocal folds as the equivalent of violin strings, the closest comparison is that of a passive double reed. In the larynx the vibration passes as a passive mucosal wave in the vocal folds from below upwards. Vocal pitch is proportional to the tension in the vocal folds, but inversely proportional to their length and mass. Intensity depends on the force of the air passing between the vocal folds.

The fundamental frequency (f_o) is the most common frequency (modal frequency) used in speech by an individual. The fundamental frequencies for male habitual voices may vary from 90 to 130 Hz, whereas the female range is from 170 to 260 Hz. It is widely accepted that a fundamental frequency above 155 Hz is perceived as female.[2] Apart from the fundamental frequency, the other differences between male and female communication are intonation, inflexion, gesturing and body language. Although a transsexual may appear female, a masculine voice and a prominent Adam's apple may still be a source of embarrassment.

Voice feminisation surgery

Through appropriate speech and language therapy the majority of transsexuals will achieve a satisfactorily female voice and manner. In the author's series less than one-fifth of patients request or are referred for pitch-elevation surgery. Surgery can help raise vocal pitch but will also help with problems of 'breakthrough' low-pitch voice when distracted or tired. Where surgery has been carried out, post-operative speech and language therapy will be needed to optimise surgical outcomes.

An appreciation of the function of two intrinsic laryngeal muscles allows for a better understanding of how surgery for elevating vocal pitch has evolved:

- *the cricothyroid muscle* takes its origin from the anterior surface of the arch of the cricoid and inserts into the antero-lateral surface of the thyroid cartilage. Its action is to lengthen and exert tension on the vocal cord. By elevating the arch of the cricoid the distance between the angle of the thyroid cartilage and the vocal process of the arytenoids is increased (*see* Figure 13.2)
- *the thyroarytenoid muscle* passes from the base and anterior surface of the arytenoid cartilage to the inner surface of the thyroid cartilage in the midline. The thyroarytenoid muscle shortens the vocal fold and adjusts the tension within it during phonation.

In principle it should be possible to raise vocal pitch by shortening the vocal cords or reducing their mass. Increasing the tension in the vocal cords should achieve the same result.

Advancing the vocal cord attachment

The tension in the vocal cords can be increased by exposing the larynx and advancing the anterior commisure, which is then held forward by a mini-plate (*see* Figure 13.4). The disadvantage of this technique is that the laryngeal prominence becomes more exaggerated and cannot be reduced.

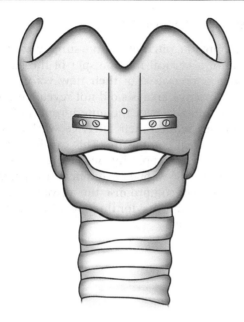

Figure 13.4   Anterior advancement of the vocal fold attachment maintained with a mini-plate.

Cricothyroid approximation

This operation is carried out through a small skin incision over the larynx. Permanent mattress sutures are placed between the thyroid and cricoid cartilages (*see* Figure 13.5). This has the effect of increasing the tension in the vocal cords much like the action of the cricothyroid muscle. A review of this procedure showed that 80% of patients were satisfied with the results and objectively 71% had gains in f_o in free speech, reading and singing, maintained at 41 months' follow-up.[3] There was, however, a narrowing of the vocal range following surgery.

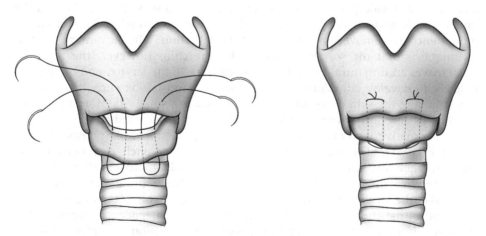

Figure 13.5   Cricoid and thyroid cartilages are approximated with mattress sutures to tension the vocal cords.

Vocal cord-shortening procedures

The initial surgical attempts at pitch-elevation surgery were directed at vocal fold shortening by way of a vertical midline split of the larynx (laryngofissure approach). Patients were appreciative of their new voice because of increased 'breathiness', however, objective analysis did not reveal an increase in f_o.

Surgically stripping the mucosa over the anterior ends of the vocal folds and suturing them together can reduce their effective working length by creating a web at the anterior laryngeal commisure. This can be carried out through a laryngofissure approach, or endoscopically (*see* Figure 13.6). The anterior one-third of the vocal folds needs to be webbed to duplicate the female working length. Unfortunately a large web may compromise the airway at the glottis. Although high success rates have been published for this operation,[4] other authorities have not been able to reproduce these.

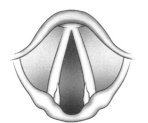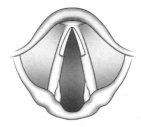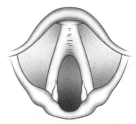

Figure 13.6 Anterior webbing technique to reduce the working length of the vocal folds.

Thyroid chondroplasty

Thyroid chondroplasty (or 'laryngeal shave') is the surgical reduction of the laryngeal prominence ('Adam's apple') to give the neck a feminine contour. Two techniques are widely used. The first technique uses a small incision high in the midline neck. Scissors are passed through a soft tissue tunnel and the laryngeal prominence is removed without direct visualisation. The advantage of this technique is that the scar is hidden under the chin. However, the resection often leaves an unnatural 'open book' appearance to the larynx, and the patient is likely to develop adhesions between the skin and larynx such that there is 'puckering' of the skin on swallowing. There is also a small risk of detaching the vocal cords anteriorly, with an associated risk to the voice and airway.

The alternative is to place the small incision in a suitable skin crease directly over the larynx. If a cricothyroid approximation (for pitch elevation) is also planned, then the same incision can be used. This approach allows for the dimensions of the larynx to be measured accurately for maximal and safe removal of the laryngeal prominence (*see* Figure 13.7). The soft tissues are closed in layers so that there is little risk of skin tethering to deeper structures. Unless there is a history of hypertrophic or keloid scar formation, the incision is not easily visible after a few weeks.

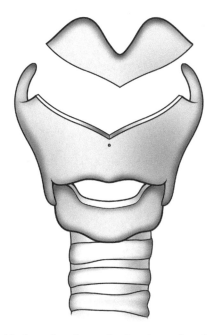

Figure 13.7 Thyroid chondroplasty (reduction of 'Adam's apple).

Discussion

There are no long-term results available for any of the surgical techniques described for pitch elevation. One reason for this may be that surgery for pitch elevation is far from ideal. The ideal surgical procedure would shorten and reduce the bulk of the male vocal cords with appropriate pitch elevation maintained for life. It would also be carried out endoscopically to avoid scars. Further surgical advances need to be made in the field of laryngology before this is possible. In addition, surgeons and voice therapists need to work more closely and be encouraged to improve the quality of their analysis of surgical outcomes.

References

1 Hirano M. *Histological Colour Atlas of the Human Larynx.* San Diego: Singular Publishing group, Inc: 1993.
2 Wolfe VI, Ratusnik DL, Smith FH and Northrop G. Intonation and fundamental frequency in male-to-female transsexuals. *Journal of Speech and Hearing Disorders* 1990; **55**: 43–50.
3 Kanagalingam J, Georgalas C, Wood GR *et al.* Cricothyroid approximation and subluxation in 21 male-to-female transsexuals. *Laryngoscope* 2005; **115**: 611–18.
4 Gross M. Pitch-raising surgery in male-to-female transsexuals. *Journal of Voice* 1999; **13**: 246–50.

Part 4

Surgical treatments for born males

14

Breasts

Dai M Davies and AJ Stephenson

The breast

The adult female breast is often the most outstanding secondary sexual characteristic. In transsexual females the presence of developed breasts may impair appearance and be at odds with feelings of masculinity. The absence of developed breasts acts similarly in transsexual males.

Breast augmentation: history

In 1895, Czerny reported the reconstruction of a female breast, by transplanting a lipoma from a patient's flank to the breast of the same patient, with 'good results'.[1] Subsequent efforts at augmenting and reconstructing breasts were for many years plagued by complications.

Subcutaneous petrolatum injection for local soft tissue reconstruction was reported by Gersuny in 1900. Enthusiasm for the injection of petrolatum and paraffin reached a peak of popularity in 1911, before enthusiasm was tempered by reports of severe late complications including local necrosis, paraffinomas and non-malignant metastases to lymph nodes.[2]

Subsequently, silicones were investigated as a possible injectable material for soft tissue augmentation, with initially favourable laboratory results.[3] Medical grade silicones were used by both medically qualified and non-medically qualified practitioners, and were admixed with other materials, including industrial silicone and oils. Some of these mixtures were intended to produce 'permanent fixation' in the tissues via an inflammatory reaction. When used in the breast, complications included multiple abscesses, sinuses, local tissue necrosis, painful breast masses, acute pneumonitis and death.[4–6]

By 1965, the US Food and Drug Administration (FDA) limited silicone injections to eight named investigators. It did not permit liquid silicone injection for breast augmentation.[3] Complications in transsexual patients who have sought intramammary silicone augmentation and other foreign liquid injections include acute pneumonitis, multiple abscess and sinus formation.[4,6,7]

Management of the complications of injected breasts, by subcutaneous mastectomy with excision of involved parts of the underlying pectoralis muscle, has been reported in multiple patients. Subsequent formal breast augmentation in these patients has had poor results.[2,3,5]

Local, de-epithelialised pedicled flaps and free dermis-fat grafts have been used to augment breasts.[1] There are reports of breast reconstruction using autologous latissimus dorsi by pedicled transfer as well as transverse rectus abdominis myocutaneous (TRAM) flaps, deep inferior epigastric artery perforator (DIEP) flaps and others, by free tissue transfer. These are established methods of breast reconstruction after mastectomy. There are no reports of their use for primary cosmetic breast augmentation.

Formal prostheses – of Ivalon sponge – were used from 1951. In 1962 Cronin and Gerow used a silicone envelope filled with silicone gel.[1,8] This basic prosthesis design has since been modified by many manufacturers. Alterations have included coating the outer shell in a sponge to improve tissue adherence, filling the shell with saline instead of silicone, allowing the implant size to be adjustable after insertion for tissue expansion, and including a separate adjustable saline-filled bladder as well as the silicone gel to allow expansion or adjustment.

In 1982, connective tissue disease was first linked with silicone breast implants. Gel 'bleed' of silicone gel through the outer envelope was identified. Shell modifications were made, to reduce the rate of gel diffusion. In 1992, the FDA restricted the use of silicone gel-filled implants, but allowed the continued use of saline-filled, silicone-walled implants. In 1994, implant manufacturers agreed to pay 4.25 billion US dollars to women with breast implants, as part of a class action settlement. The UK Department of Health concluded that there was no reason to ban silicone implants. In 1998 the Independent Review Group, commissioned by the UK Department of Health to review the possible health risks associated with silicone gel breast implants, concluded that there was no evidence of abnormal immune response to silicone breast implants and no epidemiological evidence for any link between silicone gel implants and any established connective tissue diseases.[9]

There had been similar concerns about carcinogenicity and teratogenicity of silicone breast implants. These have not been substantiated. The incidence of breast cancer in women with silicone breast implants is lower than in the general population.[9] In 2005, the FDA again licensed silicone gel breast implants for cosmetic use.[10]

Current preferences for prosthesis design are for cohesive silicone gel-filled implants. These replicate the feeling of breast tissue better than saline-filled implants. Their silicone envelope has a textured outer surface to reduce the incidence of capsular contracture. They may be of a round or a more anatomical, teardrop, shape.

Breast differences

The male thorax is wider than in the female. The amount of breast tissue in the male breast is less than in the female breast, although in the male breast tissue is still present. The underlying pectoralis muscle is more developed in the male, contributing to the male breast contour. The female nipple and areola complex is qualitatively the same as in the the male, but larger.[11] It is generally felt to be more laterally placed in females, although this is disputed by Kanhai et al.[12]

Selection

Although hormonal treatment does increase breast size in a similar pattern to that seen in female pubertal mammogenesis, this increase stops after approximately 18 months of treatment, and is generally disappointing.[13]

Kanhai, studying patients who subsequently underwent augmentation, recorded a mean increase in chest circumference from 91 cm before hormone therapy to 93 cm during the first 18 months of treatment.[14] In patients who did not request augmentation, an increase from 94 cm to 102 cm was reported.

Between 66% and 90% of patients want augmentation after hormone therapy.[14,15] Some patients who may initially have had satisfactory size breasts find that following weight gain their breasts do not increase in size. They may then request first or further augmentation.

Referral for either mastectomy or breast augmentation should, in accordance with the Royal College of Psychiatrists guidelines, be from a multidisciplinary gender clinic.[16] Referral with written support, from a specialist psychologist or psychiatrist and with an independent second opinion from a medical gender dysphoria specialist or gender dysphoria specialist chartered psychotherapist, is required to ensure that the proposal for surgery is appropriate. Surgery is normally suggested when hormonal approaches have been exhausted, and after at least 2 years of real life experience.

Implant choices

Silicone-walled implants are available with saline or silicone gel filling.

Saline-filled implants may form detectable wrinkles or ripples in the envelope. These may lead to rupture of the implant. This partly explains the high rate of deflation in saline-filled implants. Saline-filled implants have been associated with a lower incidence of capsular contracture, and are round shaped.

The viscosity of the silicone gel content of silicone gel-filled implants can be varied by the manufacturer. Implants with a higher viscosity or more 'cohesive' gel have a more firm consistency. Even after rupture of the outer silicone envelope, they maintain their shape. The more solid gel content is liable to fracture during traumatic insertion or with subsequent trauma.

Silicone gel-filled implants may be round shaped or may be anatomically shaped or teardrop in profile, more closely mimicking the natural breast shape. An anatomically shaped implant may be an advantage where there is little soft tissue cover in the upper pole of the breast and the implant is placed in a submammary position.

Placement

The prostheses may be placed between the breast tissue and the pectoralis major muscle, or beneath the pectoralis major muscle.

Placement above the pectoralis major leaves less covering soft tissue, so the cranial edge of the implant may be more visible. Placement below the pectoralis major is more painful post-operatively, and is more likely to result in cranial and lateral prosthesis displacement unless the pectoralis is released from its insertion infero-medially.

Access

The approach to the subpectoral or submammary plane for implant placement may be via the inframammary fold, the axilla or a peri-areolar route via the inferior margin of the areloa.

The peri-areolar route accesses the subpectoral or submammary plane, either directly through the breast tissue or between the skin and breast tissue from the areola margin to the inframammary fold.

Size

The most common reason for dissatisfaction with augmentation is inadequate breast size. In Kanhai's series from Amsterdam, 68 of 107 patients were satisfied with their initial augmentation.[17] Twelve were satisfied with subsequent augmentation(s), of which the average size was 265 ml. Eighteen remained dissatisfied, feeling their breasts were too small. Nine remained dissatisfied for other reasons, of which only one was because the breasts were too large. Of the 27 who were dissatisfied, five underwent further augmentation elsewhere.

In Kanhai's series, the average implant size rose over a 17-year period from 165 ml to 287 ml, with a range in 1999 from 225 ml to 450 ml. The average size of implant did not differ between the 80 satisfied and 18 dissatisfied patients, nor did pre-operative and post-operative bra sizes.

Kanhai recommends aiming for a breast size larger than that indicated by the patient, to avoid disappointment.[12]

Ratnam in Singapore had previously reported a range of 180 ml to 300 ml, with a mode of 225 ml.[18] The available skin envelope generally limits the maximum practical size of implant that may be used to around 370 ml in the case of a submuscular placement in a first-time augmentation.

Author's preferred technique

The senior author's (DMD's) preference is to engage the patient in selecting the implant size, by trying different sized implants in a sports bra that they aspire to fill. A textured, round, silicone gel-filled implant is placed in a subpectoral position via an inframammary fold scar, as a day case under general anaesthesia. Careful haemostasis under direct vision is important, particularly of the medial perforating vessels from the internal mammary vessels.

Dissection towards the midline, with partial release of the insertion of the pectoralis major inferomedially and avoidance of excessive lateral dissection, keeps the implants medial, to create a satisfactory cleavage.

As the male chest is wider, with more laterally placed nipples, and as implants are designed for the female chest which is more narrow, care should be exercised to avoid placement of the implant too medially in relation to the nipple.

Complications

The most common early complication of breast augmentation is haematoma.
The implants may be malpositioned and may be palpable.[19]

Nipple-areolar sensation may be altered. Although this will often resolve, it may not.

Infection is an uncommon early complication, which will require the implant to be removed before being replaced, usually at least 3 months later.

The most common later complication is capsular contracture (11% in Kanhai's series).[12]

Once an implant is placed, a capsule of scar tissue forms around it, and may contract. This may go unnoticed by the patient, may alter the shape of the breast and may become painful. Capsular contracture is treated by open surgical release of the capsule (open capsulotomy) or removal of the capsule (capsulectomy), possibly with repositioning of the implant in a submuscular position.

Other than capsule contracture, Kanhai reported immediate and long-term complications in a further 11%, including haematoma and synmastia (medial confluence of the breasts).

Trauma to a submammary implant may result in necrosis of the overlying soft tissue and extrusion of the prosthesis.[19]

As discussed, patients may be disappointed with the breast size achieved by augmentation. Subsequent ptosis may require correction,[14] and reduction may be requested.[20]

As breast implants do have a finite life, limited by rupture, some surgeons recommend implant replacement after 10 or 15 years. Suspected rupture may be investigated by either ultrasound or magnetic resonance imaging, but regular screening of asymptomatic implants is not justified.

Breast cancer

Breast cancer has been reported in four male-to-female transsexuals – one 10 years after orchidectomy and estrogen therapy,[21] two at 5 years after,[22] and one at 14 years later.[23]

Acinar and lobular formation occurs in transsexuals treated with progestagenic anti-androgens and feminising estrogens such that histologically they become indistinguishable from the natural female breast.[12]

It is suggested that breast cancer develops in men with hyperestrogenicity and androgen deficiency.[24] This is the hormonal picture produced by castration and estrogen therapy.

Hyperestrogenity has been linked to increased risk of male breast cancer, and the *BRCA2* gene is implicated in male breast cancer.[25,26] Male breast cancer appears to be associated with a family history of breast cancer, particularly in first-degree relations.[25] Accordingly, male transsexual patients should be followed up for the development of breast cancer.[21]

References

1   Rees TD (1977) Plastic surgery of the breast. In: Converse JM (ed). *Reconstructive Plastic Surgery*. Philadelphia: WB Saunders; 1977.

2   Ortiz-Monastero F and Trigos I. Management of patients with complications from injection of foreign materials into the breasts. *Plastic and Reconstructive Surgery* 1972; **50**: 42–5.

3 Wustrack KO and Zarem HA. Surgical management of silicone mastitis. *Plastic and Reconstructive Surgery* 1979; **63**: 224–9.

4 Chastre J, Basset F, Viau F *et al.* (1983) Acute pneumonitis after subcutaneous injections of silicone in transsexual men. *New England Journal of Medicine* 1983; **308**: 764–5.

5 Parsons RW and Thering HR. Management of the silicone-injected breast. *Plastic and Reconstructive Surgery* 1977; **60**: 534–8.

6 Fox LP, Geyer AS, Husain S *et al.* Mycobacterium abscessus: cellulites and multifocal abscesses of the breasts in a transsexual from illicit intramammary injections of silicone. *Journal of the American Academy of Dermatology* 2004; **50**: 450–4.

7 Doney IE and Ranson DL. Unusual breast findings in a transsexual. *American Journal of Forensic Medicine and Pathology* 1987; **8**: 342–5.

8 Ruberg RL and Smith DJ. *Plastic Surgery a Core Curriculum*. St Louis: Mosby; 1994.

9 Department of Health. *Silicone Gel Breast Implants. The Report of the Independent Review Group*. London: Department of Health; 1988.

10 Moynihan R. FDA panel approves one make of silicone breast implant in the US. *British Medical Journal* 2005; **330**: 919.

11 Montagna W and MacPherson EE. Proceedings: some neglected aspects of the anatomy of human breasts. *Journal of Investigative Dermatology* 1974; **63**: 10–16.

12 Kanhai RC, Hage JJ, Bloemena E *et al.* Augmentation mammaplasty in male-to-female transsexuals. *Plastic and Reconstructive Surgery* 1999; **104**: 542–51.

13 Ortenriech N and Durr NP. Mammogenesis in transsexuals. *Journal of Investigative Dermatology* 1974; **63**: 142–6.

14 Kanhai RC. Augmentation mammaplasty in male-to-female trans-sexuals: facts and F figures form Amsterdam. *Scandinavian Journal of Plastic and Reconstructive Surgery and Hand Surgery* 2001; **35**: 203–6.

15 Hastings D. Postsurgical adjustment of male transsexual patients. *Clinics in Plastic Surgery* 1974; **1**: 335–44.

16 Royal College of Psychiatrists. *Consultation on good practice guidelines for the assessment and treatment of gender dysphoria*. Open consultation document. RCPsych guidelines. London: Royal College of Psychiatrists.

17 Kanhai RC. Long-term outcome of augmentation mammaplasty in male-to-female transsexuals: a questionnaire survey of 107 patients. *British Journal of Plastic Surgery* 2000; **53**: 209–11.

18 Ratnam SS and Lim SM. Augmentation mammaplasty for the male transsexual. *Singapore Medical Journal* 1982; **24**: 107–9.

19 Bellinger CG and Goulian D. Secondary surgery in transsexuals. *Plastic and Reconstructive Surgery* 1973; **51**: 628–31.

20 Kaczynski A, McKissock P, Dubrow T *et al.* Breast reduction in the male-to-female transsexual. *Annals of Plastic Surgery* 1989; **23**: 323–6.

21 Pritchard TJ, Pankowsky DA, Crowe JP *et al.* Breast cancer in a male-to-female transsexual. A case report. *Journal of the American Medical Association* 1988; **259**: 2278–80.

22 Symmers WS. *British Medical Journal* Carcinoma of breast in trans-sexual individuals after surgical and hormonal interference with the primary and secondary sex characteristics. 1968; **2**: 82–5.

23 Ganly I and Taylor EW. Breast cancer in a trans-sexual man receiving hormone replacement therapy. *British Journal of Surgery* 1995; **82**: 341.

24 Thomas DB, Jimenez LM and McTiernan A. Breast cancer in men: risk factors with hormonal implications. *American Journal of Epidemiology* 1992; **135**: 734–8.

25 Sasco AJ, Lowenfels AB and Pasker-de-Jong P. Review article: epidemiology of male breast cancer. A meta-analysis of published case-control studies and discussion of selected aetiological factors. *International Journal of Cancer* 1993; **53**: 538–59.

26 Thorlacius S, Tryggvadottir L, Olafsdottir GH *et al.* Linkage to BRCA2 region in hereditary male breast cancer. *Lancet* 1995; **346**: 544–5.

15

Genital surgery

James Bellringer

History

It can be argued that genital surgery to males to alter their sexual role goes back many thousands of years, with numerous well-documented examples of eunuchs created by bilateral orchidectomy. It is recorded, for example, that Alexander the Great took at least one eunuch as a sexual partner. It is unlikely that all of these people chose to be surgically castrated, but for some it may have been a free choice. This practice continues today in India, where there is a group of biological males who are brought up in the female role, and who are surgically castrated in adolescence. The penis and scrotum are usually removed with the testes. Many of these people work as 'female' prostitutes, and usually live in communities with others who have undergone castration.

Current practice

In modern medicine, the first recorded attempt at a male-to-female gender reassignment probably took place in Germany in the 1930s, where a patient underwent bilateral orchidectomy, penile amputation, and construction of labia. There was no attempt made to create a vagina. The Moroccan surgeon, Georges Burou set up a clinic in Casablanca in the early 1950s, where he subsequently performed many hundreds of these operations. He described his technique in a lecture given in 1957 and illustrated by his own hand drawings. It is probable, however, that the operation had already been performed before 1957 in Britain, as it is described in a textbook of plastic surgery published in 1954 by the group based in East Grinstead.[1] Clitoroplasty became established in the early 1990s, when various techniques were described for producing a sensate clitoris based on the dorsal neurovascular bundle of the penis.

Genital surgery in male-to-female transsexuals may consist of several components, not all of which are requested by any individual patient. These are:

- bilateral orchidectomy
- amputation of the penis (with creation of new urethral orifice)
- labioplasty
- vaginoplasty
- clitoroplasty.

Bilateral orchidectomy

This procedure is often requested by patients as a first stage prior to continuing to further genital surgery at a later date, but may in some patients be the only operation desired. The most usual approach is an incision through the midline raphe of the scrotum; this has the advantage of avoiding possible damage to the blood supply to the scrotal skin, which might be needed later. The scrotum is usually otherwise left intact. The disadvantage of orchidectomy is that it usually results over time in a diminution of the scrotal skin, which may compromise subsequent vaginoplasty or labioplasty. If the latter are contemplated, orchidectomy is more usually done at the time of other surgery.

Amputation of the penis

Amputation of the penis is normally performed as part of labioplasty with or without vaginoplasty. A few patients request removal of male genitalia with no attempt at feminising surgery, but this is unusual, and arguably does not fall within the realm of gender reassignment, as these patients often express the desire to continue to live in the male role.

The penile skin is usually incised circumferentially in the coronal sulcus (as for a circumcision). If the skin is to be used for the vaginal skin inlay intact, the penis may than be everted, and the corpora cavernosa and urethra separated from the skin. Alternatively, the skin may be detubularised, usually by a ventral incision, and the skin dissected off the underlying structures. The urethra is mobilised away from the cavernosa, and may be divided. The bulbospongiosus muscle is removed from the proximal portion of the urethra and surrounding spongiosus, which can then be separated from the two corpora cavernosa. The corpora cavernosa can then be removed. There is debate as to whether complete removal is required; it requires little extra dissection, but leaving it in place does not lead to adverse side-effects. The current practice of the author is to leave the short stumps of erectile tissue in place, and aim to place any neoclitoris over them in an attempt to create 'natural' female anatomy.

The reconstruction of the urethra in a manner that resembles 'natural' female anatomy presents a significant challenge. The male urethra passes through a 90° bend after passing through the perineal membrane, and is covered by erectile tissue, especially posteriorly. If any length of urethra is left intact, there will always be the tendency for urine to be directed forwards, even to the extent that the stream in the sitting position may be directed out of the front of a conventional toilet pan. The simple reconstruction involves amputation of the urethra in the area of the bulbar urethra, but often the direction of the subsequent urinary stream is significantly forward, and the residual erectile tissue remains, with the complication that it tends to engorge during sexual arousal, with consequent narrowing of the neovaginal introitus. It also carries a significant rate of urethral stenosis post-operatively. Spatulation of the urethra gives a wider anastomosis to the perineal skin, with a lower stenosis rate. Furthermore, the epithelium of the urethra is moist, which is closer in appearance to the epithelium of the female vulva in this area. Some surgeons preserve most of this epithelium to optimise the cosmetic appearance. The erectile tissue may be removed, although this risks compromise to the urethral epithelium, or the cut edges may be under-run to reduce the risk of bleeding. Furthermore, the large amount of corpus spongiosus posterior to the urethra proper has significant erogenous sensation, which can be useful for future sexual function. The current practice of the author is to excise much of the tissue posterior to the new meatus, and under-run the cut edges. This gives an acceptable result in terms of both subsequent meatal stenosis and engorgement of the remaining erectile tissue. Sexual function appears no worse than in patients in whom the erectile tissue was left intact, and is often superior, as they do not find the vagina obstructed by the erect corpus spongiosus.

Labioplasty

Even if some of the skin is used for vaginoplasty, there is normally sufficient scrotal skin available after orchidectomy to permit the construction of labia. The penile skin may also be used in some areas, especially if it is not being used for a neovagina.

After removal of the penis and testes, there is a natural tendency for the remaining skin to form bilateral mounds that resemble labia majora. Patients who have undergone radical excisional surgery for tumours of the male genitalia look superficially similar to females in the standing position. Construction of labia that can stand up to more detailed scrutiny, for example during sexual activity, is more difficult. There are a number of problems; firstly, anteriorly, where the penis was removed, there tends to be a gap between the labia majora. Secondly, the skin of the perineum resembles poorly the epithelium of the vulva around the urethra and vagina, being dry and keratinising rather than moist. Thirdly, there is the question of creating realistic labia minora.

From the point of view of the anterior gap, this is most usually managed by the creation of a clitoral hood, associated sometimes with incisions to allow the upper end of the labia majora to come more towards the midline. Alternatively, a 'cosmetic clitoris' can be made out of a fold of skin, although in patients reviewed by the author, this is a less satisfactory alternative. A clitoral hood may be formed by making an inverted 'U' incision. The skin is reflected downwards, and the inner part is closed on itself, before the outer skin is closed over the top. This usually achieves a satisfactory hood, and also brings the upper ends of the new labia majora closer together.

The different epithelium of the natal female vulva is most easily replicated by using the epithelium of the urethra. Schrang in Wisconsin (personal communication) recommends keeping as much of this as possible to cover the area between the labia majora anterior to the urethral meatus. This requires careful dissection to remove the majority of the erectile tissue from the epithelium, and carries the risk of devascularisation and tissue loss. The current practice of the author is to leave a strip of urethra opened out between the urethral meatus and clitoris, which can look very realistic. A potential long-term complication of leaving this epithelium exposed is the incidence of squamous carcinoma in the urethral epithelium, which has been described.

The labia minora present a significant surgical challenge. In scrotal inlay techniques, these are formed by suturing the scrotal skin to the lateral border of the penile skin flap above the urethral meatus. The drawback is that, even when there may appear to be an excess of skin left at the time of the operation, this usually flattens out greatly with time, and is usually far less evident later. Furthermore, the new labia minora do not extend as far forward as the clitoris in most instances, unlike the natal female, and the scrotal skin component, including as it does the dartos muscle, tends to be rather thicker than is desirable. An approach which gives much superior long-term results is to leave 1 cm or so of the prepuce attached to the glans penis when the latter is dissected out for the clitoris (*see* below); these are then folded on either side of the clitoris where they can look very similar to natal female labia. Furthermore, they will usually have some erogenous sensation. This approach is clearly not suitable in patients who have previously undergone circumcision, and may compromise the amount of skin subsequently available for vaginoplasty. Finally, some semblance of minora may be achieved by careful positioning of the urethral flap in the penile skin of the anterior vulva. Some tension on this area produces folds in the adjacent penile skin, which can look reasonably like labia minora. This avoids any compromise over the skin available for subsequent vaginoplasty, but the labia produced in this way are seldom as large as those of the natal female.

Vaginoplasty

Creation of a neovagina has two components: firstly the creation of a cavity for the vagina within the male pelvis/perineum, and secondly providing an epithelial lining for that cavity.

Fortunately, there exists within the male pelvis a natural plane for the creation of a neovagina. During fetal life, the peritoneum comes down to the cloacal membrane. The rectum and anus develop behind this double layer, while the urogenital structures develop anteriorly. In the female, these differentiate into vagina, uterus and bladder, while in the male they become the prostate, seminal vesicles and bladder. The space between the double layer of peritoneum, which is known as Denonvillier's fascia, is obliterated but the layers can be easily separated, allowing a tissue plane suitable for a neovagina to be created. This fascia is closely applied to the posterior surface of the prostate and terminates at the perineal body, a tendinous structure in the perineum to which many of the small muscles of the perineum are attached. If the perineal body is divided, the posterior leaflet of Denonvillier's fascia can be found over the posterior aspect of the prostate and incised. It is then possible to open the space between the two layers, and the space for the vagina is created. The upper limit of this cavity is the pelvic peritoneum, which will freely peel off adjacent structures allowing more than adequate depth in the majority of patients. It is usually necessary to divide part of the levator ani muscle on each side of the neovagina to permit greater width, especially for colonic implants.

The epithelial lining of the vagina may be derived either from skin, or from intestinal mucosa. Skin tube vaginoplasties may be formed from the skin of the penis and scrotum, or from free skin grafts from other areas, such as the thigh. Rarely, myocutaneous flaps based on the gracilis are used. The simplest skin tube is a penile inversion. In this operation, the penile skin that remains after excision of the urethra, corpora cavernosa and glans penis, is used intact to create a new vagina. The distal end of the tube is closed with sutures, and this tube is inverted into the previously created cavity. It is normally necessary to mobilise the skin of the anterior abdominal wall over the pubis and lower abdomen to reduce the tension on this flap. The connective tissue at the back of the new vagina usually also needs to be divided. Penile skin is in many ways the most satisfactory lining for the new vagina, as it is extremely elastic, and does not bear any hair. Where penile skin is inadequate, most often because of a previous circumcision, it becomes necessary to use other sources of skin. The scrotum is close to hand, and is elastic, but it is also hair bearing, which can lead to hair continuing to grow in the neovagina. This skin may be used as a free graft (and some surgeons try to remove the hair follicles from it before introducing it into the cavity), or may be used as a vascularised pedicle. In this latter case, the viability of the long (18 cm) skin graft is maintained by small branches of the posterior scrotal arteries, which run into the back of the graft. The skin may then be formed into a tube, which is inverted to form the vagina. A disadvantage of using this skin flap is that it is necessary, in order to preserve the blood supply, to leave a significant amount of fat attached to the skin. This fat may reduce the adherence of the skin to the walls of the cavity, and is associated with subsequent vaginal prolapse. Finally free skin grafts may be used; these are best harvested from non-hair-bearing skin. Usually a length of skin is formed into a tube around a mould and inverted. Many surgeons use these grafts to augment penile inversions where the skin from inversion alone is inadequate. They carry a significantly higher risk of graft failure.

It is the author's practice to reserve colovaginoplasty for cases where primary skin tube vaginoplasty has failed. Other surgeons offer it as a primary technique. A suitable length of gut is mobilised on its vascular pedicle. The most common segment used is the caecum, but sigmoid colon is also used, as occasionally is ileum. The literature would suggest that sigmoid colon is the most satisfactory bowel segment[2] but sigmoid is used principally because it is nearby and available. Caecum is probably a more satisfactory option.[3] The mobilisation is usually performed at an open laparotomy, but laparoscopic techniques are increasingly popular, and have the advantage of reducing the abdominal scarring and post-operative recovery time. The segment is then passed through the pelvic floor (using the cavity described above), and the open end is sutured to the perineal skin. Colovaginoplasties usually offer extremely good vaginal depth, although there is an incidence of stenosis at the suture line between the skin and the colonic mucosa. Since the colon also continues to produce mucus, most patients notice a significant discharge. In the long term, there is an incidence of defunction colitis in the colonic segment.

Clitoroplasty

Creation of a sensate clitoris was first described in 1980[4] but the original technique, using blood supply through the urethra, has been superseded by techniques using the neurovascular bundle on the dorsum of the penis.[5] Earlier, some surgeons produced a small skin fold in an attempt to improve the cosmetic appearance, but this had no true sensation, and is not particularly realistic. The sensate clitoris uses parts of the glans penis, which can be isolated on its neurovascular pedicle. These nerves and vessels lie in the tissue between Buck's fascia and the tunica albuginea which surrounds the corpora cavernosa, and runs along the dorsum of the penis. The commonest part of the glans to use is the dorsum, which is immediately adjacent to the vessels, although some surgeons prefer to use the tissue from the ventral part of the penis, which is usually more sensitive. After the tissue is freed on its pedicle, the pedicle may be folded under the suprapubic skin, and the neoclitoris is sutured to the skin. Normally, a clitoral hood is made out of the surrounding skin. The long folded pedicle is at risk of occluding the vessel, with subsequent loss of the neoclitoris, but the author's experience is that over 95% survive and are sensitive. Despite this, only some 75% of patients are able to reach orgasm.

Complications

Unfortunately, the nature of surgery is such that complications happen, regardless of the skill of the surgeon and anaesthetist and any precautions taken to avoid problems. Male-to-female gender reassignment surgery (GRS) is a major and long operation on the pelvis and perineum, carried out with the patient in the 'lithotomy' position. It carries the risks common to any such procedure. These include deep vein thromboses and pulmonary emboli, chest infections, and cardiac events. These can be minimised by the use of heparin injections, anti-embolism stockings, and careful anaesthesia. They cannot be eliminated. In addition to these general risks, there are complications specific to the procedure itself.

The first group of complications is that caused by damage to bodily structures during the dissection, particularly that carried out to create the cavity for the neovagina. As described earlier, this dissection relies on entering a tissue plane between the layers of fascia at the apex of the prostate gland. If this tissue plane is missed, or if an instrument passes out of the correct plane, the neighbouring structures are at risk of damage.

Anteriorly, these structures are the urethra, prostate, and bladder. Injuries to the urethra are rare, and fortunately a small hole may almost always be closed without sequelae. It is not unusual to make a small cut into the prostate, and whilst this can cause a small amount of bleeding, it is seldom the cause of any problems. In the author's experience, injury to the bladder is very rare, although it is certainly possible that small holes in the posterior wall of the bladder may occur more frequently than is clinically apparent. The normal management for a small hole in that part of the bladder next to the cavity would be to leave a catheter in the bladder for 5 to 7 days. This is the normal protocol for the male-to-female GRS patients, so such injury is unlikely to become obvious. In the event that a larger hole or tear is made this could be sutured from without, and would be expected to heal without complication so long as catheter drainage was maintained post-operatively.

The rectum, however, is far less forgiving of injury and is more at risk than the anterior structures. Failure to enter and stay in the correct plane at the apex of the prostate carries a high risk of a tear in the rectal wall. This may be sutured safely if the bowel preparation has left the rectum clear and essentially clean but there is an incidence of subsequent breakdown of such repair, with the formation of a fistula into the neovagina. If the surgeon is not confident in the integrity of any repair, it is probably best to perform a temporary loop colostomy to allow the rectum to heal without the risk of fistula formation. In addition to damage obvious at the time of surgery (and it is the author's practice to inspect the anterior rectal wall carefully at the conclusion of the dissection to exclude any small hole) the rectum also appears to be at risk of invisible injury. This appears to lead to weakness of the rectal wall after the operation, with late fistula formation. The mechanism for this weakness is not known, but it is speculated to be a vascular phenomenon. The author has seen spontaneous breakdown of the rectal wall up to 5 weeks after surgery and also cases of perforation of the rectum by dilators. This would be very unusual if the strength of rectal wall were normal.

Fistula formation is a shattering complication for the patient (and the surgeon). Fortunately, most fistulas close if the rectum is defunctioned by formation of a colostomy, but formal repair is occasionally necessary.

Complications resulting from bleeding may be seen during the first few days after surgery. The corpus spongiosus is a structure surrounding the urethra, made up of sinusoids that give it erectile function. This tissue must be cut when the urethra is shortened, and post-operative bleeding may occur from the cut edge. This usually responds to pressure being applied on the post-operative ward, but occasionally it is necessary to return to theatre to resuture the cut edges.

A small number of patients also develop haematomas. These occur typically under the labia on either side and may require surgical evacuation. The blood which collects there may come from the cavity (although this is rare because of the pressure of the vaginal pack), the tissues of the labia, or occasionally from the clitoral pedicle. In the last case, careful bipolar diathermy is required to stop bleeding while maintaining the integrity of the clitoral blood vessels.

Another group of complications arises when the blood supply to the new skin flaps fails or is inadequate. The flaps used all have an identifiable blood supply, but this can be damaged during the dissection, or may be compromised by subsequent dissection. The neurovascular pedicle to the neoclitoris is the longest and potentially most at risk because the pedicle has to be folded away under the suprapubic skin at the end of the procedure. Accurate dissection is required to preserve the small blood vessels of the pedicle in the first place, but any twisting during positioning of the neoclitoris can result in loss of blood supply to the neoclitoris. The loss of the clitoris is seldom dramatic and immediately obvious (it doesn't 'drop off'), but typically by 6 weeks post-operatively, the clitoris is no longer visible. Fortunately, in some of these cases the nerves are preserved, with preservation of some of the sexual sensation to the area. The scrotal skin flaps used for scrotal inlay seem to be relatively hardy, and loss of this skin is very rare, although the author has seen a case where the skin was largely lost secondary to infection and an ill judged revision procedure in which the blood vessels were probably divided.

Similarly the penile skin flap seems relatively immune to failure of blood supply. In some instances it may well be that the skin is able to function as a free skin graft, which gives 'insurance' against loss of blood supply. Some apparently dead penile skin is occasionally seen to slough off at around 2 weeks in some patients, but in the author's experience so long as dilation is maintained there are seldom any sequelae. It is likely that sufficient islands of epithelium survive for the cavity to 'fill in' any gaps. If dilation is not maintained, however, some loss of depth and width is probable.

Loss of blood supply to the labial flaps can result in necrosis. Fortunately, this seldom affects the whole of the flap and is usually confined to the apex, which is at the back of the new vulva. Loss of skin here is fairly common, resulting in small gaps at around 3 weeks. Most of these gaps close spontaneously, although some require subsequent revision.

Two further complications which are seen fairly commonly are the result of problems with healing. If the vaginal skin tube does not 'stick' to the walls of the cavity, it will subsequently prolapse and need to be reattached. This complication seems to be confined to the use of scrotal flaps, and is presumably the result of having a layer of fat between the scrotal skin and the cavity wall. Its incidence has been reported in up to 15% of cases. The author has found that this is reduced by early mobilisation and the use of a gauze pack soaked in 'Proflavine' lubricating antiseptic cream This cream can be observed to leak out into the cavity, and the author believes that it is responsible for causing an inflammatory reaction which helps to cause adhesion of the flap. Other surgeons sprinkle antibiotic powder into the cavity prior to placement of the skin tube, which may have a similar effect. The vault of the vagina can also be sutured to the walls of the cavity.

The other common complication, which is a result of the healing process, is stenosis of the new urethral meatus. Despite all attempts to ensure that the epithelium of the urethra and the skin of the flap to which it is sutured are approximated accurately, there would appear to be a risk of subsequent scarring of the anastomosis with the formation of a stenosis. Rates of up to 30% are reported. Stenosis causes a progressive slowing of the urinary stream, followed by urge incontinence and in some cases urinary retention. Treatment is by dilation of the stenosis, or formal meatoplasty, in which a new and wider meatus is fashioned.

In addition to the complications outlined above, there are fairly frequent minor problems. Development of granulation tissue within the neovagina and at the introitus is common, and is the result of gaps between the skin edges at the end of surgery. These gaps usually epithelialise without any problem, but sometimes the gap is kept open by granulation tissue. This tissue bleeds easily and produces a serous fluid that almost always becomes infected, leading to bleeding (classically on dilation or intercourse) and an offensive vaginal discharge. Treatment is by removal of the granulation tissue. This can usually be achieved in clinic using silver nitrate sticks, but sometimes requires examination under anaesthesia, with the granulations removed by sharp dissection or diathermy.

Infections of the labial tissues are common; most are superficial and respond to physical washing. Occasionally antibiotics are needed. Rarely, a deeper collection forms and requires drainage. Such collections may result in unsatisfactory scarring that compromises the cosmetic result. Fortunately, the use of antibiotic prophylaxis reduces the incidence of such deeper collections.

Although the cosmetic and functional results are usually good, some patients find some aspect of the vulva unsatisfactory. Particularly with penile inversion techniques, there is a tendency for the skin at the back of the neovagina (the 'fourchette') to be pulled forward, and in some patients this may partially cover the vaginal introitus. Treatment is very simple – the skin may be incised backwards as an episiotomy, and sutured open. The cosmetic result after this is often enhanced, and penetration and dilation made very much easier. The neolabia are occasionally also a source of dissatisfaction. If too much skin is left they may become pendulous, and even lead to discomfort in underclothing or on sitting. The excess skin may easily be excised. With care it is sometimes possible to augment any labia minora at the same time.

In patients whose scrotal skin has been used in the neovagina, hair continues to grow. This hair growth is seen even after attempts at depilation during surgery, probably because hair has a 4 month growth cycle and some follicles that are inactive at the time of surgery are missed by depilation and subsequently become active. The only reliable way of avoiding hair in the neovagina is to depilate the scrotum by electrolysis or laser before surgery. Such depilation will take a minimum of 4 months because of the growth cycle, and must be completed at least 2 weeks before surgery takes place.

Fortunately, in most patients hair growth is not a major problem; in one series of 250 patients it was only mentioned by three patients, one of whom had undergone a colovaginoplasty. Nevertheless, the hair in the neovagina can form uncomfortable hairballs in the vaginal vault that need to be removed because they cause bleeding, discharge and pain. This may require general anaesthesia, but can usually be done without anaesthetic.

Many patients devise quite interesting methods for hair removal; one patient known to the author uses a crochet hook. In the author's experience, the use of depilatory cream in the neovagina has been very disappointing, and may cause severe skin reactions. Therefore patients with significant hair growth on a scrotum which will subsequently be needed in reconstruction should be advised to undergo depilation prior to surgery.

Post-operative care

Traditionally, patients have been nursed lying flat in bed for 5 days post-operatively, often on a fluid only diet, presumably to allow for maximal adhesion of the vaginal skin tube to the walls of the cavity by avoiding any movement.

In the author's unit, this approach has been dropped, and patients are mobilised from the first post-operative day. Unexpectedly, this change resulted in a halving of the prolapse rate. Similarly, giving a normal diet from day one has not been accompanied by a higher rate of other complications, and made the whole post-operative experience more tolerable for patients.

On the fifth day the vaginal pack is removed, and dilation taught. It is very important that this is carried out or supervised by an experienced person. Incorrect dilation causes problems. In the author's unit, two perspex dilators of 2.5 and 3 cm diameter are used, and these appear suitable for the vast majority of patients. A few patients move up to larger dilators after the initial few months; some because they have a 'well endowed' male partner who exceeds the large dilator. The reason for using a larger dilator in other patients is less obvious, and appears to be personal choice.

Dilation is usually taught with the patient lying supine, with the head and shoulders propped up on pillows. A mirror is a great aid to teaching. The patient will often find that it is best to locate the introitus with a finger prior to inserting the dilators. The shaft of the well lubricated dilator should be held essentially horizontal, and the dilator pushed gently forward without twisting or forcing until it reaches the vault of the vagina. Some resistance may be felt at the level of the pelvic floor muscles, and it is helpful if the patient can relax as if to open their bowel or pass urine at this point. For this reason, it is best to empty bladder and rectum before dilating. Mistakes can be messy! Initially, it is common for some blood to appear on the tip of the dilator when it is withdrawn; this usually gradually settles down within a few weeks. The author usually recommends using the smaller dilator essentially as in/out, and then leaving the larger dilator in place for 20 minutes. For the first 2 months dilation should take place three times a day. Thereafter, the frequency can normally be reduced. Since no two patients are the same, a certain amount of 'try it and see' is needed. One of the daily dilations is dropped. If the subsequent dilation is still relatively easy, the new frequency can continue. If the next dilation is very hard, the original frequency needs to be restored for a little longer. Most patients get down to weekly dilation by about 1 year.

In the first month or so, it is sensible to keep the inside of the new vagina clean by douching to remove any blood or spare lubricant. A dilute solution of antiseptic such as Betadine can initially be used, but in the longer term physical cleaning of the vagina can probably be satisfactorily achieved using plain water. This avoids the possibility of allergic reactions to the antiseptic. The skin of the neovagina is especially sensitive to allergens, and it is wise to restrict any cleaning agents to an absolute minimum for fear of sensitisation.

Superficial infection of the suture lines is also fairly common in the first few weeks. These can safely and effectively be treated by washing in warm water. Baths should be taken as often as possible, as they are usually very effective at achieving cleaning of the labia. Some patients also find it easiest to dilate in the bath, and this is worth trying in patients who are finding dilation difficult. Adding salt or antiseptics such as Betadine and Dettol to the bath water has not been shown to be of any additional benefit.

Sexual function

There are few studies of sexual function in post-operative male-to-female transsexual patients. One problem is that sexual activity may vary dramatically between patients. Probably a third of patients express their sexual orientation as lesbian. This is a significantly higher proportion than most populations. Many older patients are not sexually active at all, or indulge in masturbation only. Studies concentrating on heterosexual penetration as an end point therefore miss a lot of the sexual activity enjoyed by these patients. Furthermore, the size of the vagina in lesbian and chaste patients has a different importance to that of those who express their sexuality as heterosexual female, and who wish to have penetrative vaginal intercourse with men.

Provided there has been adequate skin initially, and dilation has been performed rigorously, the majority of patients have a vagina wide enough for penetration by an erect penis. Because the skin tube does not lubricate itself, most need to use additional lubricant (as do a lot of born women).

Some report more than adequate lubrication during sexual arousal. This fluid presumably comes from the prostate and urethral glands in response to stimulation. Indeed, some patients report significant discharge of fluid at around the time of orgasm; because the bulbo-spongiosus muscle is removed, this fluid dribbles out, rather than being forcefully ejaculated. Lack of depth is a more common problem than inadequate width, although some patients, especially those of Afro-Caribbean descent, find that the width of the vagina is limited by the angle between the inferior pubic rami and the symphysis pubis. The majority of such patients cope by choosing sexual positions where penetration is not deep enough for the penis to hit the end of the skin tube and cause pain to both partners.

Lesbian patients use either fingers or smaller dildos to avoid problems. Most report satisfaction with their neovaginas, although the author did have one patient who complained that her girlfriend was unable to insert a clenched fist.

Some patients ask for lengthening procedures; currently colovaginoplasty is the only reliable way of achieving this. Even after colovaginoplasty, there are some patients who find the vagina of insufficient capacity for intercourse; the reasons for this are not well understood.

Accepting that there are inaccuracies resulting from incomplete reporting of orgasmic function, a reasonable estimate is that some 85% of patients are able to attain orgasm after the operation. Whilst this is more common in patients in whom the clitoris is sensitive, it is by no means exclusive to that group. Patients who underwent surgery prior to the development of the sensate neoclitoris are not anorgasmic. Stimulation of the residual tissue of the corpus spongiosus around the urethral stump is usually reported as pleasurable. Some patients report orgasms from vaginal penetration alone, even when that penetration occurs during 'routine' dilations. As much seems to depend on the mood of the patient as the presence of a sensitive clitoris.

Almost all patients report that their orgasms are different to before the operation. Some claim to be able to differentiate between 'clitoral' and 'vaginal' orgasms. Some report multiple orgasms which they did not experience before their surgery. Much of this increased satisfaction with their sexual function is presumably a result of their being able to have sex as women, freed from what they considered an unsatisfactory penis (most pre-operative transsexuals do not want anyone to see their genitalia, let alone stimulate them), but it seems improbable that their surgery has had no physical effects.

Some patients find that intercourse is limited by length or width of the neovagina. Inadequate depth is usually the result of limitations brought about by limited skin at initial operation, and is very difficult to treat. If it is a significant problem to the patient, a colovaginoplasty is normally required. Inadequate width may be the result of skin tube narrowing, which may be improved by dilation, sometimes under anaesthetic. There are a small number of patients in whom the width is restricted by the angle of the pubic rami on either side. This is more common in Afro-Caribbean patients, who tend to have narrower bony pelvises than Caucasian and Asian people.

References

1 Gillies HD and Millard DR. *The Principles and Art of Plastic Surgery*. Butterworth; 1958.
2 Hensle TW, Shabsigh A, Shabsigh R, Reiley EA and Meyer-Bahlburg HF. Sexual function following bowel vaginoplasty. *J Urol*. 2006; **175**(6): 2283–6.
3 Woodhouse CRJ. Personal communication.
4 Rubin SO. A method of preserving the glans penis as a clitoris in sex conversion operations in male transsexuals. *Scand J Urol Nephrol*. 1980; **14**(3): 215–7.
5 Fang RH, Chen CF, Ma S. A new method for clitoroplasty in male-to-female sex reassignment surgery. *Plast Reconstr Surg*. 1992; **89**(4): 679–82.

16

Advice for patients undergoing vaginoplasty and vulvoplasty

James Barrett

Things to do before you come into hospital

Sort out the sorts of thing usually required before a short holiday, such as:

- someone to look after pets
- someone who can check up on your home
- getting plenty of books and magazines to read while you are in hospital (and also for when you are recovering at home)
- stocking up on videos or DVDs to watch
- arranging for someone to do your shopping for you, or sign up for internet shopping or home delivery with a supermarket.

Things to buy to use at home after your operation

- Lots of aqueous lubricant for dilation.
- Lots of tissues (for cleaning up after dilation).
- 'Wet ones' or baby wipes (for use as above).
- Disinfectant wipes (optional).
- Panty liners.
- Senna tablets or similar in case of constipation.

Suggested list of what to bring with you to into hospital

- Books, magazines, personal stereo, headphones and CDs.
- A small quantity of loose and comfortable clothes.
- Night clothes, dressing gown and slippers.
- Wash kit and towel, tissues.
- Panty liners (more comfortable than hospital dressings).
- Cash: for phone cards, newspapers etc.
- Fruit squash to give some flavour to the water and also supply a few calories. to sustain you while you are on clear fluids only.
- Biscuits to sate a light appetite post-anaesthesia.
- Baby wipes for cleaning up after dilation at the end of the stay.

In hospital

Arrival

- Book in at Admissions and go to the ward.
- Be introduced to any other gender reassignment surgery patients on the ward, who can give hints.
- Unpack till first baseline nursing observations are made.
- Visit the hospital shop.

Day 2

- Receive first dose of Picolax – the effect starts an hour or so later with regular toilet visits for the next few hours.
- Walk, sleep, read, listen to CDs, chat with people.
- Be visited by the clinical nurse specialist and your surgeon.
- Sign consent form.
- Receive second dose of Picolax and first injection of heparin.

Day 3

- Wash your hair for the last time in several days.
- Give the surgical area a close shave.
- Fill in menu cards for day 4, choosing 'small' meals.
- Be measured for TED (compression) stockings.
- Be given a hospital gown to wear.
- Change into gown and stockings, remove jewellery, cosmetics (including nail polish) and underwear.
- Hand over valuables for safekeeping.
- Talk to the anaesthetist, be measured for endotracheal tube, discuss analgesia.
- Be taken to theatre, have intravenous lines sited.
- Wake up in the recovery room.
- Fall asleep again and be taken back to the ward.

On waking

- Take sips of water to avoid vomiting.
- After several hours, try larger sips, maybe try eating biscuits.
- Become aware of huge dressing, tight and quite uncomfortable.
- Become aware of the urinary catheter and two surgical drains.
- Experience observations taken every hour.

Day 4

- Possibly eat a little.
- Be visited by the surgeon, to change the dressings to a smaller one.
- Drains are removed.
- Discuss pain relief, which may include weaning off patient-controlled analgesia.

- Sleep in the afternoon, if visitors allow, and then have dinner.
- In the evening, try sitting with your legs over the same side of the bed as the catheter.
- Perhaps try standing up and walking a few steps, carrying urine drain bag.

Day 5

- Carry on with the eating, sleeping, reading, getting bored.
- Towards the end of the day, bowel movements may resume.
- Perhaps switch to a leg bag for the catheter.

Day 6

- Bowel movements should resume today if they haven't already; remember to wipe backwards and upwards.
- Try going for longer walks.

Day 7

- Continue to recover.

Day 8

- Have catheter and vaginal packing removed.
- Nurse will introduce the smaller (2.5 cm diameter) dilator; this is kept inside for five minutes. Fluid runs out as it is removed. This is a liquefied lubricant, iodine-based disinfectant and blood.
- Blood is to be expected for a few days, as it takes a while for the internal bleeding to stop. The actual amount of blood is very small.
- The clinical nurse specialist will later introduce the larger (3 cm diameter) dilator and when it is part way in, will let you take over. This is kept *in situ* for ten minutes.
- Dilating occurs three times a day. This can be before meals as an *aide memoire*.
- Once your first dilation is out of the way, baths or showers recommence.
- In the evening you will do your second dilation, unaided.

Day 9

- Eat, sleep, read, dilate, go for walks.
- Remove TED stockings.

Day 10: discharge

- Receive discharge kit (Betadine douches and pessaries, painkillers, lubricant, inpatient certificate).

Post-operative care at home

- Bath or shower at least once a day, taking special care to ensure that the surgical site is kept thoroughly (but gently) cleaned.
- Use the Betadine douches and pessaries as directed.
- Change panty-liners twice a day, or more frequently if needed.
- Some bleeding and a creamy discharge at the suture line is perfectly normal. Keep the area clean and dry.
- Initially, the suture lines may become inflamed and sore. This indicates that they are healing, but unfortunately, makes it difficult to sleep or sit down.
- It may help to place a pillow or cushion between the legs when sleeping.
- If there are problems sitting down, extra cushions on seats may help.
- Take painkillers as and when you need them.
- Avoid constipation by the judicious use of mild laxatives.

Dilation

- Set aside specific times of day for this. Allow about half an hour each time.
- It requires five tissues, 'wet ones' or baby wipes, a mirror, lubricant, both dilators, plus an incopad mat to absorb the leakage that comes out after the dilators are removed.
- Set things out on your bed, so that they are readily to hand. Lie back (keeping your shoulders flat), lubricate the small dilator and insert. Dilate as in hospital.
- Afterwards, wipe yourself with a tissue, then clean up with a wet one or baby wipe, then dry off with another tissue.
- Thoroughly clean and pack away the dilators.
- Dilation with the larger dilator is slightly painful for the first few days, particularly when the suture lines are inflamed. This will ease as the general swelling reduces and the inflammation disappears.
- It may help to empty the rectum a short while before dilating.

Part 5

Surgical treatments for born females

17

Breasts

Dai M Davies and AJ Stephenson

There is a paucity of literature about surgical management of the breast in the female-to-male transsexual patient. The aim of mastectomy and chest-contouring surgery in the female transsexual patient is to remove breast tissue and redundant breast skin, to contour the chest by feathering out the adjacent fatty tissue and to convert the female nipple–areolar complex to the male appearance.[1]

Referral for either mastectomy or breast augmentation should, in accordance with the Royal College of Psychiatrists guidelines, be from a multidisciplinary gender clinic.[2] Referral with written support from a specialist psychologist or psychiatrist and with an independent second opinion from a medical gender dysphoria specialist or gender dysphoria specialist chartered psychologist is required to ensure that the proposal for surgery is appropriate.

Surgery is normally timed after a year of real life experience. However, once masculinising hormones are started, many changes, including voice deepening are irreversible, so breasts are inappropriate and may hamper progress with full real life experience. Exceptionally, earlier mastectomy may be appropriate.

The choice of procedure depends on breast size and the preferred method of the surgeon.[3] In the small breast, of B cup or less, with thick skin of good elasticity, a periareolar incision around the inferior half circumference of the areola, with short lateral extensions if necessary, may be used for the mastectomy. This is usually combined with liposuction to optimise the breast contour. Excess skin may be removed as a ring from around the areola, and the areola may be reduced in size. This peri-areolar approach minimises the visibility of scarring. It is, however, difficult to achieve the correct amount of reduction by this approach, which may over-reduce the breast and cause a depression and tethering of the nipple–areolar complex that is not usually correctable. Repositioning the nipple and areola complex to a more lateral, male position is not usually possible without more conspicuous scars.[3]

Where the breast is larger than a B cup, or if the skin elasticity is poor, as is the case with most patients, the breast is removed as an ellipse, retaining skin and some breast tissue from the upper part of the breast.

It is usual to attempt to place the scar in the inframammary crease. This reduces the conspicuity of the scar. The nipple and areolar complex is reduced in size and repositioned as free graft overlying the lateral border of pectoralis major. This option is more predictable than the peri-areolar approach. Patients are usually happier with overall result (*see* Figures 17.1 to 17.5 in the plate section).

Patients should be aware that not all breast tissue is removed in a mastectomy. In view of the potential for breast cancer, although long-term androgen therapy does not appear to increase the chances of pre-malignant or malignant-associated changes in breast tissue,[4] breast awareness and monitoring for breast cancer, in accordance with national guidelines, should be offered to female transsexual patients.

Author's preferred technique

The senior author's (DMD's) preferred technique is as above, according to breast size and skin quality, under general anaesthetic with an overnight stay after surgery. It is preferred that mastectomy is not combined with phalloplasty. Hormone therapy is not stopped for this surgery.

Complications

The most common complication after mastectomy is haematoma.

If the nipple–areola complex is to be repositioned as a free graft, the graft is more likely to fail in smokers, although the senior author has had only one graft loss in over 300 free nipple grafts.

Scars can become hypertrophic or keloid, both of which respond best to early scar management, by massage, silicone ointment or sheeting and steroid injection in the earlier stages.

'Dog ears', where skin bunches up at the end of ellipse excisions, can be excised if they fail to subside satisfactorily.

At follow-up, at around 6 months, any adjustments required can be planned. These can usually be done under local anaesthesia.

Choice of surgeon

The results of breast surgery in gender reassignment are judged primarily on the cosmetic outcome. A gender dysphoria clinic will usually have an association with a surgeon with experience of gender reassignment breast surgery. It is helpful for patients – and referring clinicians – to be able to see different surgeons' results, which will inform both the choice of surgeon and patient expectations.

References

1 Gilbert DA. Transsexual surgery in the genetic female. *Clinics in Plastic Surgery* 1988; **15**: 471–87.
2 RCPsych guidelines
3 Davies D. *Chest Reconstruction for Female to Male Trans People*. London: FTM; 2002.
4 Burgess HE and Shousa S. An immunohistochemical study of the long-term effects of androgen administration on female-to-male transsexual breast: a comparison with normal female breast and male breast showing gynaecomastia. *Journal of Pathology* 1993; **170**: 37–43.

18

Phalloplasty

David Ralph and Nim Christopher

History of modern phalloplasty surgery

Phalloplasty is the surgical technique of penile reconstruction. Modern phalloplasty surgery reflects the development of surgical techniques in plastic and reconstructive surgery. The three most significant developments were the discovery of the tubed or pedicled flap, the advent of microsurgical techniques and free flaps, and thirdly the use of inflatable penile prostheses for erectile dysfunction.

The pedicled flap came about as a result of treating severe maxillofacial injuries during World War I. The concept was developed independently by surgeons in different countries. Filatov from Russia published in 1917 and Sir Harold Gillies in England in 1920.[1] The principle was that suturing the two long sides of a skin flap into a tube reduces the infection rate and increases the vascularity and survival of the pedicle. This allowed more reliable and cosmetic reconstruction of head and neck trauma with reliable skin from distant sites.

The tubular shape of the pedicled flap lends itself to phalloplasty. In 1936 Nikolai Bogoraz from Russia published the first report of phalloplasty using this technique.[2] His patient was a 23-year-old man whose jealous wife had inflicted a traumatic penile amputation. For rigidity Bogoraz implanted a piece of rib cartilage inside the tubed pedicle flap, and the phalloplasty was completed in multiple stages. The urethra was made from tubularised scrotal skin.

Maltz (1946) and Gillies (1948) brought about the next development. This was to make the urethra and phallus simultaneously from the abdominal pedicle flap, using a tube within tube technique (as described later in the text).[1,3] This was also a multistage operation, using delayed pedicle transfer to reduce the risk of graft loss. This Gillies phalloplasty was the standard technique for the next 30 years. It gave a reasonably aesthetic phallus, but there was no cutaneous sensation and, because of hair and poor blood supply, many problems with the urethra.

The second major development was the provision of high precision lenses and operating microscopes by Carl-Zeiss in the 1970s. This allowed the development of free myocutaneous and fasciocutaneous flaps. The phallus could be constructed completely at the donor site with its own blood supply, and could then be transplanted using microsurgical vessel anastomosis to the pubic area. The aim was to use thin non-hair-bearing donor skin with cutaneous nerves to get the best phallus and urethra. In 1978, Chang described the radial forearm fasciocutaneous free flap. This has become a workhorse flap in reconstructive surgery because of its versatility. Chang and Hwang (1984) published the first report of the radial forearm flap phalloplasty for penile trauma using a tube within tube technique for the urethra.[4] This phallus could develop sensation. The reliability of this flap and its excellent aesthetic properties allowed the radial forearm flap phalloplasty to supplant the Gillies phalloplasty as the procedure of choice. The main drawback with this flap is the very visible donor site defect. A number of modifications of the flap design have occurred since, to address this.

The third development of note was the use of the inflatable penile implant by Scott and Bradley in 1973, for treating men with erectile dysfunction.[5]

Before then, a variety of solid and semi-malleable artificial prostheses had been used. Biological alternatives, much as in phalloplasty surgery, had been cartilage, bone and other naturally stiff tissues implanted into penises and phalluses for rigidity. The problem for phalloplasties was that both the lack of cutaneous sensation and the rigidity of the prosthesis meant that erosion was very common.

The hydraulic nature of the inflatable prosthesis meant that in the flaccid state there was little pressure on the phallic tissues, so erosion was less common. The free flap phalloplasty's ability to develop cutaneous sensation also meant the patient was able to feel when something was going wrong, so that the problem could be rectified before it was too late.

The original inflatable prostheses were not very reliable, but the current models are good. American Medical Systems 700CX model and the Mentor-Porges Titan models are the latest incarnations. They come with antibiotic coatings and the ability to adsorb antibiotics onto the surface respectively. This has reduced the infection rate dramatically.

There are two main areas that currently need improvement. The reconstructed urethra still causes the most complications. The use of tissue engineering so a pseudo-urethral tube might be grown from the patient's own tissues would probably help. The donor site defect is becoming less unsightly, with the use of colour- and hair-matched skin and the use of new dressings to improve cosmesis. Again, tissue engineering may provide a more aesthetic solution.

For the future, there is the possibility of cadaveric penile transplantation. The technical expertise to do this already exists. Any surgeon who can do a free flap phalloplasty will have no problems performing a penile transplant. This has not happened because immunosuppressant drugs are not yet safe enough for long-term use in an essentially non-life-threatening condition.

Surgical stages

We divide the various components of phalloplasty surgery into four groups or stages, as listed below:

- *stage 1*: construction of the phallus
- *stage 2*: construction of the neo-urethra
- *stage 3*: cosmetic tidy-up; this includes glans sculpting, insertion of testis prosthesis, insertion of reservoir for inflatable penile prosthesis and tidy-up of scars
- *stage 4*: insertion of cylinders and pump of inflatable penile prosthesis.

Each stage can consist of one or more operations. Depending on the exact phalloplasty technique used, some of the stages can be combined, resulting in fewer operations. The important point of the staged approach is that the neo-urethra must be completed before any prosthetic devices are inserted. If there are problems with the urethra then infection may set in, resulting in a prosthesis infection and the loss of the prosthesis.

Extra procedures such as hysterectomy, vaginectomy and clitoroplasty can be incorporated in stages 1, 2 and 3. Because these require extra surgical expertise and operative time this may not be practical for all centres.

Some centres insert the cylinders in stage 3 and the pump and reservoir in stage 4. Others insert all three components of the inflatable penile prosthesis and testis prosthesis at the same operation, that is to say, combining stages 3 and 4. The order of component insertion is not very important. We will discuss the choice of penile prosthesis in the surgery section.

The ideal phalloplasty

The ideal phalloplasty is one where the phallus, neo-urethra and erection ability or device are constructed in one procedure, with good functional and cosmetic result and with minimal donor site morbidity. This is not currently possible. Most centres will implant the prosthesis separately to the phallus construction, to minimise infection problems.

Types of phalloplasty

Modern phalloplasty techniques consist of three classes of surgery.

- local flaps
- pedicled flaps
- free flap transfer and microsurgical vessel anastomosis.

There is also a special category of mini-phalloplasty or metoidioplasty (or sometimes metatoidioplasty). This is not really a flap-type of phalloplasty. The clitoris is converted into a small penis and there is no donor site to worry about.

A little preliminary background on skin flaps is useful. For a phalloplasty, skin and subcutaneous fat is needed to give the new phallus bulk. Sometimes the underlying deep fascia or muscle, or both, are incorporated because the blood supply runs in it. Occasionally, vascularised bone is taken with the flap for rigidity.

The size of the skin flap that can be taken depends on the type of blood supply. A random subcutaneous blood supply with no axial feeding or draining vessels is limited to a flap length not greater than the width at the base of the flap still connected to the patient. This is known as a random flap. If there are axial vessels, then the flap can be longer than the base because the blood supply extends the whole length of the flap. These flaps can be much longer than the width at the base. They can be formed into pedicled flaps (like a suitcase handle), where the blood supply and venous drainage is polarised into the ends of the pedicle. Later, one end of the pedicle can be transplanted elsewhere to establish a new blood supply. The pedicle can be gradually transferred in a stepwise fashion. Alternatively, the skin of the pedicle base can be incised and mobilised still in continuity with the blood supply, and tunnelled to the correct location, having disconnected the distal end. These local and pedicled flaps are not usually sensate.

A free flap has a named artery and vein or veins, and sometimes some nerve supply as well. The whole flap containing skin, fat and sometimes fascia, muscle or bone is disconnected from the donor site and transplanted using microsurgical arterial, venous and nerve anastomoses. This dedicated blood supply gives the free flap a huge advantage when compared to the local or pedicled flaps in terms of tissue survival and shrinkage due to ischaemia. There is also the possibility of developing touch sensation to the flap when the nerves are connected to local sensory nerves.

Local flap phalloplasty

The simplest local flap is the pubic flap. Three sides of a 12 cm square flap are incised with the base and blood supply at the clitoral area. The flap is raised and contains skin and subcutaneous fat. Some defatting may be required before the flap can be rolled into a tube with the skin on the outside. The abdominal defect is closed by primary closure, by mobilising the abdominal skin. The phallus is insensate but hairy. It will need regular shaving. The neo-urethra is constructed either separately or at the same time.[6] One disadvantage for patients is that they lose their pubic hair. An advantage is that all the scars are easily concealed by their underpants.

If the flap is made narrower and shorter, and the phallus made inside out with the fat on the outside, then a urethra is made. The fat on the outside may be covered with a split skin graft to form the phallus. Later, this urethra can be extended to the native urethral meatus. This latter technique is rarely used because the urethra is very hairy and prone to infection. Also the phallus is not cosmetically very realistic. An alternative is not to create a neo-urethra but rather to insert a temporary stiffener into the blind-ending urethra to have intercourse.[7]

The extended groin flap is based on the superficial epigastric and superficial circumflex vessels. Because the blood supply is axial, the length of the flap can be much longer than the width. The flap is positioned in a diagonal fashion along the inguinal region, extending laterally past the iliac crest. Incisions are made along the two long sides, and a tube made by suturing the two edges together skin side out, so it looks like a suitcase handle. Later, the lateral end is disconnected, to form the tip of the phallus. The medial end is de-epithelialised to create a long vascular pedicle. The phallus is then tunnelled under the skin to end up in the pubic area, retaining the blood supply via the same vascular pedicle. This kind of phallus is often very large but not very cosmetic. If there is enough skin then the infero-lateral 3 to 4 cm of the flap can be tubed, fat side out, into a urethra using the tube-in-tube method. A tissue expander can be inserted under the skin beforehand to expand the usable skin to allow this. The donor site defect is closed, usually by primary closure.

Another way of making the urethra is to skin graft the deep surface of the 'suitcase handle' and tube it over later. This results in a quite thin phallus with urethra. This method is used by some surgeons in the US. The urethra for the pubic phalloplasty is usually constructed from the inner labial non-hairy skin. This is tubed on a long pedicle and tunnelled up the phallus. The blood supply is based on the clitoral vessels. Unfortunately, the meatal opening does not reach the tip of the phallus. The labial tube is not long enough unless the phallus is quite short. Extending the meatus to the tip involves using free grafts of skin or buccal mucosa, which are then tubed over in two stages. The blood supply of these multisegment urethras is not reliable, and the stricture rate is high. Some patients choose to void sitting down instead.

Pedicled flap phalloplasty

The classic example is the Gilles phalloplasty. One or two suitcase handle-type pedicles are created using the 'love handles' area in the lateral abdominal wall, where there is ample non-hairy skin. After some weeks, when the blood supply has polarised to the ends of the pedicle, the distal end is disconnected and reattached nearer the pubis, to establish a new source of blood supply. The process is repeated every 6–8 weeks, until the bases of the pedicles are on the pubis. The neo-urethra is formed from the opposing skin between the two pedicles.

Alternatively the urethra can be made, as in the extended groin flap, as a tube within a tube at the original donor site. This is a long series of operations, and because of ischaemia there is a risk of losing the whole pedicle or shrinkage every time there is a pedicle base transfer.

Free flap phalloplasty

The commonest free flap in use today is the radial forearm flap. A large piece of skin and subcutaneous fat is marked out with the urethral strip over the medial aspect of the forearm, where the skin is least hairy. Only a strip of skin on the extensor aspect of the forearm is left. The flap is raised with the radial artery and associated subcutaneous veins and nerves under tourniquet. The urethral strip is tubed over a catheter or stent. The rest of the flap is wrapped round to form the phallus. The phallus is disconnected from the arm and transplanted to the pubic area.

Using microsurgical techniques, the radial artery is anastomosed to either the inferior epigastric or the femoral artery. The flap veins are connected to the long saphenous veins and its branches and the cutaneous nerves of the flap to the ilio-inguinal, genito-femoral or sometimes one of the dorsal clitoral nerves. There are many design variations of this flap. Some allow for the pseudo glans to be constructed as well.

Other flaps in use are an ulnar artery-based flap, latissimus dorsi flap, deltoid flap, lateral thigh flap, fibula flap and many others.[8-11]

For flaps from distal extremities like the forearm and lower leg, it is important to ensure that there is a second artery that can adequately supply the distal limb before harvesting the flap.

The latissimus dorsi flap can incorporate muscle for bulk.

The radial and fibula flaps can incorporate bone, which can give rigidity to the phallus. The radial bone segment does not include the complete circumference of the radius bone so there is an increased post-operative risk of pathological radius fracture. The fibula bone segment contains the whole circumference of the fibula and has fewer donor site problems.

The deltoid flap often does not have enough skin to make the neo-urethra, which has to be constructed by other means. Usually bilateral lateral thigh flaps are needed to construct a phallus with neo-urethra, which increases surgical complexity and time.

The radial flap has the thinnest skin, the most reliable anatomy, a long vascular pedicle with a large-calibre artery and is relatively straightforward to harvest. A flap big enough to include skin for the neo-urethra and phallus is always possible. For these reasons it remains the most popular phalloplasty flap in current use. The main disadvantage of the forearm flap is the donor site defect. This is covered with either a partial- or a full-thickness skin graft. A full-thickness skin graft looks better, feels softer and grows hair. This hair may help conceal what is a very noticeable defect.

Metoidioplasty

This procedure essentially converts the female clitoris into a mini-phallus. Full sexual sensation is preserved. It is most successful in thin patients with little pubic or labial fat and a very hypertrophic clitoris. The mini-phallus is not long enough for penetrative sex except in the very unusual circumstance of a massively hypertrophic clitoris. It is also not very wide. This procedure comprises clitoral lengthening, urethral advancement to the tip of the mini-phallus and the formation of a neo-scrotum.[12,13] The patient may choose any combination of these components.

Clitoral lengthening involves dividing the suspensory ligament of the clitoris at the pubis and mobilising the crura. For further length, the 'urethral plate' has to be divided and mobilised off the crura, so the mini-phallus can be positioned more anteriorly. Unfortunately, this makes the neo-urethral surgery more difficult because a second urethral segment has to be constructed to get the meatus to the tip of the mini-phallus. As with any neo-urethra, the more segments it has, the higher the complication rate. For patients for whom voiding is more important, a one-stage urethral advancement without clitoral lengthening is performed.

The simplest urethral advancement is the one-segment version. A flap of anterior vaginal wall is elevated and brought forward to cover the native meatus. Parallel longitudinal incisions on both sides of the 'urethral plate' are made to the ventral groove of the glans clitoris, which has to be wide enough to tube over a 14 French urethral catheter (*see* Table 18.1). The size of meatus that can be made depends on how hypertrophied the glans clitoris is. If it is large enough and has a deep ventral groove, then a bigger size 16 French catheter could be used.

Table 18.1   Catheter sizes: the cross-sectional area rises exponentially with the French size. Thus even a 1 size difference in French size gives a significant change in flow, as flow is proportional to cross-sectional area

French (F)	Circumference (mm)	Area (mm²)
8	8.5	5.7
10	10.4	8.6
12	12.6	12.6
14	14.8	17.3
16	16.7	22.1
18	18.8	28.3

The bigger the meatus the less likely are urethral problems, because lower meatal resistance decreases voiding pressure in the proximal half of the urethra. As meatal size goes down, resistance goes up and the voiding pressure in the proximal urethra goes up with it. This neo-urethra has a relatively thin wall when compared to the thick and vascular corpus spongiosum in biological males. Proximal neo-urethra can develop severe ballooning or a fistula, or the meatus can split to become wider, to equalise the pressures. Thus glans clitoris size is a very important factor for neo-urethral construction.

There are a number of two-segment urethral advancement techniques, depending on clitoral size. Some were developed from hypospadias repair techniques in children. Others were developed specifically for this group of patients. In all of them the available meatal size is an important factor for success. Needless to say, this is a highly specialised form of surgery.

The neo-scrotum may be fashioned in a number of ways. A simple V–Y plasty of the labia majora to drop it inferiorly will create bilateral pouches lower down. Sometimes the labia majora are sutured together across the midline to create a pouch. Tissue expander prostheses can be implanted temporarily to expand the labia majora. Testicular prostheses are inserted later.

In summary, metoidioplasty can in some centres be a one-stage operation. The more complex the neo-urethra or neo-scrotum, the more likely it is the patient will require two or maybe even three stages. The bigger the clitoris, the more likely is a satisfactory outcome.

Referral criteria

The recommended criteria are that the patient has successfully lived in a male role and has been on androgen therapy for at least one year. The referral should be made by two of the gender identity clinic specialists, taking into account the patient's mental, emotional and physical ability to withstand major surgery of this nature. This is derived from the Harry Benjamin criteria used by most centres.[14]

Assessment in clinic

When we assess patients for phalloplasty surgery, it is important to find out what the patient wants.[15] Most want to void standing up, from the tip of the phallus if possible. A large percentage of patients are interested in having the ability to have penetrative sex. Some just want to have a good cosmetic-looking phallus. Along with all these it is important to discuss the donor site defect, possible complications and the number of operations needed. Information on post-operative recovery time and time off work is essential. This will give them some sort of time-scale to work to. This kind of surgery, even if funded by the public health sector, is still expensive for the patients. They have to take into account lost earnings, travel and accommodation costs and time spent recovering from somewhat painful surgery.

The age and medical history of the patient are also important. Those over 45 years, particularly if they are smokers or have existing cardiac or vascular disease, will not be good candidates for free flap phalloplasty, due to poor-quality vessels. Those over 60 years will have poorer skin blood supply irrespective of which phalloplasty technique is used. They have to be watched very carefully post-operatively. Those with poor perineal hygiene have a very high risk of prosthesis infection. Testicular and penile prostheses are contraindicated. Patients with severe eczema or psoriasis are likely to have problems with the skin disease forming in the neo-urethra. This would cause rapid urethral stenosis. They may decide not to have a neo-urethra or may undergo a first-stage neo-urethra to see what happens before deciding whether to proceed further. Patients with tattoos in the donor site have to be warned that the phallus will be tattooed as well. We try to arrange the skin flaps in such a way as to pick the best aesthetic position of the tattoo on the phallus.

If a free flap phalloplasty is chosen the feeding vessels must be confirmed to be intact, usually by a vascular Doppler ultrasound examination. If the flap is from a distal limb, then the remaining artery must be shown adequately to perfuse the distal hand or foot on its own. A typical clinical test is the Allen test for the upper limb. Both the radial and ulnar arteries are occluded by digital compression at the wrist. The patient makes a fist a few times till the hand goes white as the veins empty. The compression on the ulnar artery (assuming a radial artery flap is planned) is released while still occluding the radial artery. The hand should pink up within a few seconds. This confirms that the ulnar artery is adequate to supply the hand. Patients who have had fractures of the distal limbs must all have a vascular Doppler ultrasound examination anyway, to check both the arteries and the veins. Extensive scarring from suicide attempts on the forearm may preclude the use of a forearm flap, particularly if the cuts were very deep or involved any vessels.

If some form of abdominal local or pedicled flap is chosen, the patient's abdomen should be carefully examined for scars that might interfere with the blood supply of the flap. Such scars may limit the choice of flap that can be done. A transverse hysterectomy scar may preclude a one-stage pubic phalloplasty. The pubic flap can still be marked out, lifted up and replaced to see if the blood supply is adequate. If this flap survives, the pubic phalloplasty can be completed 6 weeks later.

Some patients ask for an 8–9 inch (20–23 cm) phallus under the mistaken conception that this is a normal size. This misassumption comes from adult films and magazines. The average stretched penile length in Europe is about 12–12.5 cm, and this is generally what we try to achieve with a phalloplasty.[16] Erect length in biological males is very closely correlated to stretched length, which is only slightly less. Patients are warned that the final result is unpredictable and depends on their skin elasticity and amount of subcutaneous fat. Some phalluses will elongate and some will get smaller. In order to get a neo-urethra with lower chance of complications and a meatus nearer the tip, some patients deliberately select a smaller phallus size, particularly if an erection device is not required.

A small number of our patients request a smaller procedure without a full-size phalloplasty. Their main concern is the donor site morbidity. For these patients we offer a mini-phallus or metoidioplasty. The best results for this operation are in thin patients with little pubic or labial fat and a significantly hypertrophied clitoris from testosterone therapy. If neither of these two conditions is fulfilled, they are advised that the outcome is likely to be poor.

We feel it is important for new patients to meet those who have completed or nearly completed the same type of phalloplasty. There are many practical matters that only a patient who has had the surgery can adequately describe. We show all patients a selection of phalloplasty pictures, in progress and completed. For those interested in operative details we also have short video clips of key parts of the phalloplasty surgery. To give an unbiased view they are shown poorer results and complications as well as good ones, so they will have as much information as possible before deciding. Some patients require many consultations before reaching a decision. It is very important for the patient to be absolutely sure what they want before we agree to start the phalloplasty surgery. Some thought needs also to be given to any associated surgery such as mastectomy, hysterectomy, vaginectomy and clitoroplasty, and how to fit these into the phalloplasty operative sequence.

Preparation for surgery

As with all patients who undergo major surgery, some general points need to be reinforced.

Smokers should stop smoking for at least 2 weeks prior to admission. Giving up smoking would be better; however 2 weeks' abstinence is enough to improve lung function and particularly the ability of the lung to expel mucus using mucosal ciliary action. Smoking increases vascular risk, especially thrombosis of the small vessels with free flap surgery.

Patients should attempt to be close to their ideal body weight, to reduce risk with the possible exceptions listed later.

Most patients undergoing phalloplasty nowadays will be under 40 years of age. They will be unlikely to be on other medication apart from androgens. If they do have pre-existing cardiac disease, hypertension, diabetes or any other systemic diseases, then these should be optimised prior to surgery.

For pubic or extended groin flap phalloplasty, we do need a reasonable amount of subcutaneous fat with the skin or the phallus is very thin.

If the patient is already overweight, then losing about 15 kg will allow us to perform less defatting of the flap, and because the skin will be looser it will also allow easier closure of the abdominal defect.

If the patient is very thin, then putting on 7–14 kg is advisable. Once the phallus is made, the weight can be lost. The fat in the phallus fortunately appears to be very resilient to weight loss from dieting. If the phallus has too little fat then it will remain floppy until the erection device is inserted.

If the forearm is very hairy, especially on the ulnar side where the urethra would be made in a radial forearm flap phalloplasty, then pre-emptive laser hair removal is advisable. This only works well in those with pale skin, and dark hair may preclude some patients from having this kind of phalloplasty. Laser hair removal can also be done on the abdominal skin prior to pubic phalloplasty, but many patients wait till after the phalloplasty so it is not essential. No blood should be taken from the potential donor forearm in order to preserve the veins.

If an urethroplasty is being planned or an erection device is being inserted, then a urine culture should be taken to confirm it is sterile. Any infection is treated with appropriate antibiotics and the urine retested and confirmed to be clear prior to proceeding with surgery. For erection device surgery, the patients also need to have an antiseptic shower or bath immediately pre-operatively. We recommend Hibiscrub™ for our patients, and all start Naseptin™ intranasal antibiotic cream, to clear *Staphylococcus aureus* from the nose pre-operatively. The latter continues until the surgical wounds have healed, usually in 1 or 2 weeks. The surgical site is shaved in theatre and a five to ten minute skin scrub with antiseptic is also performed. These precautions reduce the infection rate.

If skin grafts are being harvested from the buttocks for forearm coverage, we advise patients to bring slip-on shoes, as bending over to tie laces will be difficult for about 3 weeks. Sometimes a soft cushion to sit on is useful, as after urethroplasty or penile implant insertion it is a little uncomfortable to sit for a few days. Loose-fitting clothes to go home in are a must, as there will be a lot of bulky bandages and padding to protect the new phalloplasty, penile implant or urethroplasty.

Phalloplasty surgery

The actual surgical technique varies from centre to centre but the essentials remain the same. We will describe in pictorial form a pubic phalloplasty, an extended groin flap phalloplasty, a radial forearm flap phalloplasty and some of the variants of metoidioplasty (*see* plate section). Some of the urethroplasty, glans sculpting, neo-scrotum formation and penile implant surgery will also be demonstrated.

Pubic phalloplasty

For a public phalloplasty, the base of the flap is at the root of the clitoris and is 12 cm wide. The length of the flap is usually 1–2 cm with an extra 1–2cm for the glans (*see* Figure 18.1, plate section). Extra marks are placed to allow accurate apposition of the sutures. Once defatted the flap is tubularised to form the phallus. The lower abdominal skin is mobilised and brought down and lateral hip skin flaps are raised and rotated inwards to fill the remaining gap (*see* Figure 18.2, plate section). If there is a transverse hysterectomy scar then the flap needs to be raised first and replaced to see if there is an adequate blood supply before forming the phallus 6 weeks later. Insufficient blood supply leads to flap necrosis within a few days (*see* Figure 18.3, plate section). These patients are offered a radial artery phalloplasty instead once the necrotic tissue has been debrided.

Extended groin flap phalloplasty

In the extended groin flap phalloplasty, the tissue is taken from the inguinal and iliac crest area and tubularised. The proximal inguinal skin is de-epithelialised to form a vascular pedicle. The whole phallus and vascular pedicle is tunnelled under the skin to reach the pubic area (*see* Figure 18.4, plate section). These phalloplasties are large, bulky and not particularly cosmetic.

Radial forearm flap phalloplasty

For a radial forearm flap phalloplasty, the skin is marked on the non-dominant arm. Usually, the urethral segment is 4 cm wide to prevent stenosis and the length is 2–3 cm longer than the phallus to allow tunnelling of the urethra down to the side of the clitoris. The phallus is 12–14 cm long and 11 cm in circumference at the tip (wrist) and 13 cm in circumference at the base (elbow). The urethral segment is placed on the ulnar aspect of the forearm (*see* Figure 18.5, plate section). The urethral portion is tubed fat side outside over a stent and the phallus portion is then wrapped around with the skin side outside to form the phalloplasty. This is transplanted to the pubic area (*see* Figure 18.6, plate section). The forearm is covered either with split thickness (*see* Figures 18.7, 18.8, plate section) or full thickness skin graft (*see* Figures 18.9, 18.10, 18.11, plate section). The end result of a stage 1 radial artery phalloplasties is shown in Figure 18.12 (plate section).

Urethroplasty

The labial urethroplasty going partway up the phallus has already been described, as has the use of buccal and other grafts to extend the urethra to the tip (*see* Figure 18.13, plate section). A better solution is to do a radial artery urethroplasty to reduce urethral segmentation. A strip of skin with radial artery and supporting veins is harvested and tubed over a stent. This is implanted in the phallus and connected to the usual blood vessels. This urethra extends from the tip of the phallus to near the clitoris. The donor site scar is much smaller and on the inside of the forearm and so less noticeable (*see* Figure 18.14, plate section). Other forms of distal urethroplasty use the Gillies technique. A strip of skin on the lower abdominal wall is incised on the two long borders, and a urethra formed over a stent by suturing the long borders together. The skin has to be relatively hairless, and one end has to be near the base of the phallus. The phallus is then split and sutured fat side down, to encompass the neo-urethra. After a few months the phallus and neo-urethra is gradually lifted in stages from the distal end, and the phallus reformed with the neo-urethra inside. The blood supply of the neo-urethra should be mostly from the phallus rather than the abdominal wall by this time. Part of this neo-urethra may be lost due to ischaemia at any time.

The join-up urethroplasty operation is the same whichever distal form of urethroplasty is performed. A small anterior vaginal flap is raised to divert the urine stream at the native meatus. The antero-lateral walls are formed of the labia minora, and the native meatus is thus extended to the opening of the distal urethra.

Formation of neo-scrotum

If the labia majora are large and there is sufficient space between the thighs, testicular prostheses can be inserted directly (*see* Figure 18.15, plate section). Tissue expanders can be used to make more space. The problem with these methods is that the scrotal contents look perfect side by side in the operating theatre with the legs in the lithotomy position, but once the patient is standing or walking the testes move to lie vertically one on top of the other, so often one testis moves to the base of the phallus and the other to the bottom of the labia majora. Using smaller-sized prostheses can help. Some patients just have a single testis or single pump as there is always enough space for one item. An alternative is to create a more anteriorly placed scrotal pouch that sits in front of the thighs rather than between them. To do this the inferior poles of the labia majora are disconnected and rotated up to the base of the phallus to form an anterior pouch. This results in a more male-looking scrotum (*see* Figure 18.16, plate section).

Glans sculpting

If the glans is not preconstructed as in some free flap phalloplasties, the preferred technique is the Norfolk method. A distally based circumferential skin flap is raised and folded over to form a thick rim. The raw surface under the rim is then skin grafted (*see* Figures 18.17, 18.18, plate section). Split skin graft can be used, though we prefer full-thickness skin graft from non-hairy skin, labia minora or vaginal mucosa. This gives the phallus a circumcised appearance. Some centres offer tattooing of the pseudo-glans.

Choice of penile prosthesis

Because the phallus only consists of skin and fat, any prosthesis has a risk of extrusion or erosion. Therefore any inflatable prosthesis has an advantage over a semi-rigid prosthesis since in the flaccid state there is little pressure on the skin. Hage advocated the one-piece inflatable (Dynaflex) and recommended the use of a Dacron™ or synthetic sheath to create an extra protective layer around the prosthesis to simulate the function of the tunica cavernosum.[17] He also recommended that the base of the prosthesis be surgically fixed to the inferior pubic ramus to allow reliable penetration. The one-piece inflatable had the reservoir, inflatable cylinder and pump all incorporated together. The problem with the Dynaflex™ prosthesis was that it was still quite stiff even in the flaccid state. Secondly, the deflation mechanism involved bending the shaft of the prosthesis to initiate deflation. This could cause problems during intercourse if the phallus bent accidentally. The Dynaflex has since been discontinued. The current preferred model is the three-piece inflatable, where the reservoir, cylinder and pump are all separate.[18] This allows for greater contrast between flaccid and rigid states (*see* Figures 18.19a, 18.19b, 18.20a and 18.20b, plate section).

The body forms a protective non-elastic fibrous capsule around all prosthetic components. The reservoir has to be left fully inflated for about 4 weeks, so that the capsule forms in maximal dimension to allow complete deflation of the cylinder later. We also recommend putting a large testicular prosthesis into the neo-scrotum a few months previously. The pump of the penile prosthesis will then fit into the capsule of the removed testicular prosthesis. The pump can be manipulated easily in this space. This alleviates the problem of the pump being trapped in an unfavourable position by the fibrous capsule, which might occur if it were put into a virgin neo-scrotum. The cylinder also needs to be cycled regularly early on to prevent a tight fibrous capsule forming.

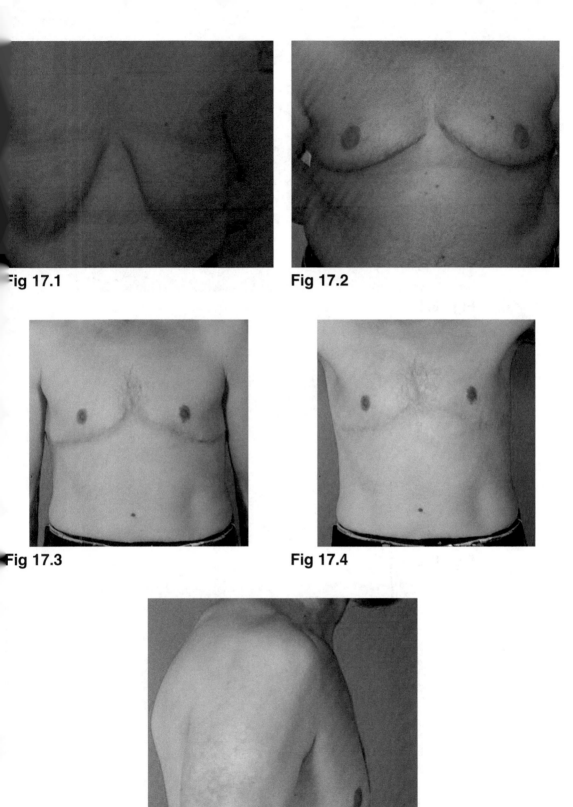

Fig 17.1

Fig 17.2

Fig 17.3

Fig 17.4

Fig 17.5

Figures 17.1 to 17.5   Pre and post operative views, ellipse mastectomy method

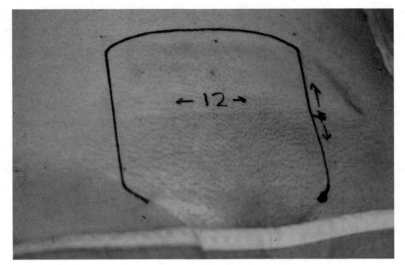

Fig 18.1

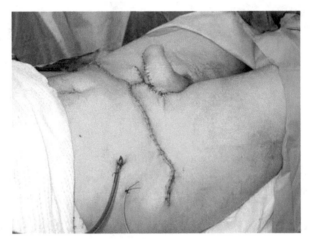

Fig 18.2

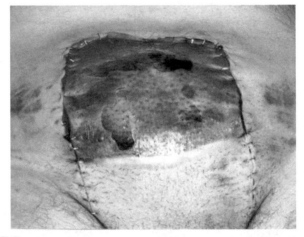

Fig 18.3

Figure 18.1 Pubic phalloplasty flap dimensions (cm)

Figure 18.2 Pubic phalloplasty abdominal closure

Figure 18.3 Necrotic pubic flap with transverse hysterectomy scar

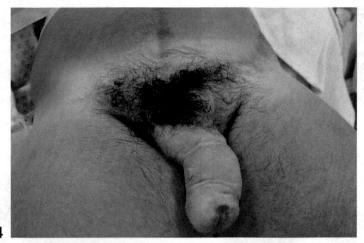

Fig 18.4

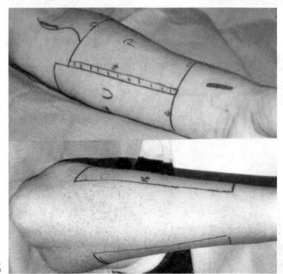

Fig 18.5

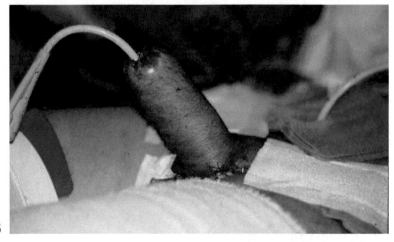

Fig 18.6

Figure 18.4 Extended groin flap phalloplasty

Figure 18.5 Forearm markings (cm). Showing flexor and extensor aspects for radial artery
        phalloplasty

Figure 18.6 Radial artery phalloplasty transplanted to pubic area

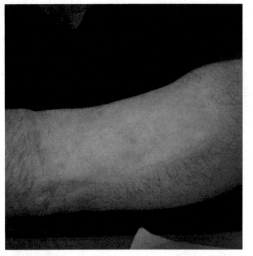

Fig 18.7

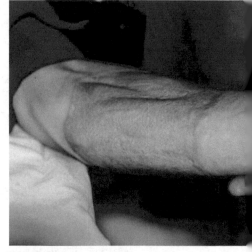

Fig 18.8

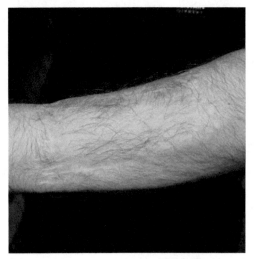

Fig 18.9

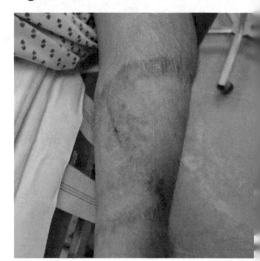

Fig 18.10

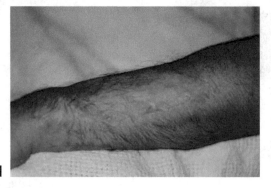

Fig 18.11

Figure 18.7   Forearm with split thickness graft
Figure 18.8   Forearm with split thickness graft
Figure 18.9   Forearm with full thickness graft
Figure 18.10 Forearm with full thickness graft
Figure 18.11 Forearm with full thickness graft

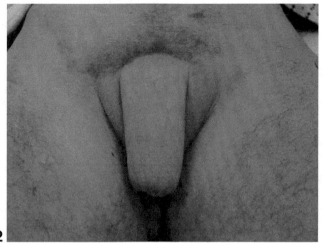

Fig 18.12

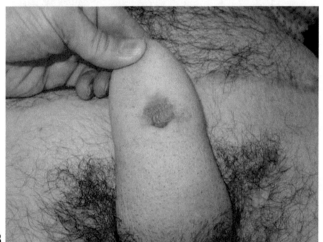

Fig 18.13

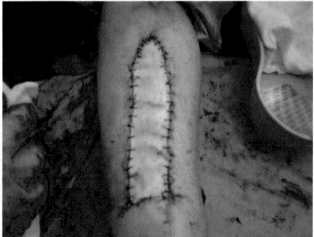

Fig 18.14

Figure 18.12 Radial artery phalloplasty stage 1

Figure 18.13 Labial urethroplasty in pubic phalloplasty showing meatus partway up phallus

Figure 18.14 Skin graft on radial artery urethroplasty donor site

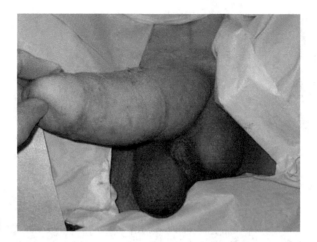

Fig 18.15

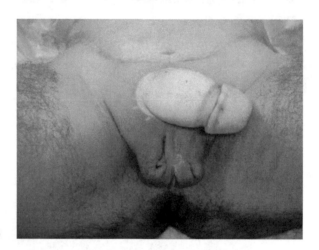

Fig 18.16

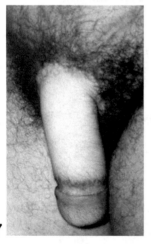

Fig 18.17

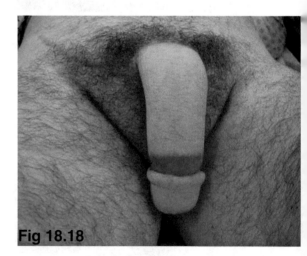

Fig 18.18

Figure 18.15 Testes prosthesis inserted directly into labia majora in a very large pubic phalloplasty

Figure 18.16 Anterior scrotal pouch formation

Figure 18.17 Glans sculpting – full thickness skin graft

Figure 18.18 Glans sculpting – full thickness labial graft

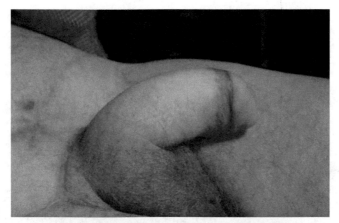

Fig 18.19 a

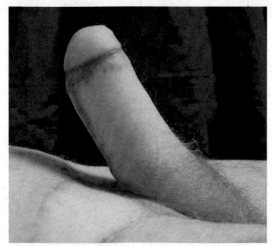

Fig 18.18 b

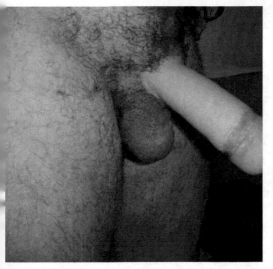

Fig 18.20 a

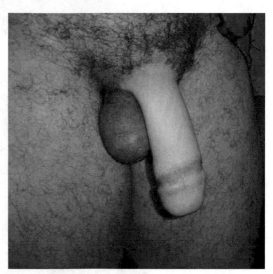

Fig 18.20 b

Figure 18.19a   Flaccid pubic phalloplasty

Figure 18.19b   Erect pubic phalloplasty

Figure 18.20a   Flaccid radial artery phalloplasty

Figure 18.20b   Erect radial artery phalloplasty

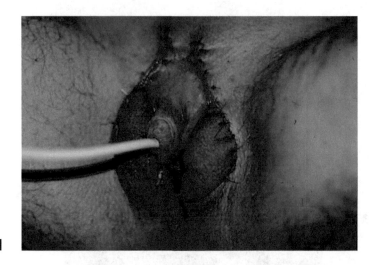

Fig 18.21

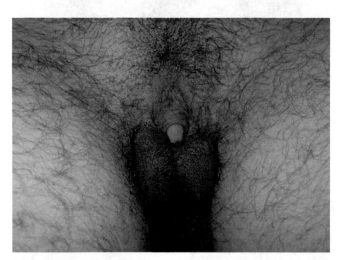

Fig 18.22 a

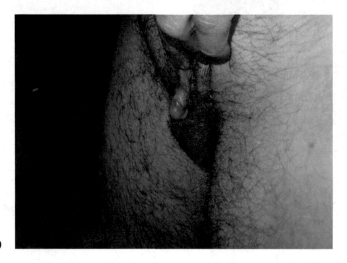

Fig 18.22 b

Figure 18.21   Metoidioplasty - urethral advancement & V-Y plasty for neo-scrotum

Figure 18.22a Front view of metoidioplasty

Figure 18.22b Side view of metoidioplasty

Metoidioplasty

A typical metoidioplasty performed in our unit consists of a urethral advancement and V-Y scrotoplasty without clitoral release in order to reduce urethral segmentation and hence worse complications (*see* Figure 18.21, plate section). Once healed, two small testicular prosthesis are inserted into the neo-scrotum for cosmesis. There is rarely enough clitoral length to allow the mini-phallus to clear the trouser zip in order to avoid standing up (*see* Figures 18.22a, 18.22b).

Associated surgery

Breast tissue

Nearly all patients will arrange to have a mastectomy unless they have rudimentary breast tissue. Usually this will be performed towards the end of their first year of testosterone treatment. If there is a large amount of breast tissue, then the procedure may need to be done in two stages. The best cosmetic results seem to be obtained by the concentric technique where the incision is limited to the circum-areolar line. A second circular incision is placed around this and the breast tissue excised between the two incisions. The outer circle is then sutured to the inner circle. However, excellent results are also obtained by an infra-mammary incision and nipple transplant. Often the areolar area needs to be reduced, and some patients also need a nipple reduction.

Hysterectomy and oophorectomy

This is not an essential part of surgery, but a large majority of patients choose to have it done. Advantages of having a hysterectomy are that there is no risk in the future of cervical, ovarian or uterine malignancy. There is also no need for the inconvenient reminder of female parts by having regular cervical smears. If the ovaries are removed, then androgen requirement often needs to be reduced. Many patients feel more male after the hysterectomy, since it is an irrevocable step.

We recommend a laparoscopically assisted vaginal hysterectomy if possible. If the patient has never had vaginal intercourse then it may not be possible to deliver the uterus via the vaginal canal. If open surgery is necessary, we recommend a midline skin incision so that future phalloplasty options are not compromised. Once the skin has been reflected then either a V-suprapubic or midline rectus sheath incision can be made as normal. The V-suprapubic rectus incision appears to give less pain and have a quicker recovery.

It may be more convenient to offer the patient their hysterectomy during their phalloplasty procedure. We routinely offer patients a hysterectomy during the course of a pubic phalloplasty, to reduce the number of operations needed. If they are having a free flap phalloplasty and if they are not particularly obese, we would consider doing the same. Otherwise a laparoscopically assisted vaginal hysterectomy, preferably before but possibly after the free flap phalloplasty, is the normal recommendation.

In those patients who will be wanting a mucosal vaginectomy as well (*see* below), it would be possible to do this at the same time with two surgeons, one at the abdomen and one at the perineum. If this is not possible, then as much vaginal mucosa as possible is removed before closing the vaginal vault. When closing the vaginal vault, the sutures must go thorough the mucosa to ensure haemostasis. This results in a short vaginal canal and an easier subsequent mucosal vaginectomy.

Vaginectomy

Total vaginectomy (where the muscle and mucosa and serosa of the vagina are completely removed) is a major operation with a high risk of blood loss, bladder dysfunction and bladder and bowel perforation. This kind of surgery was originally designed to remove malignancy, and the the risks were thus felt acceptable.

A much safer procedure for patients is a mucosal vaginectomy where these risks are significantly reduced. The vaginal mucosa is lifted off the muscle layer by a mixture of sharp and blunt dissection, taking care to remove every piece of mucosa. The vaginal opening is then closed making sure the pelvic wall muscles are sutured together for support. The vaginal cavity collapses down and is obliterated. The longer the vagina the more likely it is to have bladder dysfunction post-operatively. Most patients are fine within 3 weeks, but occasionally some patients require prolonged suprapubic or intermittent self-catheterisation until the bladder regains function. Patients are also warned of the potential need for a covering colostomy if there is a rectal perforation with gross faecal contamination. If a good bowel clear-out is performed pre-operatively, there would be minimal faecal contamination and any rectal defect can be closed primarily without a covering colostomy.

The advantage of a mucosal vaginectomy is that the patient gets a male-type perineal appearance. A disadvantage is that there may be reduced sexual sensation because of the loss of sensate vaginal mucosa at the introitus, as well as the potential complications mentioned earlier. Unless the patient is very keen to have this done, we do not advocate it as a routine procedure. If they are having a neo-urethra construction then part of the anterior wall of the vagina is used for the neo-urethra, resulting in a very small vaginal opening which is not obvious.

Clitoroplasty

The hypertrophied clitoris is important for sexual sensation in most but not all patients. Depending on patient preference there are a number of procedures that can be done. For those patients that do not want it visible on the outside, the clitoris can be buried under the skin or inside the neo-urethra. Burying the clitoris in the neo-urethra gives rise to problems. The urine flow becomes very turbulent and there is a relative restriction to the flow of urine. Some patients experience pain as the urine jet hits the clitoris. For these reasons we do not offer this any more. Instead the clitoris is de-epithelialised and then buried under the skin. The raw surface sticks to the underlying tissues and sexual sensation is retained.

An alternative is to circumscribe the glans of the clitoris and some hood skin, and mobilise the crura leaving the neurovascular bundle intact. The glans can then be moved further down the perineum so that it lies beneath the neo-scrotum and therefore is relatively hidden but functional. It is also possible if the crura are long enough to place the clitoris on the base of the phallus ventrally for sexual stimulation during intercourse. If sexual sensation is very important, or the patient is not too bothered about it being on the outside, then we leave the clitoris untouched exactly where it is.

Post-operative care

Patients are discharged as soon as their wounds are suitable for self-, district or practice nurse-care. This does depend on individual patient circumstances. We recommend keeping most skin suture lines dry for about a week. This is long enough for the skin surface to heal over. Sutures and staples are usually removed at 10 days. Most skin sutures are subcuticular and therefore no removal is needed. Sutures on the phallus tend to be left for about 3 weeks, that is to say long enough to ensure the subdermal layer is strong enough to stop the phallus splitting open.

Skin grafts need to be kept covered and immobile for 5 days. After that the graft is reviewed to see if it has taken. It is exposed for a few hours and then covered to prevent it drying out. The exposed time is increased daily. Split skin donor sites can normally be left exposed after 5–7 days once they are dry. It is important to arrange physiotherapy for the forearm or other donor site in free flap phalloplasty. It can take 6–12 weeks to regain reasonable function, so early physiotherapy input is essential.

Catheter management is the bane of patients' lives. After urethroplasty, urethral catheters usually stay in for 1 or 2 weeks, depending on individual surgeons' preferences. Catheters are necessary to act as stents to keep the neo-urethra patent. However, they become colonised with bacteria within 2 weeks, and can cause mechanical irritation to suture lines and hence fistulae. Accordingly they should only be in for the minimum length of time needed. Some surgeons insert additional suprapubic catheters to divert the urinary stream while the neo-urethra is healing. Because the neo-urethra often does not have urine flowing through it until the join-up urethroplasty, the distal urethra has a tendency to shrink from disuse. We advise our patients to dilate the distal urethra with a 16F or 18F catheter on a weekly basis until the join-up urethroplasty.

Dealing with complications

There are complications common to all procedures, and some specific to a particular procedure. The most common complications are with the neo-urethra, whether it is a full phalloplasty or a urethral advancement in a metoidioplasty. There are two complications of note, namely stricture (narrowing) and fistula (urine leak). Other less severe complications are recurrent urinary tract infections, hairballs and stone formation. These last three are more likely to occur if a stricture is present.

Strictures form because of relative ischaemia in the tissues, which therefore contract and narrow. If there is a relative weakness in the urethral wall upstream, then a blow-out or fistula might occur. If the stricture is short then simply excising it and doing a spatulated anastomotic urethroplasty is the preferred treatment. The neo-urethra is not as forgiving as a native urethra, so if there is any sign of tension, a two-stage urethroplasty is recommended. In the first stage, the stricture is opened and a buccal mucosa or other suitable graft is applied to the sides of the urethra. The graft has to be wide enough to tube over later. Buccal mucosa grafts shrink by about 30%, so to accommodate this the initial graft must be bigger than seemingly necessary. After 3–6 months, no further shrinkage will occur and it becomes safe to tube the urethra again.

If there is a fistula, any downstream narrowing needs to be repaired first. The fistulous tract is excised and the urethral wall closed. To ensure success, at least one or two other layers of tissue need to be interposed between the fistula repair and the skin sutures. There is no point trying immediately to repair a fistula since the tissues are very friable and the repair will break down. We recommend waiting for 3 months first. It is worthwhile waiting because about half the smaller fistulae will close of their own accord as long as there is no distal obstruction.

The use of hair-bearing skin for neo-urethral construction causes many problems. The hair harbours infection. It can form large hairballs and can also form urethral calculi. Hairiness requires repeated cystoscopy to remove the hair and debris. If there is relative distal obstruction, then the proximal neo-urethra becomes grossly distended. This gives rise to much worse post-micturition dribbling than normal. All neo-urethras will suffer from a degree of post-micturition dribbling because the neo-urethra does not have the bulbo-cavenosus muscle to squeeze the last few drops of urine out after voiding.

With a free flap phalloplasty, the worst problem is an arterial thrombosis. The phallus will be cold and white and there will be no arterial signal on vascular Doppler ultrasound. In the immediate post-operative period immediate exploration and thrombectomy is the only way to save the phallus. If this happens long after the surgery when the patient has gone home, then usually the phallus cannot be saved. If there is partial blood flow, treatment with thrombolytic agents like streptokinase or tissue plasminogen activator may save the phallus.[19]

A more common problem is venous thrombosis. Usually more than one vein is connected to anticipate this possibility. If one of the smaller veins becomes thrombosed, then a small area of the phallus will become cool and swollen with a purple or blue discoloration. This area can be excised later. If a larger vein is involved, most of the phallus is affected. Exploration and thrombectomy of the vein is one treatment. An alternative is to use medical leeches to reduce the venous congestion in the skin until the thrombus is dispersed naturally.

There are usually very few problems with a pubic phalloplasty. If there is a transverse hysterectomy scar, then the flap may not survive so an alternative phalloplasty needs to be chosen. If there is a problem, it is usually with the lateral hip skin flaps used to close the abdominal defect. They join at the base of the phallus, which is the furthest point from the base of the lateral flap and the blood supply. The skin here may become ischaemic and break down. As it heals it may pull the phallus up. If so, the tethered phallus needs to be released and dropped down later.

The skin grafts on the forearm or other donor site may not survive. If so, the dead tissue needs to be debrided. Once healthy granulation tissue appears, the area can be regrafted with split skin. If tendon is exposed, then it needs to be kept moist and covered as soon as possible or else the tendon may break down. Very rarely, the hand becomes ischaemic. Severe pain may be a sign of a compartment syndrome. This will need urgent surgical decompression to prevent muscle death and a contracture.

Testicular and penile prostheses can get infected. If they do they need to be removed and a new prosthesis replaced after a few weeks, when the tissues have healed. The typical signs are redness, inflammation, pain and sometimes fluctuance if a lot of pus is present. It can be difficult to distinguish between a superficial skin infection and a deep prosthesis infection, so antibiotics should be started in all cases. A deep prosthesis infection will not settle, but a skin infection should get better within 48 hours. Erosion of the penile prosthesis often happens in the presence of infection. Occasionally, it occurs because the implant is too big. Typical signs of impending erosion are whitening of the skin, sometimes accompanied by a blister. Treatment is urgent exploration to shorten the prosthesis before erosion occurs. Once erosion has occurred the patient should be treated as for an infected prosthesis.

Mechanical failure of the penile prosthesis presents as inability to cycle the pump. We usually replace all the components in one procedure, as often there is more than one problem.

Outcome

The most comprehensive review of outcome after gender reassignment surgery was by Pfafflin and Junge in 1992.[20] They reviewed three decades of surgery with about 3700 male and 1300 female patients from 86 published studies being considered. They reported a global percentage of satisfactory results from 71.4% for males and 89.5% for females in the early reviews, increasing to 87% for males and 97% for females in the last review, which contained only follow-up studies of the last decade. The criteria used were as follows:

- increase in subjective satisfaction
- mental stability
- socio-economic stability
- partnerships and sexual experience.

All the criteria were significantly improved, even after the first intervention, which was the 'real-life test' and hormone therapy. Results for female patients were better in spite of the more complex surgery and poorer cosmetic and functional outcome.

There are few studies relating to the cosmetic and functional outcomes of phalloplasty itself. The most common problems are urethral complications such as fistulae and strictures. The frequency of these ranges from 30% to 90% for multi-segment urethras.[6,21,22] Attention to surgical technique is the most important factor here. There are some reviews on the appearance of the glans sculpting, favouring the Norfolk technique using split skin graft.[23] Our own unpublished data, in contrast, seem to favour full-thickness grafts. The group from University of Gent in Belgium has published some data on voiding function after phalloplasty, which show no significant changes in uroflowmetry.[24] However, 79% of patients had post-micturition dribbling.

Both the Belgian and Dutch groups report on penile prosthesis use in phalloplasty. Hage in Amsterdam advocated the use of one-piece inflatables instead of semi-rigid prostheses to prevent erosion.[17] The Belgian group reported that of 25 patients having a three-piece inflatable prosthesis, 5 underwent revision for complications, and after 1.8 years of follow-up, 23 still had a functioning prosthesis. With the one-piece inflatable, which has been discontinued since, the results were similarly good.[18] Other groups report an explant rate with the three-piece inflatable of 2 out of 20, which is comparable.[23] There are no specific data on sexual use, satisfaction or cosmesis.

References

1 Maltz M. *Evolution of Plastic Surgery*. New York: Frobin Press; 1946, pp. 278–9.
2 Bogoraz NA. Plastic construction of penis capable of accomplishing coitus. *Zentralblatt für Chirurgie* 1936; **63**: 1271–6.
3 Gillies HD and Harrison RJ. Congenital absence of the penis with embryological considerations. *British Journal of Plastic Surgery* 1948; **1**: 8–28.
4 Chang TS and Hwang WY. Forearm flap in one-stage reconstruction of the penis. *Plastic and Reconstrive Surgery* 1984; **74**: 251–7.
5 Scott FB, Bradley WE and Timm GW. Management of erectile impotence. Use of implantable inflatable prosthesis. *Urology* 1973; **2**: 80–2.
6 Bettocchi C, Ralph DJ and Pryor JP. Pedicled pubic phalloplasty in females with gender dysphoria. *BJU International* 2005; **95**: 120–4.
7 Noe JM, Birdsell D and Laub DR. The surgical construction of male genitalia for the female-to-male transsexual. *Plastic and Reconstructive Surgery* 1974; **53**: 511–16.
8 Fang RH, Lin JT and Ma S. Phalloplasty for female transsexuals with sensate free forearm flap. *Microsurgery* 1994; **15**: 349–52.
9 Felici N and Felici A. A new phalloplasty technique: the free anterolateral thigh flap phalloplasty. *British Journal of Plastic Surgery* 2005; Aug 9 (Epub ahead of print)
10 Hester TR, Hill HL and Jurkiewicz MJ. One-stage reconstruction of the penis. *British Journal of Plastic Surgery* 1978; **31**: 279–85.
11 Kaplan I and Wesser D. A rapid method for constructing a functional sensitive penis. *British Journal of Plastic Surgery* 1971; **24**: 342–4.
12 Perovic SV and Djordjevic ML. Metoidioplasty: a variant of phalloplasty in female transsexuals. *BJU International* 2003; **92**: 981–5.
13 Hage JJ. Metoidoioplasty. An alternative phalloplasty technique in transsexuals. *Plastic and Reconstructive Surgery* 1996; **97**: 161–7.
14 Meyer W III, Bockting W, Cohen-Kettenis P *et al.* The standards of care for gender identity disorders – sixth version. *International Journal of Transgenderism* 2001; **5**(1). www.symposion.com/ijt/soc_2001/index.htm.
15 Hage JJ, Bout CA, Bloem JJ *et al.* Phalloplasty in female-to-male transsexuals: what do our patients ask for? *Annals of Plastic Surgery* 1993; **30**: 323–6.
16 Ponchietti R, Mondaini N, Bonafe M *et al.* Penile length and circumference: a study on 3,300 young Italian males. *European Urology* 2001; **39**: 183–6.
17 Hage JJ. Dynaflex prosthesis in total phalloplasty. *Plastic and Reconstructive Surgery* 1997; **99**: 479–85.
18 Hoebeke P, de Cuypere G, Ceulemans P *et al.* Obtaining rigidity in total phalloplasty: experience with 35 patients. *Journal of Urology* 2003; **169**: 221–3.
19 Noordanus RP and Hage JJ. Late salvage of a 'free flap' phalloplasty: a case report. *Microsurgery* 1993; **14**: 599–600.
20 Pfafflin F and Junge A (1992) *Sex Reassignment: thirty years of international follow-up studies after SRS – a comprehensive review, 1961–1991*. English translation (1998) available on the internet www.symposion.com/ijt/pfaefflin/1000.htm.

21 Rohrmann D and Jakse G. Urethroplasty in female-to-male transsexuals. *European Urology* 2003; **44**: 611–14.

22 Jordan GH, Rosenstein DI and Gilbert D (2002) Phallic construction 2002: current concepts and future directions *Growth, Genetics and Hormones* 2002; **18**: 3.

23 Fang RH, Kao YS, Ma S and Lin JT. Glans sculpting in phalloplasty–experiences in female-to-male transsexuals. *British Journal of Plastic Surgery* 1998; **51**: 376–9.

24 Hoebeke P, Selvaggi G, Ceulemans P *et al.* Impact of sex reassignment surgery on lower urinary tract function. *European Urology* 2005; **47**: 398–402.

Part 6

Post-operative psychological
follow-up

Relationships

James Barrett

Post-operative romantic and sexual relationships are complex matters but ones in which a number of seemingly discrete life situations can be distinguished, and from which useful generalisations can be drawn.

The first useful generalisation is that pre-operative relationships are rarely unaltered by gender reassignment surgery. They are usually either strengthened or destroyed, destruction seeming as common as enhancement despite all pro-testations by partners that such surgery is welcome and unreservedly supported. Surgical nurses have often had to support patients whose boyfriends have dumped them immediately after gender reassignment surgery. Often the situa-tion surprises neither nurses nor patient. One assumes that the partners con-cerned must have experienced well-contained gynaeandrophilia. They seem to have been content in a relationship with a woman with a penis, even if the sexual involvement of the woman's penis was always a possibility rather than an actuality. The loss of the possibility seems to end their interest.

The second useful generalisation is that although there is some change in sexual orientation with gender reassignment surgery this is not a very marked effect. More usually, sexual drive (particularly autogynaephilic drive) is reduced.[1]

Post-operative male-to-female patients find themselves making relationships in a number of possible contexts. One is that where the partner clearly knows of the change of role and subsequent gender reassignment surgery. Another is that where such knowledge is suspected but not definite. A third is that where the partner clearly suspects nothing and believes the patient to be a born female.

In the first, where the partner clearly knows the circumstances, a problem for the patient is that of knowing the motivation of the partner, especially if he is male. Patients may wish for a heterosexual man, but fear an androgynaephilic suitor.

A reasonable tactic in these circumstances is for the patient to go out for a meal with the man concerned, and talk about things. If after 20 minutes the man has exhausted the patient's gender reassignment surgery as a topic of conversation and moved on to unrelated but preferably mutual matters, the signs are good. On the other hand if after 40 minutes nothing else has been discussed, there is the strong suggestion that it is this aspect of the patient, and no other, that appeals to the man in question.

The other contexts seem to have in common the problem of how to tell the person concerned of the role change and subsequent gender reassignment surgery.

It seems unwise to impart this information in a bar or pub. The person told it will have been drinking, probably on an empty stomach, and thus might be unpredict-able. They will already have paid for their drink and hence will have no reserva-tions, if at all shocked, about putting down their unfinished drink and walking out.

Better, perhaps, to impart this news in a restaurant. Particularly after the first course has been eaten and before the main course has arrived. The surprised person will be less likely to be drunk and less likely abruptly to leave, since to do so would squarely place the bill for the first part of the meal on the remaining diner. The surprised person would have been looking forward to the main course, and may decide to eat it and then settle the bill and leave without any pudding or coffee. The time taken to eat the main course may be the time needed for them to reason that they really liked the woman before this news was imparted, and that it ought not to change things very much.

Those post-operative patients who are particularly attractive and convincingly feminine may paradoxically encounter a greater degree of relationship difficulties. Those involved with them, unaware of their change of role, behave as if a knowledge base appropriate to the apparent sex is present. The next case illustrates this.

Case report: missing mores

NB benefited particularly well from a change of gender role, gaining in confidence at work and becoming an attractive and very successful business executive. Gender reassignment surgery consolidated her role, and she thrived in individual and employment terms.

NB wanted a boyfriend, and found that despite physical attractiveness and personal charm there were problems. She quickly discovered that men were frightened of her when they realised she earned vastly more than they did. She learned to initially conceal this aspect of her life. Despite this tactic, though, she found it difficult to make a relationship with a man. Being born male, in her teenage years she had never blundered through the mechanics of finding a boyfriend as had her born female peers. She had never herself sought to gain a girlfriend, as to have done so would have felt disturbing, despite her then male social status. In her later female role she was unclear whether it was all right for her to ask men out, or to take their phone numbers and subsequently to call them. She worried whether she would seem disturbingly forward by so doing.

NB reported that her female friends were all unaware of her change of gender role. She was scared to ask their advice for fear of evoking situations where she would be compelled to lie to them or give herself away. What advice she had obliquely sought had proved unhelpful. She reported that her friends had either been attached so long they had forgotten how they made their relationship, or were single and seemingly no more able than she to get a boyfriend.

Many post-operative relationship problems derive neither from physical post-operative status itself, nor from the social or psychological complications that go with such status. Rather, they are ordinary relationship problems encountered unusually late in life, as the following illustrates.

Case report: 'stage of life' sexual and relationship difficulties

LW reported at a post-operative follow-up appointment that she had problems with achieving orgasm with her (male) sexual partners. LW climaxed perfectly well with masturbation but not with a partner. It seemed that her born female peers had given her the impression that an easy orgasm was quite usual in sexual intercourse.

   LW's situation seemed to be typical of a late teens to early 20s woman, but she was in her mid-30s. Standard advice to teach her partner to masturbate her (and perhaps vice versa) seemed applicable, along with the observation that she simply might not yet have fallen in love with someone, the falling in love bit tending as it does to render the loved person particularly attractive. It was felt LW might learn faster than a woman in her late teens, by virtue of greater psychological maturity. She was not easily able to talk to friends about such matters, even those who knew of her earlier gender reassignment surgery, partly because such a stage of life was all a long time ago for them. It did occur to LW that those friends who were said to be orgasmic with absolutely anyone might also enjoy eating anything. She concluded that a lack of dietary discrimination would not be seen as a badge of honour and neither ought a similar lack of discrimination in sexual responsivity.

After gender reassignment surgery any problems with personality will not usually resolve, save for the extent expected by time alone, as the following illustrates.

Case report: relationship problems unaltered by role change and gender reassignment surgery

GC was a secondary transsexual whose earlier relationships (including a marriage) had always been characterised by her great dependency. She underwent gender reassignment surgery in her middle 50s, and passed very well thereafter as a middle-aged woman.

   The gender reassignment surgery did not change her personality. She remained very clingy and dependent. There followed a series of attachments to social acquaintances, often beginning with the provision of such small services as baby-sitting and childminding. Each of these attachments ended when GC became too clingy and sought too much time in the company of her acquaintances. GC's reaction to the termination of these social relationships was usually deliberate self-harm, usually by means of an overdose.

   GC tried to make a closer relationship with the daughter from her earlier marriage. Although the relationship started reasonably well, her dependency was such that in the end her daughter broke all contact with her. GC was so persistent in seeking her attention that in the end her daughter took out an injunction to prevent further contact, which GC

---

immediately broke. She was convicted, given a suspended sentence and thereafter stopped trying to contact her daughter.

GC saw part of a television documentary, which featured the intimate relationship between two young women. She reported this as having deeply affected her. She reported that such a relationship was what she wanted more than anything, and that she had always wanted it but had never previously known that this was so.

GC began to attend lesbian venues, but found that her previous problems with relationships recurred. She coincidentally won a modest prize from the National Lottery and began to pay lesbian prostitutes. GC realised that this would last only as long as her lottery win funds. Insolvency was delayed (but deepened) when she obtained a number of credit cards and spent up to the limit on each. The sexual content of the experiences seemed slight and not to be a major motivator; indeed she usually paid only for the company of the women. She reported omitting to take her customary hypnotic in order to be able to stay awake and take pleasure in the sensation of being next to the young woman sleeping beside her. GC described herself as being 'in love' with some of the women concerned; her idea of what this involved seemed rather empty of content. She felt that because she was in love with a woman it would lead them to spend their every moment in each other's company, usually doing nothing other than staying indoors enjoying the sensation of being together.

When her funds ran out GC decided to divert herself with a long-term and incomplete hobby project. She accepted that were she to accrue more funds she would be likely to return to attempting to buy friends and company.

Successful, longer-term relationships in very convincing patients may be complicated not by the feelings of the parties concerned, but by a partner's decision to keep his or her wider family in ignorance of the patient's situation. As the relationship deepens and lasts ever longer, the demands from the partner's parents for marriage and children grow the more strident. Since the Gender Recognition Act (*see* p. 261), marriage has been perfectly possible, though some churches might refuse to solemnise the marriage and thus alert the potential in-laws to some sort of difficulty. Grandchildren prove a thornier problem. Statements of irreversible infertility, while perfectly correct, seem to invite probing medical questions and treatment suggestions from relations who would never make such impolitely detailed enquiries about any other aspect of the patient's medical history (*see* 'Fertility issues', p. 285).

A particularly difficult situation is that in which the patient has contracted a relationship with a man who has remained unaware of her earlier status for a very long time. At least one such has additionally not been detected as originally male by her GP. It is hard to see how someone in these circumstances can tell the truth so late in the relationship, and it may be difficult for her to obtain an appropriate birth certificate and marry her long-term boyfriend, as to do so might prompt questions of why this is being done at this time and not earlier. It remains untested whether her concealed earlier male status would be reasonable grounds for divorcing a woman. One suspects that in a younger patient, failure to dispel the natural implication of ordinary female fertility would make this more likely.

Reference

1 Lawrence AA. Sexuality before and after male-to-female sex reassignment surgery. *Archives of Sexual Behavior* 2005; **34**: 147–66.

20

Reversion to former gender role after gender reassignment surgery

James Barrett

If gender reassignment surgery is offered to carefully selected patients, reversion to the former gender role is rare. This is fortunate, because the effects of hormonal and surgical treatment are at best difficult (and more usually impossible) to reverse.

Reversions can best be thought of as sustained returns to a former gender role, and are to be distinguished from brief returns for 'special occasions'. They seem to fall into discrete classes, which comprise the following:

- religiously motivated
- motivated by the ending of a relationship
- related to an inadequate assessment prior to gender reassignment surgery or hormonal treatment.

These will be considered in turn.

Religiously motivated reversion

Reversions in this setting have seemingly been isolated to patients who were Jehovah's Witnesses prior to contact with a gender identity clinic. The Jehovah's Witnesses' belief system specifically opposes people changing gender role and especially undergoing hormonal or surgical treatments. Patients from such a background claim (probably honestly) to feel so strongly that they ought to change their gender role that they can overrule the strictures of a faith that in other regards has won their allegiance. Some Jehovah's Witness patients have managed to change their role and remain at ease in their contact with Jehovah. It does seem, though, that the Jehovah's Witness faith is particularly hard to relinquish. Jehovah's Witness patients have reverted to their former gender role, some without overtly religious motivation and others openly reintegrating with their faith community by so doing. The same does not seem to have occurred with other faiths.

Reversion motivated by a relationship or its breakdown

This is a common reason for a reversion to a former gender role when it happens earlier in the course of a real life experience (*see* 'Relationship issues and outcomes', p. 84).

A relationship, and its breakdown, can prompt a post-operative reversion, as the following illustrates.

Case report: relationship issues and reversion to former role

SL originally changed gender role at the instigation of his then partner, a man who did not want to regard their relationship as a gay one. The rather older and emotionally dominant partner funded SL's attendance at a psychiatric practice where SL was prescribed estrogens and progesterone in association with an anti-androgenic agent. It seemed that SL had attended these appointments in clearly female attire, but that in ordinary life he presented as a rather feminine man, in accordance with his partner's wishes. The psychiatrist seemed not to have been concerned with whether SL's life outside their meetings was also in a female role, and whether SL could reasonably have been thought of as succeeding in that role.

After about 9 months, SL underwent gender reassignment surgery, without a second opinion. Not very long afterwards, the relationship with his partner broke down. SL adopted a very clearly female role and appearance for a while, hoping to rekindle his former partner's interest by so doing. When this failed he reverted to a male role, with considerable psychological instability and episodes of deliberate self-harm.

Reversion related to inadequate assessment or diagnosis

A failure to establish a proper diagnosis of transsexualism but treatment with gender reassignment surgery nonetheless results (perhaps unsurprisingly) in reversion to the former role, as the following illustrates.

Case report: reversion motivated by inadequate assessment prior to surgery

PL had always been sexually aroused by women's clothes, and the wearing of women's clothes. It seemed that a series of women with whom he made relationships could not understand or support this sexual interest, and that after a time PL began to feel that he would be better off being a woman, rather than being with one.

PL underwent a 9-month real life experience and was subsequently referred for gender reassignment surgery, all this being done by one practitioner (who noted PL to present 'awkwardly' as a woman).

After gender reassignment surgery, PL tried to live in a female role, making two very short and half-hearted sexual relationships with men before settling into a lesbian role. Over the course of 2 years in this lesbian role, he 'got butcher and butcher' until it was clear to him that he had to return to a male role. In the resumed male role, he needed considerable hormonal manipulation to achieve a male eugonadal status. He worried about the lack of a penis. This was less of a concern to the female partner he had attracted. PL withdrew a request for phalloplasty after one consultation, but continued to benefit from endocrine help.

Part 7

Legal issues

21

The Gender Recognition Act 2004

Stephen Whittle

Transsexual people are now part of our social environment. Hormonal and surgical reassignments are regularly sought, and it is estimated that in the major centres in the UK, around 300 genital reconstructions are performed annually. Social attitudes have changed considerably since the early 1990s, when transsexual people first started to campaign for their rights to 'respect and equality'. Now many people have friends, neighbours and work colleagues who are transsexual people.

However, when faced with a transsexual person many people are challenged because of their lack of knowledge of the reality of transsexual people's lives and, in particular, what transsssexual people's bodies are like.

The Gender Recognition Act 2004 (GRA) came into force in April 2005. It affords full legal recognition to a transsexual person's acquired gender.

The GRA enables transsexual people to apply for 'gender recognition'. Those born in the UK can obtain a new birth certificate. In order to qualify, transsexual people have to show that:

- they have been diagnosed as having gender dysphoria, or
- they have had gender reassignment surgery, and
- they have lived in their acquired gender role for at least 2 years, and
- they intend to do so permanently for the remainder of their life.

Gender recognition will mean that transsexual people must be treated as of their new sex for all legal purposes, including family relationships, employment, welfare benefits, health and social care.

The award of a gender recognition certificate is not dependent upon particular surgical processes having happened. This recognises reality. Not every transsexual person will undergo all possible surgery. This might be for reasons of personal choice or for health reasons. Patients may have been living in their acquired gender role for 4 years or more before the first surgical intervention. The Act is designed to enable such people to have their rights acknowledged once their commitment is evident. As such, we have a world in which some legal women have a penis, and (more commonly because of the limitations of surgery to make a penis) some legal men have a vagina. Clearly established in their new gender role, and often indistinguishable from those born to that role, these people are arguably better termed 'transman' than 'female transsexual' and 'transwoman' rather than 'male transsexual'

There are estimated to be 15 000 transsexual people in Britain, of whom around 6000–8000 are now living permanently in their new gender role. Within

6 months of implementation of the Act, over 800 transsexual people were awarded Gender Recognition Certificates (GRCs) under the fast-track provisions of the GRA. This provision recognised that many people had much earlier changed their gender role and undergone gender reassignment surgery. It was seen as just for them to take precedence.

From October 2005, the first applications for a legal change of gender using the standard-track application process were processed.

How the Gender Recognition Act works

The Act enables transsexual people to apply for 'gender recognition'. There were, as outlined above, initial fast-track provisions designed to enable those who have been living in their acquired gender role for many years to obtain gender recognition promptly. The standard track, which came into force in October 2005, enables those who have more recently started the process of gender reassignment to be recognised, for all legal purposes, in their new gender.

In order to qualify, a transsexual person has to provide documentary evidence of the requirements of the Act, as given above.

The Act creates panels of lawyers and doctors who can award a GRC to successful applicants who are over 18 years of age and unmarried. A GRC affords them legal recognition in their acquired gender for all purposes. They will be able to obtain a new birth certificate if their birth was registered in the UK, and marry someone of the opposite gender.

It is the GRC that provides the full legal recognition, not the new birth certificate. If a person's birth was registered overseas they will still have full UK rights in their acquired gender.

Marriage, civil partnership and the family

The GRA enables marriage and civil partnership for transsexual people in their acquired gender once they have obtained a GRC.

In order to benefit from a GRC, a transsexual person must not be married or in a civil partnership at the time of the application (unless they are applying using the Overseas Process which provides recognition on the basis of the trans person having already had legal recognition and formed a legal relationship in another jurisdiction where that jurisdiction's requirements are at least as strict as the GRA's requirements.). If a transsexual person is in a pre-existing marriage or civil partnership they cannot be awarded a full GRC, but instead, if they meet all the other requirements, they will receive an Interim Certificate. The Interim Certificate does not afford legal rights in the acquired gender, but it will enable a quick and easy annulment of a marriage or civil partnership. This will then lead to a full GRC being awarded. If the couple then intend formally to continue their relationship, a mechanism has been created whereby an award of nullity is made by the court, which will then provide a formal transfer from Interim Certificate to full GRC. If the couple have prepared well, they could then proceed immediately to a registrar's office and have a marriage or civil partnership enacted (whichever is the opposite of their former arrangement) on the same day.

Full legal recognition does not affect anything that happened previously, including anything between the application being made and the GRC being issued. As a result, prior marriages and obligations, such as financial maintenance on an earlier divorce, will continue. Any obligations to children remain. A transsexual person remains the father or mother of a child despite their own change of gender role.

Some transmen in relationships with women have a paternal role, their partners having become pregnant through donor insemination. There are mechanisms by which transman parents can be afforded some legal rights to continue in a paternal role should the relationship later end or the partner die. For those whose partners have had children by fertility treatment from a licensed clinic, the easiest route will be to get married once a GRC has been issued, and then jointly to adopt the children.

Some have used informal networks to assist their partner in conceiving a child, and have retained contact with the child's biological father to the extent that he has a parental responsibility agreement. In this setting it will be necessary to obtain his agreement and take the 'step-parent' adoption route. This circumstance is rare.

More common are those couples where both care for children who have resulted from either partner's earlier relationship. The step-parent route is likely to be used in these situations. It is generally recognised that even where children have been living with an unmarried couple for many years, the courts are unwilling to allow joint adoption until the marriage has lasted 1 or 2 years. It has yet to be seen whether the courts will take into account the earlier unmarried status having been unavoidable.

Welfare benefits

Many areas of life may be affected by a person obtaining a GRC. It must be remembered that no one will be forced to apply for a GRC, but that the decision may have practical as well as emotional consequences. At one point these included a possible change in status from single parent status to cohabiting couple, with a resulting decrease in benefit entitlement. From December 2005, though, the award of a GRC to one half of a couple resulted in the relationship automatically changing status between a cohabiting couple and a civil partnership. This leads to no change in financial arrangements.

Pensions

Pension rules are many and varied. From 2005, state pension ages were regularised to remove any sex differences in benefits, phased in over a 15-year period.

Until full regularisation, the differential between male and female benefit ages means that where those born male would previously have been made to wait until aged 65 to receive their state pension after being awarded a GRC, they became able to receive it at 60. Because the GRA is not retrospective, if they were over 60 at the time of the GRC being awarded, their pension entitlements would only be from the date of the GRC. They would not receive any back payment.

Similarly there were some born females who when awarded a GRC had already been receiving their state pension because they had passed the age of 60. When awarded a GRC their pension entitlement ceased (though any already received benefit was not claimed back). They were required to wait until aged 65 to recieve further pension payment. For these people this was particularly harsh. Many had given up work on the assumption they would receive this pension. They had faced a choice between trying to find work again or foregoing until they were 65 their legal right to a GRC.

People whose birth dates cause them to fall in the phasing in period of regularisation are assessed on a sliding scale system so complex as to require advice from the pensions authorities.

Employment law prior to the Gender Recognition Act

Until the Act came into force, transsexual people were held to be of their birth gender for employment purposes. Popular prejudice made life very miserable for many transsexual people. Employment discrimination in particular was rife, principally around the time when a person changed gender role and commenced living in their new gender. Research in 2002 demonstrated that 10% of transsexual people faced such harassment in the workplace that it amounted to a criminal offence.[1] Some employers had been prejudiced, leading to several significant cases in the employment tribunals and senior courts. Other employers found it difficult to balance the rights of the transsexual person against what they saw as the needs of other employees or clients what might be termed the 'I don't mind, but of course they will' syndrome. This was despite clear employment legislation in this area since 1999.

In 1999 the Sex Discrimination (Gender Reassignment) Regulations 1999 (SDGRR) clarified UK employment law relating to transsexual people. The Regulations amended the Sex Discrimination Act 1975 and prohibited workplace discrimination against people who were 'intending to undergo, are undergoing or have undergone gender reassignment'.

Again, in 1999, the Court of Appeal determined that transsexualism was an illness within the terms of the NHS Acts, and that, as such, gender reassignment should be regarded as any other medical treatment when considering workplace absence and sickness payments.

With the added impact of the Gender Recognition Act and, in particular, the ability to obtain full legal recognition regardless of surgical status, there ought to be a considerable change of attitude from employers.

The impact of gender recognition for employment

In January 2005 the Women and Equality Unit of the Department of Trade and Indusrty (DTI) produced new guidelines for employers: *Gender Reassignment: a guide for employers.*[2] This addressed many of the legal questions. Personnel officers still have to deal with day-to-day practical issues, some of which may be challenging.

Transsexual people still retain the workplace protection of the SDGRR but, when a person has obtained a GRC, they must also be regarded as of their new gender for the workplace. This includes access to those facilities and services accessible to others of the same gender. For example, a person who was born female but who now permanently lives as a man is to be regarded as man for the purposes of sex discrimination. That is to say, just as it is illegal to discriminate against a man because he is black or homosexual, it is illegal to discriminate against a man because he happens to be transsexual. The situation is less legally clear-cut if the individual is between a change of role and the award of a GRC.

The 'toilet question'

The toilet question has proved a major challenge for employers. There have been numerous cases where employers have insisted that until transsexual people have had full gender reassignment surgery they use either the toilets of their birth sex or the disabled facilities. There were concerns raised that there could be men pretending to be transsexual women to gain access to the female facilities. This appears to be something to do with crimes perpetrated by men, not transsexual people. Access to services by transsexual people should not be limited because of other people's misunderstanding and stereotypes.

Most transsexual people who have not completed all gender reassignment surgery will avoid using facilities where people are usually fully unclothed or shower together, for fear of harassment and ridicule. However, once a person has obtained a GRC and legal recognition, it would be unlawful to insist they use separate facilities.

My own experience of advising on these questions has led me to believe that there are simple solutions. I would recommend that all toilet and changing facilities should be maintained to a high standard to ensure all employees feel comfortable and safe when using them. Regarding changing rooms, the assumption that all staff want to get undressed in front of each other is, in itself, discriminatory. There will be employees who for personal, religious or health reasons prefer privacy. Simple curtained or cubicle changing areas should be provided for all who want to take advantage of them.

Privacy protection

Section 22 of the Gender Recognition Act provides for very high levels of privacy protection, making it a criminal offence with a fine of up to £5000 for any individual who has obtained the information in an official capacity to disclose that a person has a GRC. This includes:

- employers or prospective employers, or
- a person employed by such an employer or prospective employer
- and generally covers all industries and services, excepting the police and courts when investigating or prosecuting a crime.

It is a strict liability offence, so there is no room for pleading 'reasonableness' as a defence. Permission to make further disclosure can be sought from the transsexual person, but there is no obligation under the Act for them to give that permission, or to even disclose that they have obtained a GRC.

Section 22 is likely to be the most problematic area of the Act for employers and service providers. Some people will already be known to be transsexual. Others will have been 'invisible' within the system for many years. Any of these could present with a GRC requesting that their legal situation, particularly relating to pension provision, be regularised.

There should be a prima facie assumption that a transsexual person has the protection of section 22 of the Act. Employers and service providers should assume that a transsexual person has obtained a GRC unless their paperwork discloses otherwise. All staff should be made aware that a person's transsexual history should not be passed on, not even to line managers, since that could incur a criminal conviction. It would be good practice for all employers and service providers dealing with known transsexual people to let them know what is happening to their confidential information, if only to reassure them that their privacy is being protected.

Healthcare providers' obligations regarding privacy for transsexual people

Most healthcare providers have extensive and detailed notes on a transsexual person's history. Healthcare providers are expected to protect client confidentiality where possible. From the start of a therapeutic relationship they are expected to be open and honest about the limits of confidentiality so that clients can make informed choices about the disclosure of personal material.

A healthcare provider does have a limited exemption to the section 22 privacy rules. It is worth reprinting in full section 5 of The Gender Recognition (Disclosure of Information) (England, Wales and Northern Ireland) Order 2005:

1   Disclosure for medical purposes
2   It is not an offence under section 22 of the Act to disclose protected information if:
    a   the disclosure is made to a health professional;
    b   the disclosure is made for medical purposes; and
    c   the person making the disclosure reasonably believes that the subject has given consent to the disclosure or cannot give such consent.
3   'Medical purposes' includes the purposes of preventative medicine, medical diagnosis and the provision of care and treatment.
4   'Health professional' means any of the following:
    a   a registered medical practitioner;
    b   a registered dentist within the meaning of section 53(1) of the Dentists Act 1984;[3]
    c   a registered pharmaceutical chemist within the meaning of section 24(1) of the Pharmacy Act 1954[4] or a registered person within the meaning of article 2(2) of the Pharmacy (Northern Ireland) Order 1976;[5]
    d   a registered nurse;
    e   a person who is registered under the Health Professions Order 2001[6] as a paramedic or operating department practitioner;
    f   a person working lawfully in a trainee capacity in any of the professions specified in this paragraph.

However, this disclosure is quite limited. It clearly does not include administrative and support staff. Healthcare providers need to ensure that they are confident that consent has been given by the transsexual person. It might be that healthcare providers are approached by a transsexual person with a GRC and are asked to have their records purged of their relevant history. There are good reasons why transsexual people get worried in this situation. One sees letters that begin 'this nice young woman is a male transsexual' on referal for an investigation on an ingrown toenail.

If a transsexual person refuses consent for further disclosure, then healthcare providers should investigate why they will not provide it, and also explain to the transsexual person why they feel that in the circumstances disclosure would be in their best interest.

It would also be appropriate, in my opinion, for a provider to say that in certain circumstances it would be an unreasonable risk to undertake treatment without disclosure, and that they would not refer the patient for that treatment without appropriate consent. My own view is that I would prefer healthcare providers to know, but only when relevant.

There has been bad practice in the past, and the GRA provides an opportunity for healthcare providers to reassess their views of transsexual patients and accept that after transition most of them wish to be recognised as of the gender they have felt themselves to be for a long time. Now their patients will be able to enforce that legally.

Conclusion

The GRA is 'state of the art' legislation. In particular, the lack of enforced sterilisation, the lack of specific surgical requirements and the privacy protection it affords exceed any legislative, judicial or administrative process provided in any other jurisdiction other than in South Africa, where the GRA was duplicated. To that extent, it is hoped that the GRA will resolve most of the problems of nearly all transsexual people living and working in the UK and South Africa.

References

1 Whittle S. *Employment Discrimination and Transsexual People, Report to the Gender Identity Research and Education Society, 2002*. www.gires.org.uk (accessed 16 November 2006).
2 Women and Equality Unit, DTI. *Gender Reassignment: a guide for employers*. London: Department of Trade and Industry; 2005. www.womenandequalityunit.gov.uk/publications/gender_reassignment_guide05.pdf (accessed 16 November 2006).
3 1984 c. 24.
4 1954 c. 61.
5 S.I. 1976/1213 (N.I. 22).
6 SI 2002/254.

22

Military service

Stephen Whittle

Many transsexual people have served or are serving, although not openly, within the armed services. Research undertaken by Captain George Brown MD of the United States Air Force, in the mid-1980s, whilst an active duty military psychiatrist at an air force base situated in the mid-western United States, showed that it is likely that

> the prevalence of transsexualism in the armed services may actually be much higher than in the civilian population.[1]

There are historical as well as contemporary examples of transsexual people who have served their country in the forces, both in and out of combat. One notable historical example was Sir James Barry, who served in the British army for more than 40 years and who became colonial medical inspector-general in South Africa. He was discovered on death to have been born a biological female.[2] More recent examples have included Jan (née James) Morris,[3] Roberta (née Robert) Cowell,[4] Christina (née George) Jorgensen,[5] Robert (née Joyce) Allen[6] and Renee (née Richard) Richards.[7] The question cannot be one of whether transsexual people serve in the armed services, but whether on discovery of their transsexualism they should be discharged or allowed to continue to serve but as members of their acquired gender.

Transsexualism and homosexuality

Lesbian women and gay men will still be discharged from some armed services if their sexuality becomes known to their commanding officers. Increasingly, though, the recognition by the courts of the privacy rights of homosexual people has caused some armed services to operate a 'don't ask, don't tell' policy.[8] Since decisions of the European Court of Human Rights in the late 1990s, technically homosexual people are entitled to have their rights to their sexuality fully respected within the armed services of Europe.[9] However, work by Bruce Bartley showed that even after the court decisions the responses of forces throughout Europe varied from full integration (Netherlands) to severe, although informal, sanctions that would result in dismissal (France).[10]

It could be argued that asserting one's gender role can never constitute unacceptable behaviour, as gender role is an integral part of a person's sense of self, does not involve harassment or coercion of others and does not have any relationship to sexual behaviour. Theoretically if a transsexual person transgresses acceptable sexual role mores, then one could expect them to be dealt with using the regulations that currently exist. That is to say, if there are sanctions against homosexual behaviour in the armed services, and a transsexual person participates in lesbian or gay sexual activities in their new gender role, then the mechanisms that are in place could be used. However, this is made difficult by the nature of the transsexual persons's body. The question of what being homosexual means can be formulated either through 'attraction to the same sex' or 'participating in sexual activity with the same sex'. More commonly, transsexual people prefer partners of the opposite gender, but the same sex. These relationships are identified both inside and out as heterosexual, but in terms of biological relationship are homosexual, particularly if prior to full genital reassignment surgery. Similarly, those transsexual people in gay or lesbian relationships will be having hetereosexual sexual activity.

Those analyses of sexual orientation in the armed services have singularly failed to address the relevant questions as regards transsexualism, which involves gender role transition and has little, if anything, to do with sexual activity.

Some states provide within their birth and death certification legislation a provision for the amendment of or reissuing of the birth certificate of a transsexual person so that it reflects their new gender status. This enables that individual to obtain full legal rights in their new status such as the right to marriage. Thus, apparently, a transsexual person would be able to serve in the armed services of these countries in their new gender role. Certainly there appears to be no bar to transsexual people serving in the other uniformed public service groups such as the police, fire service and paramedical services. Where there have been actions pleading unfair dismissal from any of these services in Europe and the USA, they have been found to constitute illegal sex discrimination.[11,12]

The question of service in the armed services has been different. In the Israeli Defence Force, transsexual people openly perform their national service in their acquired gender role, regardless of operative status. (The author has met several transsexual people serving in their new gender role on visits to Israel). Similarly, since the decision of the European Court of Justice in *P* v. *S and Cornwall County Council* (1994),[13] the UK military states that being transsexual is no bar to joining the forces. There are several examples of transsexual people who have transitioned on the job and retained their appointment,[14,15] but to date there is no knowledge of any openly transsexual person being recruited. However, these two countries are the exceptions rather than the rule,[16] though it has recently been reported that Thailand has ended bars to transsexual people serving.[17]

In the USA, the United States Military's policy regarding transsexual people is quite straightforward. The specific disqualifying regulation, common to all service branches, which bars appointment, induction and enlistment of transsexual people reads:

Section IX. GENITOURINARY SYSTEM
Genitalia

The causes for rejection for appointment, enlistment and induction are:

Major abnormalities and defects of the genitalia such as a change of sex, a history thereof, or complications (adhesions, disfiguring scars etc) residual to surgical correction of these conditions.[18]

There have been very few cases concerning transsexuals serving or applying to serve in the US forces. In the case of *Doe* v. *Alexander*,[19] Doe, a post-surgical reassignment male-to-female transsexual, brought a suit for damages following rejection of her application for admission as an officer into the Army Reserves in 1976. The court held that it was particularly ill-equipped to develop judicial standards for commenting on the validity of judgments concerning medical fitness for the military.

In *Leyland* v. *Orr* et al[20], a 15-year veteran of the US Airforce/Airforce Reserve made the promotion list to Lieutenant Colonel just prior to gender reassignment surgery. Following a review board hearing she was discharged from the service. She filed for relief in the Southern District Court of California, alleging the discharge was invalid for a variety of constitutional reasons. The trial court found the Airforce had acted in an arbitrary and capricious manner in their handling of the matter, but failed to rule on what should be done, preferring instead to refer back to the parties for resolution. Leyland appealed, and the Ninth Circuit Court of Appeals ruled that a discharge on the ground of physical unfitness after gender reassignment surgery did not violate regulations requiring individual assessment of a person's ability to perform for medical reasons, given expert testimony that sex reassignment *'invariably impairs ability to perform'* (my italics). It should be borne in mind that this case took place in 1987, and that medical opinion has since altered in relation to gender reassignment treatment. It is unlikely that medical testimony would now hold that such treatment invariably impairs ability to perform complex jobs, or hold leadership positions.

Interestingly, the regulations only cover genital surgery. Therefore the situation of the female-to-male transsexual man who does not undergo genital surgery is not covered. Most (female to male) transsexual men do not undergo genital surgery because of the limited and expensive nature of such surgery and its consistent failure to be effective. However in the case of *Von Hoffburg* v. *Alexander*, a service woman who married a transsexual man, who was legally recognised as male, was dishonourably discharged as it was held that the relationship disclosed her alleged homosexual tendencies.[21] This seems a very illogical state of affairs, since though her husband was a legal male he was held for the purposes of army regulations to be a biological female. Again, it must be considered that if this case was heard today a very different result would be achieved.

Just as many pre-reassignment transsexual people have served in combat zones, the Transgendered Veterans Association in the USA claim to have several post-operative transsexual members who were called up from the reserves to serve in the US forces in the Gulf Conflict. More recently, Royal Air Force pilot Caroline Paige (née Eric Cookson) changed gender role and underwent gender reassignment surgery while continuing to serve.

Particular issues in relation to military life

Certain questions are often raised whenever the participation of transsexual people in the armed services is being discussed. These are: morale and unit effectiveness; the services are in loco parentis; communal living; and security implications.

Morale and unit effectiveness

Accepting that a high state of discipline, morale and unit effectiveness is essential to create and maintain an operationally efficient and effective fighting force, the question then arises as to how transsexual people might affect this. As has been seen, transsexual people have always served and often reached high rank. These people were not open about their transsexualism and therefore it must be presumed that the unit continued to be effective. But there is the evidence of those who have continued to serve during assessment of the syndrome, where there has been no report of a breakdown of unit effectiveness. Furthermore, in the non-military uniformed services, transsexual people have been able to openly serve and to participate as full and valued members of the service.

Though individuals may not like the fact that someone is transsexual, it is on a similar basis that they do not like people of a different race, skin colour, or sex. In the RAND report,[22] which discussed the possibility of ending discrimination against homosexuals in the US military it was emphasised that in police and fire departments where homosexuals were allowed to serve:

> Anti-homosexual sentiment does not disappear. However heterosexuals generally behave towards homosexuals more moderately than would have been predicted based on their stated attitude.

Implementation is most successful where the message is unambiguous, consistently delivered and uniformly enforced. Leadership is critical in this regard. Training that emphasised expected behaviour, not attitudes, was judged most effective. Thus what is important is that others are disciplined not to act upon feelings that they may have to discriminate against other individuals, and that they are told that within a disciplined force they are expected to rise above their personal prejudices. A force where people are expected to put their lives at risk, often for things that may be of no personal concern, must encompass a high discipline level. That discipline level is such that individuals are expected to respond to orders, and to perform appropriately. This aspect of military life is what can be called upon to ensure that what is expected of all ranks is an allegiance to the principles of service life, and in fields of combat it is essential that prejudice against 'innocent' civilian populations is controlled amongst soldiers. Therefore it is essential for the leadership of the armed services to ensure that non-discriminatory behaviour is practised, and that unit discipline is controlled and maintained through education and expectation.

It is only logical that if the armed services now recognise and prohibit discrimination on the grounds of race or sex, which were seen as immense problems in the past, the next step must be prohibition of discrimination on the grounds of an individual's transsexualism – another feature of a person that is literally only 'skin deep', and which does not impair their ability to function and do their job.

The case of Sister Mary Elizabeth of the Order of Elizabeth of Hungary, (née Joanna Clarke) illustrates the questions surrounding the issues of discipline problems. Sister Mary Elizabeth served 17 years as a male in the US Navy and Naval reserve, becoming an Antisubmarine Warfare Electronics technician. At that time she did not disclose that she was going to seek reassignment treatment. After discharge in the early 1970s she changed her gender role and underwent gender reassignment surgery. In 1975 she took a job with the Army

Reserves as a supply technician, and was promoted to staff training assistant 30 days later. She had been completely open about her gender reassignment, disclosing it to the recruiter, Colonel A Walford of the 49th medical battalion prior to completing her enlistment papers. On all forms she always gave her prior name and medical history.

In June 1977 she was recommended for promotion to warrant officer with full disclosure of her status. One month later she was charged with immoral sexual activities and fraudulent enlistment. Her enlistment was voided, but not before a full evaluation at the US Naval hospital in Long Beach whereby her final report found her to be:

> disqualified only on the basis of the present wording of AR 40–501, qualified both physically and mentally to perform the duties of her rank and position. Recommend full retention. (Reported in a letter to the author, 5 June 1996).

The story was broken by the *Los Angeles Times* on 14 September 1977 under the title 'Transsexual Wars with Army'. An investigation was ordered and though all allegations of misconduct were cleared, the army retained its position that transsexual people were not sociologically or psychologically suited for military service. Her final discharge, after an appeal which was settled out of court by the army,[23] was honourable with credit for time served. Throughout the period of her army career, her fellow soldiers knew of her status and there were apparently no problems.

The services are in loco parentis

The services have a responsibility for the morale, welfare and best interests of those young people they recruit. However, transsexual people would answer that they are of no risk to children or young people. The main aim in undergoing gender reassignment is to 'blend in' and be the woman or man you really are according to your gender identity. Transsexual people are just like other adults – a full range through all the walks and interests of life.

Transsexual people now participate in all walks of life. They are involved in nursing, teaching and child care along with many professions. There are now estimated to be between 5000 and 12 000 post-surgical reassignment transsexuals in the UK, and many more living the real life experience in their new gender role. Thus many people, and the children of many people, now know a trans-sexual as either a family member, a work colleague, or a neighbour. This does not appear to cause problems to most people. Thus, if acting in loco parentis, services chiefs must remember that a parent allows a child gradual independence, and does not attempt to protect a child from the realities of the world into which they will grow. In an armed force this is even more important, the young people involved may end up in all sorts of cultural and social environments, and must be prepared for the full range of people they might meet and with whom they must negotiate. If this training is poorly done, then the lives of those young people may well be put at risk. Secondly, those same chiefs must remember that they are also in loco parentis to transsexual service people, and it is not appropriate to throw somebody out of their home and their job for merely having a now easily treated condition that will enable the individual in fact to function more efficiently than before, to be much happier in themselves, to form longstanding relationships, and to perform their job effectively and probably better than they were previously doing.

Communal living

The special conditions of service life that require individuals to live in close proximity to one another are used by some to argue that it would be inappropriate to retain homosexual or transsexual people in the armed services because young people might be unhappy to share close quarters with them. Evidence of services where homosexual people are allowed to openly serve clearly proves this not to be the case. This would seem to be true with transsexual people, who are no more of a sexual threat than any other adult. Furthermore, following the initial period of the real life experience, when some do have an androgynous appearance, after hormone therapy and surgery, most transsexual people look no different from other members of their gender group. There is no need for others to know of their transsexualism, apart from those who need to know for social (someone forming a longstanding relationship with the transsexual person), administrative or medical reasons. They will not be viewed as a sexual threat, and the issues of the priority of privacy between men and women need not become an issue.

Security implications

In the past, transsexual people were only vulnerable to pressure or improper influence because of the legal limbo which insisted that they are female for some purposes and male for others. Increasingly, as transsexual people are afforded legal recognition and social recognition (regardless of whether they are 'out' or not), they are able to be open to their family, friends and colleagues. The biggest reason for transsexual people keeping their past a secret must be the fact that merely for being a transsexual they could lose their jobs at any time. Thus, details had to be withheld from employers or potential employers. However, one of the main results of the recent removal of the stigma that existed has been providing legal protection to the transsexual person in the workplace, enabling them to inform employers of the basic facts, just as a partially deaf person might disclose that they were hard of hearing and needed to wear a hearing aid. Families will of course know of their status. It is impossible to hide it in the way a homosexual might hide their sexuality.

Thus the transsexual person can be discreet, but also able to have a high security rating as long as employment discrimination is removed.

Increasingly, civilian personnel are performing many of the duties previously undertaken by members of the armed services. To refuse to retain transsexual people within the forces is likely to mean that personnel could find themselves facing a 'double value' system, whereby some workers are protected and others are not. Transsexual people, both before and after treatment, are likely to wish to prove that they are 'as good as the rest'; furthermore, research has shown that treatment in 87–97% of cases is successful.[24] Their retention, rather than threatening morale and discipline, is likely to produce a hard-working and loyal group of people who contribute a great deal to the good morale of any unit. Furthermore, the very disciplinary structure that the military services employ would enable any problems that might ensue because of the prejudices of other personnel easily to be repudiated within the structures that already exist.

The reality throughout the world is that many pre-transition transsexual people serve in both the armed services and the uniformed public services. Recently there have been increasing moves to support transsexual people in the public service areas, both socially and through anti-discrimination legislation. In a few nations this has included transsexual people within the armed services. As the issues relating to sexual orientation of armed services members are increasingly aired, and reports like the RAND report reiterate that homosexual behaviour is not a threat to unit cohesion and performance, we are likely to see issues relating to transsexual people also being aired. Transsexual people join the armed or other uniformed services for exactly the same reasons as others. Though antipathetic feelings will still exist towards them, these will be moderated in time, and they will become valued members of any such units.

References

1 Brown GR. Transsexuals in the military: flight into hypermasculinity. *Archives of Sexual Behaviour* 1988; **17**: 527–37.
2 Ray I. *The Strange Story of Dr James Barry*. London: Longmans, Green and Co; 1958.
3 Morris J. *Conundrum*. Suffolk: Coronet Books; 1974.
4 Cowell R. *Roberta Cowell's Story*. London: William Heinemann Ltd; 1954.
5 Jorgensen C. *A Personal Autobiography*. Errikson; 1967.
6 Allen R. *But For The Grace*. London: WH Allen and Co; 1954.
7 Richards R. *The Renee Richards Story: second serve*. New York: Stein and Day; 1983.
8 Belkin A and Bateman G (eds). *Don't Ask, Don't Tell: debating the gay ban in the military*. Boulder: Lynne Reinner Publishers; 2003.
9 *Smith & Grady* v. *UK* [1999] IRLR 734 and Lustig-Prean and Beckett – Application Numbers 31417 and 32377/96.
10 Bartley B. *The Role of Sexual Orientation in US and Foreign Militaries: policy and theories*. 2001, paper presented at the Conflicts and Opportunities: The Role of the Armed services in Modern Democratic Societies: Polical Studies Association Conference, Manchester, 2001. http://www.psa.ac.uk/journals/pdf/5/2001/Bartley%20Bruce.pdf
11 *Smith* v. *Salem*. Ohio, 6th Cir., No. 03–3399, June 1, 2004
12 *A* v. *Chief Constable of West Yorkshire Police* [2004] UKHL 21.
13 *P* v. *S and Cornwall County Council* [1994] ECJ.
14 Sex Change Pilot to Keep Job. *BBC News* 14 August 2000. http://news.bbc.co.uk/1/hi/world/europe/827708.stm (accessed 16 November 2006).
15 Army Transsexual puts on Brave Face. *The Express Reporter* 6 August 1998, www.pfc.org.uk/news/1998/rushton1.htm (accessed 16 November 2006).
16 Dayan A. *Serving with Pride*. UCSB: Centre for the Studies of Minorities in the Military; 2001. www.gaymilitary.ucsb.edu/ResearchResources/PressClips/news5_4_01.htm (accessed 16 November 2006).
17 356gay.com News. *Thailand OK's Gays, Transsexual Soldiers*. 10 August 2005. www.365gay.com/newscon05/08/081005thaiArmy.htm (accessed 16 November 2006).

18 General Service Regulations. Air Force AR 40-501 Chapter 2, Section IX, paras 2–14, AFR 160-45, Army AR 40–501 Chapter 2, Section IX, paras 2–14, Navy BUMED manual Chapter 2, Section IX, paras 2–14.

19 *Doe* v. *Alexander*, 510 F. Supp. 900 [1981].

20 *Leyland* v, *Orr* et al, 44 FEP 1636 [1987]; 828 F2d 584 [1987].

21 *Von Hoffburg* v. *Alexander*, 615 F.2d 633 [1980].

22 RAND Monograph Report: *Sexual Orientation and US Military personnel Policy: options and assessment*. Santa Monica, CA: National Defense Research Institute (RAND) MR-323-OSD; 1993.

23 *Clarke* v. *United States*, No 443–80C, US Court of Claims [1980].

24 Green R and Fleming DT. Transsexual Surgery Follow-Up: status in the 1990s. *Annual Review of Sex Research* 1990; **1**: 163–74.

Religious matters

James Barrett

The Jewish view

Jewish law contains 613 commandments and prohibitions, of which only a few seem pertinent to gender identity disorder. The first is detailed in Deuteronomy 22:5 which says

> There will not be a man's implement on a woman, and a man will not put on a woman's dress, because it is an abomination before HASHEM your G-d all who do these.[1]

Secondly, it is forbidden for male Jews to castrate themselves.

It is, however, accepted that violation of some laws is acceptable if life is saved: 'better to violate one Shabat so that he will be able to observe many Shabbatot' even if the violation is lifelong (as in the consumption of life-preserving drugs containing proscribed things).

Rabbi Waldenberg is considered the pre-eminent religious legal authority in Israel and in most sites outside the US (where Rabbi Feinstein is favoured). He is thought to have particular authority in medical matters. He is the only (or only major) religious authority to have addressed the question of transsexuals.

Rabbi Waldenberg maintained that the external genital organs, as visible to the naked eye, were the determinants of sexual status in Jewish law, and working from this premise made wise judgment in a case of androgen-insensitivity syndrome.

Rabbi Waldenberg noted that estrogen therapy renders male testes non-functional, and casts doubt over whether removing such non-functional organs amounts to castration. He notes also that the testes are rendered non-functional by degrees as estogens are given, implying a lack of a single castrating act. This might render the non-functionality as having arisen from a cause other than a castration.

Rabbi Waldenberg noted that in gender reassignment surgery if it happens at all, (debatable, given the preceding paragraph), patients do not castrate themselves. The surgeon does it. The question instead becomes whether male Jewish transsexuals undergoing gender reassignment surgery have been guilty of the violation of causing another (the surgeon) to transgress. It is not clear whether this would be applicable if the surgeon were anything other than another Jew.

Regarding clothing, Rabbi Waldenberg noted that a lifetime of cross-dressing without gender reassignment surgery would represent a greater violation than a more limited period of cross-dressing as part of a real life experience followed by gender reassignment surgery, since the latter would render the person female and the dressing thus no longer a violation. This would be a circumstance in which a shorter violation is acceptable to prevent a longer-term violation.

Lastly, Rabbi Waldenberg noted that preventing transsexuals from having either gender reassignment surgery or cross-dressing would, while preventing the clear violation of prolonged cross-dressing and the violation of self-castration (if his earlier arguments were not accepted), have a high chance to leading to death from suicide. He invoked the preservation of life as an accepted reason to break the Sabbath rules.[8]

The mainstream Church of England view

The mainstream Church of England does not seem to have a doctrinal position on change of gender role. It should be noted, though, that ordained Church of England priests have changed gender role and remained in their occupation. This is not necessarily well accepted by the evangelical wing of the Church of England, and it seems fair to say that the Church of England contains within it a multiplicity of opinions and managed to contain these by having no rigid doctrinal position.[1]

The Jehovah's Witness view

This faith seems to have a doctrinally based objection to both a change of gender role and gender reassignment surgery, particularly when the change is from male to female.

The Jehovah's Witness faith maintains that transvestites and those who have undergone gender reassignment surgery cannot become Jehovah's Witnesses, even if they have legally changed their gender, unless they are willing to take the painful step of reverting to their original gender. They feel that while clinical reversal is not possible, lifestyle reversion is.

The sole exception to this are those people who were born true hermaphrodites, with both male and female organs. In these circumstances it is the resposibility of the individual to prove that this is the case.

The Catholic view

The Catholic Church is opposed to any attempt by someone whose physical characteristics are unambiguously of one sex to have those characteristics altered so as to resemble those of the other sex. While it recognises the suffering caused by gender dysphoria, it does not believe that surgery or the use of hormones is the answer to that suffering. It maintains that those who are (at least physically) healthy should not be mutilated by surgical procedures: patients should be encouraged, as far as possible, to fit their self-perception to the facts about their healthy bodies and their functioning, not vice versa.

Below is a quotation from two American Catholic bioethicists, Benedict Ashley and Kevin O'Rourke, from their book *Healthcare Ethics: a theological analysis*:

> How should such cases be dealt with pastorally? The fundamental aim of the therapist, as well as of the pastoral counselor, in these cases should be to restore the patient's sense of personal self-worth. He or she must be helped

to see, as should homosexuals and those suffering from other sexual problems, that today's culture is grievously mistaken in its exaggerated stress on sexual identity and activity as a primary determinant of human worth. They must be assisted to find interests – spiritual, intellectual, and social – that will enable them to escape their preoccupation with their sexual identity and discover their more fundamental value as human persons. As for persons who have already undergone surgery, we believe they should be counseled not to attempt marriage and should be supported in their efforts to live chastely with the assistance of the sacraments and the respect and fellowship of the Christian community.[3]

The Evangelical Alliance's view

The following is taken from *Transsexuality – a report by the Evangelical Alliance Policy Commission*:[4]

We recognise that all of us are sinners, and that the only real hope for sinful people, whether heterosexual, homosexual or transsexual, is for wholeness that is to be found only in Jesus Christ. Our earnest prayer is that his love, truth, and grace would characterise evangelical responses to debates about transsexuality and in dealings with transsexual people, both now and in the future.

We affirm God's love and concern for all humanity, but believe that God creates human beings as *either* male *or* female. Authentic change from a person's given sex is not possible and an ongoing transsexual lifestyle is incompatible with God's will as revealed in scripture and in creation. We would oppose recourse to gender reassignment surgery as a normal valid option for people suffering from gender dysphoria on a biblical basis. We note, in addition, that no long-term research exists to validate the effectiveness of such surgery in effecting gender change. Rather, we believe that acceptance of the gospel of Jesus Christ affords real opportunities for holistic change in the context of non-surgical solutions. We appeal to the medical and psychiatric professions to prioritise research for the purposes of holistic treatment into the root psychological, social, spiritual, and physical causes of 'transsexuality'. This we regard as preferential to the development of technical cosmetic surgical options that remain essentially irreversible and require lifetime recourse to hormone therapy. We appeal to society as a whole to use Christian community values of love and care as a basis of thought and action.

We deeply regret any hurt caused to transsexual men and women by any unwelcoming or rejecting attitudes on the part of the church. We call upon evangelical congregations genuinely to welcome and accept transsexual people, whilst acknowledging the need for parallel teaching, wisdom and discernment, especially where children are concerned. Within the context of a loving Christian environment, we hope and anticipate that transsexual people will come in due course to accede to the need to reorient their lifestyle in accordance with biblical principles and orthodox church teaching. We urge gentleness and patience in this process, and ongoing care even following gender reorientation.

We affirm that monogamous heterosexual marriage is the form of partnership uniquely intended by God for sexual relationships between men and women. We would oppose moves within some church circles to accept or endorse sexually active transsexual partnerships where the partners are of the same biological sex as legitimate forms of Christian relationship. Additionally, we would resist church services for the marriage or blessing of transsexual partnerships on scriptural grounds, whether the partners are of the same biological sex or not.

We commend and encourage those transsexual Christian people who have determined to restore their birth sex identity as a consequence of biblical conviction, and/or who have decided to resist gender reassignment surgery. We would seek prayerfully to support their reorientation through the grace of God. We further commend and encourage those transsexual Christian people who are willing, but not yet able, to readopt their birth sex identity, but who nevertheless have committed themselves to chastity and celibacy. We affirm celibacy to be an honourable and fulfilling vocation for those whom God has not called to marriage.

We prayerfully affirm and encourage those family members who are subjected to the impact of transsexuality. We would seek to support them pastorally in coming to terms with the consequences of a declared transsexual partner, parent or other relative.

We commend the work of those organisations, pastoral workers and churches that seek to help and support transsexual people who face the traumas of loneliness, psychiatric treatment, gender reorientation and gender reassignment surgery.

We are in principle opposed to civil discrimination against transsexual people, for example in respect of human rights and employment. However, it is recognised that in practice, particular circumstances may make the continuing position of a transsexual extremely difficult whether or not he or she was in the process of transition.

Notwithstanding the arguments in favour, we nevertheless believe the case for transsexual people to be allowed to amend their birth certificates (except in those rare 'intersex' cases involving genuine medical mistake) to be fundamentally flawed, open to abuse, and tending to undermine accepted realities by condoning illusion and denial. In particular, we believe it would lead to unacceptable legitimisation of currently illegitimate 'marriage' relationships, and remove protection against deception.

The Buddhist view

Paramabandhu Groves

Buddhism originated in northern India in the fifth century BCE. The founder, Siddharta Gautama, leaving his wealthy family became a wanderer. Through intense practice, especially meditation, he attained the state of Enlightenment and became a Buddha (literally, one who is awake). The rest of his life he spent teaching others how they could become Enlightened. Many of his followers, like him, left their home and became wanderers; however, there were also many lay followers. Although becoming a wanderer was seen as a spiritually advantageous lifestyle, the Buddha made it clear that lay followers too could become spiritually attained. From an early period, the Buddha and his renunciant followers spent the rainy seasons in one place, and later this developed for some into a more settled or monastic lifestyle. Thus, the early community of Buddhists (the Sangha) included three main lifestyles: lay, the settled monastic, and those who continued to follow an itinerant lifestyle like the Buddha. Whereas the emphasis of the itinerant renunciants was one of solitude and meditation, the monastics had a greater role in teaching and spreading Buddhism. They eventually committed the oral teachings to writing, and so most Buddhist scriptures will tend to be influenced by the preoccupations of the usually male, monastic Sangha.

There are numerous formulations of the Buddha's teachings. One of the earliest and most popular is the threefold way of ethics, meditation and wisdom. The first stage involves following basic ethical precepts such as non-violence and avoiding stealing, lying and sexual misconduct. The monastic Sangha developed a much more detailed code of conduct, the Vinaya. However, much of this is about avoiding disapproval of the lay community, upon whom they were dependent for support, rather than having a purely soteriological function. Meditation, the second stage, includes practices to concentrate the mind, and those to develop greater awareness. The latter leads to wisdom, the final stage, through deeply understanding suffering and impermanence, which gives rise to peace and compassion.

From its origins in northern India, Buddhism spread throughout much of Asia. In the last half century, it has also become increasingly popular in the west. There is no one version of Buddhism, but many different expressions. Thus in examining Buddhist attitudes to transgenderism, there can be no one view. Especially around deep-rooted aspects of experience such as gender and sexuality, what may appear as a Buddhist attitude may be more indicative of the culture within which it is expressed. For example, in Thailand the Buddhist teachings failed to supplant indigenous sex/gender conceptions, leading to a consistent misreading of Buddhist scriptures.

The nearest term to transsexual in the Buddhist scriptures is 'pandaka', although this ambiguous term seems to have a wide variety of meanings including any perceived lack of maleness, such as being impotent, cross-dressing or engaging in passive homosexual acts. The attitude towards a pandaka ranges from tolerance to condemnation. The Vinaya describes cases of ordained monks changing gender and taking on the physical characteristics of women, and ordained nuns changing gender and taking on the physical characteristics of men. The Buddha was happy for these members to stay as nuns or monks with those of their new gender, and follow their respective codes of conduct. Some pandakas were recognised as being highly spiritually attained, even becoming Enlightened. However, elsewhere, pandakas are condemned, and not allowed to be ordained, or if ordained are to be expelled. In some of these instances, the pandaka is described as being highly lustful and sexually provocative. The monastic Sangha espoused chastity for both practical and spiritual reasons. The pandaka was seen as a threat to the monk's chastity, and association with a pandaka could lead to sullying the order's reputation in the eyes of the lay supporters.

Thus in traditional Buddhist society, as expressed in the scriptures, there has been a mixed response to transgender. Where there has been condemnation, this appears to be largely associated with a monastic preoccupation with maintaining lay approval and support. In contemporary western Buddhist practice outside of a monastic setting, this should be much less important. The primary focus of Buddhist practice is becoming aware of and transforming states of mind. Some strands of Buddhism assert that consciousness is already pure; that wisdom and compassion is inherent and needs to be uncovered. The main requirement for gaining realisation is having a human consciousness, and therefore being trans-sexual of itself need not impede spiritual progress. There are scriptural references to individuals who have changed their gender gaining Enlightenment, and basic Buddhist principles are just as relevant to a transsexual as to anyone else. The discrimination described above is out of keeping with espoused qualities of tolerance and kindness, which would be the most appropriate response to trans-genderism from a Buddhist perspective.

The Islamic view

The only clear, public statement about transsexuals and gender reassignment surgery in an Islamic context dates from 1987. An Iranian male patient was introduced via an intermediary Islamic scholar, from whom she had sought advice, to Ayatollah Khomeni. The Ayatollah was then a leading Shia Islamic scholar living in Iraq. He judged that she needed a clear sexual identity to carry out her religious duties, and that accordingly later gender reassignment surgery would be acceptable.[5]

The Ayatollah went on to become the Iranian Première. Under Iranian juris-diction a change of social gender role and subsequent gender reassignment surgery are legal.

This being said, it seems that Iranian social acceptance has not much followed from legal acceptability, and ordinary life in Iran for people with a disorder of gender identity is said still to be very difficult.

The Hindu view

Chetna Kang

Hinduism is an umbrella term for a number of practices that stem from a large body of books called the 'Vedas'. The Vedas are over 5000 years old, originate in India and were composed by Vedavyasa who is said to be an incarnation of God who simply wrote down knowledge that had previously been passed down orally, through a succession of disciples. It is said that he did this after he foresaw that the people of the future would not be able to retain such vast quantities of knowledge after just hearing it.

'Veda' means knowledge. The Vedas contain both material and spiritual knowledge. Some of the material topics covered include astronomy, medicine, law, mathematics, music and astrology. The spiritual teachings of the Vedas say that every living entity is made up of a gross body, a subtle body (by which is meant mind, intelligence and an everyday sense of self) and the soul. Of these three, only the soul is permanent and is therefore the real self. The soul's origin and ultimate destination is the spiritual world. The soul or real self is eternally blissful and wise. It is held that the fundamental point people have to understand in order to progress spiritually is that they are not their body or mind and the material world is not their permanent home. As long as they have desires and attachments for things in the material world their actions will result in their having to take another material body once the current one dies. What type of body they get next is determined by their desires, actions and what they were thinking of at the time of their death. If, however, they have developed such an attachment to God that all their desires and actions reflect this, and at the time of death they think of God, then they will permanently shed their gross and subtle body and return to the spiritual realm.

Developing attachment for the spiritual and hence detachment from the material might be achieved through a number of practices but mantra meditation is the main process. As one progresses, one starts to uncover the real nature of the soul and qualities such as forgiveness, tolerance, kindness, honesty, mercifulness and unconditional love manifest themselves.

According to the Vedic view God comprises aspects.

The first is 'Brahmajyoti', which describes the impersonal energy or effulgence of God, and practitioners who meditate on this and are successful go on to attain liberation and merge with the energy of God.

The second is 'Paramatma' or 'Supersoul'. This is the aspect of God that resides in every living entity alongside the individual soul.

The third is 'Bhagavan' or God the person. This is the highest level of realisation, and here the goal of all meditation, prayer or practice is to know and love God who has many names, of which Krishna, Rama and Vishnu are three.

Philosophically, gender identity is considered as being as temporary as the material body, since one's gender identity can change from lifetime to lifetime. One's physical or psychological gender identity is very separate and different from one's spiritual or eternal identity. It is held that there are no material impediments to spiritual advancement other than those we concoct in our own minds. What is considered important about gender identity is that one knows the strengths and weakness of each gender and how this can help in one's progress along a spiritual path. The Vedas describe male, female and a third or 'Tritiya' gender. Third gender includes asexuals, hermaphrodites, homosexuals and transsexuals. The Vedas describe how the third gender generally live in their own communities and are particularly talented in the area of fine arts such as dancing, drama, music, dressing etc. Historically they would often be employed to teach these subjects.

In some ways, being of third gender was also seen as a blessing for those serious about making spiritual advancement, as celibacy is strived for by the pious, who may only have intercourse to procreate. Being of third gender meant that one could potentially find it easier to be celibate. There are many historical accounts in the Vedas of personalities who were of third gender. They were never mistreated on account of their gender identity.

In summary, the gates of the spiritual world are just as open for third gender as they are for anyone else. Discrimination against those of third gender is contradictory to Vedic/Hindu theology.

References

1 *The Bible.* Deuteronomy 22:5.
2 Horton D. *Changing Channels? A Christian response to the transvestite and transsexual.* Nottingham: Grove Books Ltd; 1994.

3 Ashley B and O'Rourke K. *Healthcare Ethics: a theological analysis* (3e). St Louis: The Catholic Health Asosication of the United States; 1989, p. 316.
4 *Transsexuality – a report by the Evangelical Alliance Policy Commission*. Reading: Cox and Wyman Ltd; 2000.
5 When the Ayatollah met the transsexual. *The Independent* 25 Nov 2004.
6 Bleich JD. *Contemporary Halakic Problems*. Yeshiva University Press; 1977.

24

Fertility issues

James Barrett

Nearly all hormonal and surgical treatment in a gender identity clinic will remove the potential for fertility. This must be made clear to patients, who may wish to consider gamete banking.[1] The Human Fertilisation and Embryology Authority has not given specific consideration to the position of transsexuals or those living in an acquired gender role with regard to assisted conception treatment. However, the authority states that there is nothing in principle that would prohibit either the storage of gametes from an individual prior to gender reassignment or the provision of treatment to the female partner of a transsexual or someone living in an acquired gender, either with the previously stored gametes (sperm or eggs) of that person, or using gametes donated by a third party (or donor gametes combined with the gametes of that person). Likewise, there is nothing in principle to prohibit a surrogacy arrangement where a pregnancy is carried by a third party using embryos created with eggs or sperm of a person who has acquired a new gender identity.

The authority is of the view that as in all cases of assisted conception treatment, there is a requirement that

> A woman shall not be provided with treatment services unless account has been taken of the welfare of any child who may be born as a result of the treatment (including the need of that child for a father) and of any other child who may be affected by the birth.[2]

Further guidance on taking into account the welfare of the child is given in part 3 of the Human Fertilisation and Embryology Authority *Code of Practice*.[3]

The authority notes that there are, however, a number of complicated issues relating to the legal status of transsexuals and transgendered people with respect to children born as a result of assisted conception treatment. It is noted, in connection with this, that section 12 of the Gender Recognition Act 2004 reads thus:

> The fact that a person's gender has become the acquired gender under this Act does not affect the status of the person as the father or mother of a child.

The Act does not include the draft provision at clause 8(2) of the Gender Recognition Bill, the aim of which was to confer legal paternity on a person who had acquired the male gender and whose wife or partner had successfully received assisted conception treatment using donated sperm at a time at which that person was also legally a woman.

The authority finally notes that the permutations are manifold and the potential complications great.

Parenthood is rendered a very complicated matter because patients who change their birth certificates after having had (or adopted) children by any means remain the childrens' parent in the sex they were before they changed their birth certificate. Any children arriving (by whatever means) after the change of birth certificate will be children where the parental relationship is as the other sex.

For example, a male patient with children who changes birth certificate will remain the father of the existing children. If she goes on to marry a man (as she would be perfectly entitled to do) and that man has children whom she adopts, she would be the mother of the adopted children.

References

1   De Sutter P. Gender reassignment and assisted reproduction: present and future reproductive options for transsexual people. *Human Reproduction* 2001; **16**: 612–14.
2   Human Fertilisation and Embryology Act 1990, s.13(5).
3   Human Fertilisation and Embryology Authority. *Code of Practice* (6e). Available on www.hfea.gov.uk (accessed 16 November 2006).

Recent case law

In May 2007 the General Medical Council's Fitness to Practice Panel heard a case against Dr Russell Reid. It was claimed that Dr Reid had not adhered to the Harry Benjamin International Gender Dysphoria Association's protocols outlining how patients with disorders of gender identity should best be managed. It was contended that Dr Reid seemed often not to adhere to these protocols, sometimes to the detriment of the patients concerned.

Dr Reid seemed, more often than not, to administer hormonal treatment after one consultation in circumstances where patients had neither lived in their desired gender role nor undergone three months of psychotherapy. It seemed that Dr Reid had at times given support for the provision of gender reassignment surgery despite patients not having lived in their desired gender role for what would be regarded as a sufficient length of time (as recommended in the Harry Benjamin International Gender Dysphoria Association standards), also that Dr Reid had made no attempt to verify patients' claims that they have been so living.

There were concerns that Dr Reid sometimes advanced patients for gender reassignment surgery with a second opinion coming from someone not recognised as having any great expertise in this area, as would be required by the Harry Benjamin International Gender Dysphoria Association.

The Panel found that in all the cases it was asked to consider, Dr Reid's management had been inappropriate, had breached guidelines and had not been in the best interests of the patient. It was felt that this amounted to serious professional misconduct.

Afterword

This book has explicitly not concerned itself with questions of aetiology, but rather with practicalities.

My own view of causation, for what it is worth, is that there are probably many reasons why people present with gender identity problems. I think that some people's problems have a largely psychological origin, and others' are largely endocrine, genetic or neuroanatomical in origin.

The current diagnostic system, excluding from a diagnosis of transsexualism known genetic or hormonal abnormalities, does not seem to me to serve anyone very well. It is like the middle 20th century diagnostic view of schizophrenia, which seemed to exclude known abnormalities of brain structure or function. As technology advances ever increasing numbers of patients have detectable abnormalities of chromosomes, hormones, brain structure or function. The number diagnosed with 'psychotic illness of organic origin' or 'gender identity disorder not otherwise specified' thus grows ever greater. The management of these patients is often the same as it would have been had these findings not been present.

General psychiatrists have accepted that a diagnosis of schizophrenia is compatible with abnormalities of brain structure or function. Some would now suggest that the abnormalities must always be present to cause the diagnosis to apply.

I would suggest that an abnormality of genetic or neuroanatomical constitution or of endocrine function is compatible with a diagnosis of transsexualism. I support a practical approach based on clinical findings.

This book has captured a snapshot of a system of clinical practice at a particular time. It should be apparent that a gender identity clinic is likely to see a very wide range of people and problems. This is somewhat at odds with public and, to some extent, psychiatric perception.

Popular interest in this area has grown over the years. In the interests of producing coherent stories, particularly in a televisual setting, it has been simplest to present gender identity problems as if they consisted of nothing but transsexualism. As a result people with gender identity problems are likely to frame their difficulties in the form of a self-diagnosis of transsexualism. Local psychiatric services often co-operate in such a definition, sometimes sincerely and sometimes because it serves as a convenient label when referring the patient to a gender identity clinic.

Gender identity disorders were once viewed as always being serious mental illnesses. Over the years the pendulum has swung the other way, and it is now sometimes asserted that gender identity disorders have no such association. It seems to me that the truth lies somewhere between these polarised views.

Some would say that there are no such things as disorders of gender identity, and that those currently attracting such a label would be better viewed as unusual but perfectly normal variants of the human condition, and not the province of psychiatry.

There is merit to this perspective. It can seem particularly attractive when the gender issues appear to be unconnected to any other disorder or illness. This may become a philosophical debate, rather than anything else. In practical terms, though, it is hard to see how a state-based or insurance-based healthcare system could be expected to fund the hormonal or surgical procedures often requested if there is felt to be nothing more than a normal variant of the human condition. Those who support this stance must accept its practical consequences.

The issue becomes more clouded when one closely examines the assertion that there is no association between gender identity disorders and mental illness. Definitions of gender identity disorders in both the *International Classification of Diseases* version 10 and the *Diagnostic and Statistical Manual* version 5 specifically exclude chromosomal, endocrine disorders and mental illness as a cause for the presentations. If these exclusions apply, it is inevitable that in those not so excluded mental illnesses are rarely found. It is sometimes forgotten that a variety of mental illnesses, disorders and organic conditions can cause people to present themselves as having a disorder of gender identity, which they are likely to describe as transsexualism. Those with these other disorders are likely to present to a gender identity clinic. They will require help that may need to be much more skilled than that which would be required by those with rather straightforward transsexualism.

There are often complaints about gender identity clinics. Such complaints frequently centre on progress being delayed by an overly intrusive and bureau-cratic process, which seems to the complainant to be unnecessary. Many com-plainants say that they would have been just as well off, and probably better off, if their surgical or hormonal requests had been acceded to immediately and unquestioningly.

In some cases this is, of course, absolutely true. In others, though, careful assessment and subsequent management avoids damaging and unnecessary pro-cedures that the patients might otherwise have to live with, and regret, for the rest of their lives. It does not seem to be reasonable to abandon such careful assessment in order to temporarily facilitate some at the lifelong expense of others. I would suggest that the approach outlined in this book steers a sensible middle way between the extremes of on the one hand, radical libertarianism and on the other, patient disempowerment and medical over-control.

Index

5α-reductase deficiency, hormone
    treatment 161–2

addictions 102
affective disorders 49–51
Aiman's syndrome, hormone treatment
    160
ambivalence, gender role change 128–31
androgen insensitivity syndrome
    conditions resulting in 158–61
    diagnosis 11, 52
anorexia nervosa, diagnosis 12
armed services *see* military service
arterial thrombosis, free flap
    phalloplasty 244
artistic endeavours, occupation issues
    75–6
Asperger's syndrome 108
    psychosis 48–9
assessment/diagnosis, inadequate 258
autogynaephilia 35–7, 55

bank manager, autogynaephilia 36–7
benefits, gender role change 71–2
bereavement issues, family reactions 82
bleeding complications, genital surgery
    215
body fat distribution, hormone treatment
    173
borderline personality disorder, impulsive
    66–7
breast cancer 205
    hormone treatment 175–6, 179
breast growth, hormone treatment 172–3
breast tissue, phalloplasty 241
breasts 201–7
    access 204
    augmentation history 201–2
    augmentation selection 203
    complications 204–5, 228
    differences 202
    female-to-male patients 227–8
    implant choices 203
    placement 203
    size 204
    technique, author's preferred 204
Buddhist view 280–2

CAH *see* congenital adrenal hyperplasia
cancer
    breast 175–6, 179, 205
    gynaecological malignancy 184–5
    prostate 176–7
categorisation 17–29
    differential diagnosis 17–29
catheter management, post operative care
    243
Catholic view 278–9
challenging patients/circumstances
    55–68, 101–36
Charing Cross Clinic regimens, hormone
    treatment 171, 181
children's reactions 78–9
chromosomal abnormalities 51–2
Church of England view 278
civil partnerships, legal issues 262–3
clitoroplasty 213–14
    phalloplasty 242–3
cognition, hormone treatment 174, 182
coincidental mental illness 56, 65–7
    non-psychotic 101–2
    psychotic 102–4
communication skills
    non-verbal communication 145
    speech and language therapy 144–50
complications
    breasts 204–5, 228
    genital surgery 214–17
    mastectomy 228
    phalloplasty 243–5
complications management, hormone
    treatment 178–80
computing, occupation issues 76
congenital adrenal hyperplasia (CAH),
    hormone treatment 162–4
contentious disabilities 112
conversion disorders 102, 110–11
    fluctuating 110–11

counselling, speech and language therapy
150–1
cricothyroid approximation, voice
feminisation surgery 195
cross-checking decisions 4
cross-dressing, diagnosis 12–13

deep vein thrombosis (DVT), hormone
treatment 175
delusion mitigation, psychotherapy 94
dementia 52–3
dual-role transvestism 52
depressive disorders 49–51
deviance, sexual see sexual deviance
diagnosis 11–29
androgen insensitivity syndrome
11, 52
anorexia nervosa 12
biography 13
categorisation 17–29
chromosomal abnormalities 51–2
cross-dressing 12–13
differential 17–29, 31–53
drug history 12
examination 15–16
family issues 11
fractures 11
history 11–15
hormonal abnormalities 51–2
inadequate 258
medical history 11–15
mental state examination 15
military service records 14
occupation issues 13–14
physical examination 15–16
psychiatric history 12
pubertal development, anomalous 11
serological investigations 16
shortcomings 289
social state examination 12
verifying medical history 14–15
diagnostic confusion, mania causing 50–1
differential diagnosis 17–29, 31–53
categorisation 17–29
dilation, post operative care 217–18, 224
disabled patients 108–13
learning disability 104–8
dual-role transvestism 32–4
dementia 52
DVT see deep vein thrombosis
dysmorphophobia 37–42
androgenic effects 40–1
emerging 41–2
gender identity disorder 42

GnRH analogue 40–1
male genitals 38–40
dysphoria, gender see gender dysphoria

eating disorders 101
educational problems, male primary
transsexuals 22
eflornithine 172
employment
see also military service
legal issues 264–5
estrogens, hormone treatment 167–72
European cultural presentation, gay 57
Evangelical Alliance's view 279–80
examination
diagnosis 15–16
mental state 15
physical 15–16
extended groin flap phalloplasty 238

facial effects, hormone treatment 182
facial hair, hormone treatment 172
family issues, diagnosis 11
family, legal issues 262–3
family reactions 79–83
bereavement issues 82
gender reassignment surgery 80–3
female pseudohermaphroditism, hormone
treatment 159
female transsexuals 18–21
relationships 18–21
sexual relations 20–1
femininity, insidiously advancing 27–8
fertility 285–6
GRA 285
hormone treatment 174, 177
fetishistic transvestism 31–2
heterosexual male secondary
transsexuals 23–5
forensic settings
gender reassignment surgery 55–6
GID as a means to offend 116
life licence prisoners 114–15
patients as offenders 116
patients in 55–6
policing occupations issues 78, 117–19
Prison Medical Service 56
prison placement problems 116–17
rape 55–6
real-life experience 113–17
victims of crime 115
fractures, diagnosis/history 11
free flap phalloplasty 233–4
arterial thrombosis 244

galactorrhoea, hormone treatment 179
gender dysphoria
    hormone treatment 157–90
    psychosis 47–8
gender identity disorder
    defining 157
    dysmorphophobia 42
    as a means to offend 116
    personality disorder 65–7
    prevalence 157
    psychosis 43–7
    schizoid personality 66
    'third sex' 42–3
    views 1, 289–90
gender identity models, hormone
        treatment 158, 159
gender reassignment surgery
    declined 66–7, 134–5
    deferred 61–2, 135
    family reactions 80–3
    forensic settings 55–6
    hesitation at brink of 131–3
    orchidectomy 210
    orchidectomy, female role 90–1
    outcomes 245–6
    post operative management 170
    pre-operative relationship 88
    precipitating relationship 88–9
    real-life experience, gender role change
        71–3
    relationship pressure 25–6
    no role change 62–4
    waiting times 71–3
Gender Recognition Act (2004) (GRA)
        261–7
    fertility 285
gender role change
    ambivalence 128–31
    psychological benefit 71–2
    real-life experience 71–3
    reversion to former gender role 124–8
    schizoid personality 89
genital effects, hormone treatment 174,
        182
genital surgery 209–19
    see also gender reassignment surgery
    bleeding complications 215
    clitoroplasty 213–14
    complications 214–17
    current practice 209–14
    dilation 217–18
    haematomas 215
    hair growth complications 217
    healing complications 216

history 209
labioplasty 211–12
military service 270–1
orchidectomy 90–1, 210
penis amputation 210–11
phalloplasty 229–47
post operative care 217–18
rectal complications 214–15
sexual function 218–19
urethroplasty 238
vaginoplasty 212–13, 221–4
vulvoplasty 221–4
glans sculpting, phalloplasty 240
GnRH analogue, dysmorphophobia 40–1
gold standards, lack of 3
GRA *see* Gender Recognition Act (2004)
grief reaction, abnormal 67
gynaeandrophile man, relationship issues
        87
gynaecological malignancy, hormone
        treatment 184–5

haematomas, genital surgery 215
hair, complications, phalloplasty 244
hair, facial, hormone treatment 172
hair growth complications, genital surgery
        217
hair loss, capital, hormone treatment
        180–1
hairstyling, sexual deviance 61
healing complications, genital surgery
        216
healthcare providers' obligations, privacy
        protection, legal issues 265–7
hearing problem 109
heterosexual male secondary transsexuals
        22–6
    fetishistic transvestism 23–5
Hindu view 282–3
history
    breast augmentation 201–2
    diagnosis 11–15
    fractures 11
    genital surgery 209
    phalloplasty 229–30
    psychiatric 12
    psychosis 43
    verifying medical history 14–15
HIV/AIDS 113
homosexual dual-role transvestism
        33–4
homosexual male secondary
        transsexuals 26–8
homosexuality, military service 269–70

homosexuals 56–9
European cultural presentation 56–7
gays 56–7
lesbians 57–8
London Friend 57
religiously motivated presentation 58
hormonal abnormalities 51–2
hormone treatment
5α-reductase deficiency 161–2
Aiman's syndrome 160
androgen insensitivity syndrome
158–61
body fat distribution 173
breast cancer 175–6, 179
breast growth 172–3
CAH 162–4
Charing Cross Clinic regimens 171, 181
cognition 174, 182
complications management 178–80
contraindications 124
DVT 175
effects, hormone replacement 172–7
estrogens 167–72
facial effects 182
facial hair 172
female pseudohermaphroditism 159
female-to-male patients 181–4
fertility 174, 177
galactorrhoea 179
gender dysphoria 157–90
gender identity models 158, 159
genital effects 174, 182
gynaecological malignancy 184–5
hair, facial 172
hair loss 180–1
hormonal adjuncts 174
hyperprolactinaemia 176, 179
initiation 166–7
insulin resistance 184
lipid profile 184
liver function 176, 179–80, 183–4
male pseudohermaphroditism 159
menses 181–2
metabolic derangement 184
monitoring 177–8
negative effects 175–7
no role change 119–22
obstructive sleep apnoea 185
osteoporosis 185
polycythaemia 183
post operative management 170
practical management 157–90
pre-operative treatment regimen 171
prostate cancer 176–7

pseudohermaphroditism 159
regimens 167–70, 171, 181
Reifenstein's syndrome 160
role change without 123–4
safety monitoring 177–8
side-effects 177, 183–4
sleep apnoea 185
somatic changes 182
thromboembolic disease 175, 179
treatment protocols 167–71
voice changes 182–3
hyperprolactinaemia, hormone treatment
176, 179
hysterectomy, phalloplasty 241–2

ICD-10 see International Classification of
Diseases
impulsive borderline personality disorder
66–7
incapacity benefit 112
occupation issues 76–8
insidiously advancing femininity 27–8
insulin resistance, hormone treatment
184
International Classification of Diseases
(ICD-10), categorisation 17–18
intimate relationship issues see relationship
issues
intonation, speech and language therapy
147–8
Islamic view 282

Jehovah's Witness view 278
Jewish view 277–8

labioplasty 211–12
larynx
anatomy 191–2
development 192–3
feminisation 191–7
lavatory question
legal issues 265
occupation issues 77–8
learning disability 104–8
defining 105
implications 107
specialists 106
legal issues 261–7
civil partnerships 262–3
employment 264–5
family 262–3
Gender Recognition Act (2004) 261–7
healthcare providers' obligations
265–7

marriage 262–3
military service 269–76
pensions 263–4
privacy protection 265–7
toilet question 77–8, 265
welfare benefits 263
lesbians
bilateral mastectomy 64–5
religiously motivated presentation 58
life licence prisoners 114–15
life-threatening illness, psychotherapy 93
lipid profile, hormone treatment 184
liver function, hormone treatment 176, 179–80, 183–4
local flap phalloplasty 232–3
London Friend, homosexuals 57

male primary transsexuals 21–2
educational problems 22
male pseudohermaphroditism, hormone treatment 159
mania 50–1
marriage, legal issues 262–3
mastectomy
complications 228
female-to-male patients 227–8
lesbians 64–5
without role change 64–5
medical history, diagnosis 11–15
menses, hormone treatment 181–2
mental illness
coincidental 56, 65–7, 101–4
views 289–90
mental state examination, diagnosis 15
metabolic derangement, hormone treatment 184
metoidioplasty, phalloplasty 234–5, 241
military service 117–19, 269–76
communal living 274
ex-services patient 118
genital surgery 270–1
homosexuality 269–70
in loco parentis 273–4
morale 272–3
policy, transsexualism and homosexuality 269–71
prevalence, transsexualism 269
records, diagnosis 14
security implications 274–5
transvestism 31
unit effectiveness 272–3
models, gender identity 158, 159

monitoring, hormone treatment 177–8
motivational enquiry, psychotherapy 98–9

neo-scrotum, phalloplasty 239–40
neo-urethra, phalloplasty 243–4
non-verbal communication, speech and language therapy 145, 149

obsessive-compulsive disorder 101–2
obstructive sleep apnoea, hormone treatment 185
occupation issues 75–8
see also legal issues; military service
artistic endeavours 75–6
computing 76
diagnosis 13–14
incapacity benefit 76–8
lavatory question 77–8, 265
paramedical 78
pensions 78
personal care 78
policing 78
real-life experience 71–3
references 78
oophorectomy, phalloplasty 241–2
opinions, second 3–5
orchidectomy 210
female role 90–1
osteoporosis, hormone treatment 185
outcomes
gender reassignment surgery 245–6
phalloplasty 245–6
relationship issues 84–9

paramedical occupations issues 78
parents' reactions 83–4
patients as offenders, forensic settings 116
PCOS *see* polycystic ovary syndrome
pedicled flap phalloplasty 233
penile prosthesis
complications 245
phalloplasty 240, 245–6
pensions
legal issues 263–4
occupation issues 78
personal care occupations issues 78
personality disorder
borderline 66–7
gender identity disorder 65–7
prevalence 65
perversion, psychotherapy 96

phalloplasty 229–47
  assessment in clinic 235–7
  associated surgery 241–3
  breast tissue 241
  clitoroplasty 242–3
  complications 243–5
  extended groin flap 238
  free flap 233–4, 244
  glans sculpting 240
  history 229–30
  hysterectomy 241–2
  ideal 231
  local flap 232–3
  metoidioplasty 234–5, 241
  neo-scrotum 239–40
  neo-urethra 243–4
  oophorectomy 241–2
  outcomes 245–6
  pedicled flap 233
  penile prosthesis 240, 245–6
  post operative care 243
  preparation, surgery 237–8
  pubic 238, 244
  radial forearm flap 239
  referral criteria 235
  size 236–7
  skin grafts 243
  strictures 243–4
  surgery 238–41
  surgical stages 230–1
  thromboses, arterial/venous 244
  types 231–5
  urethroplasty 238, 239
  vaginectomy 242
  venous thrombosis 244
physically disabled patients 108–13
pitch
  speech and language therapy 146–7
  surgical voice modification 151–2
policing occupations issues 78, 118–19
polycystic ovary syndrome (PCOS) 124
  categories 165
  hormone treatment 164–6
  prevalence 164, 166
polycythaemia, hormone treatment 183
post operative care
  catheter management 243
  dilation 217–18, 224
  genital surgery 217–18
  patient advice 224
  phalloplasty 243
  skin grafts 243
post operative management, hormone
    treatment 170

pre-operative relationship, gender
    reassignment surgery 88
prevalence
  gender identity disorder 157
  PCOS 164, 166
  personality disorder 65
  schizophrenia 65
  transsexualism 261–2
  transsexualism, military service 269
primary/secondary transsexualism 18
primary transsexuals, male 21–2
prison settings
  see also forensic settings
  life licence prisoners 114–15
  placement problems 116–17
  Prison Medical Service 56
privacy protection
  healthcare providers' obligations
    265–7
  legal issues 265–7
prostate cancer, hormone treatment
    176–7
prostitute patients 59, 72
pseudohermaphroditism, hormone
    treatment 159
psychiatric history, diagnosis 12
psychological benefit, gender role
    change 71–2
psychosis 43–9
  Asperger's syndrome 48–9
  coincidental 102–4
  gender dysphoria 47–8
  gender identity disorder 43–7
  history 43
  late diagnosis 48–9
  schizophrenia, emergent 48–9
psychotherapy 91–100
  certainty, abnormal 94
  delusion mitigation 94
  identification, lost figure 95
  identification, lost relationship 95
  life-threatening illness 93
  motivational enquiry 98–9
  perversion 96
  psychodynamic models, transsexual
    symptom 93–6
  psychotherapeutic approaches 97–9
  psychotherapists' role 92–3
  radical 97–8
  sex worker 96
  supportive 97
pubertal development, anomalous,
    diagnosis 11
pubic phalloplasty 238, 244

radial forearm flap phalloplasty   239
radical psychotherapy   97–8
rape, gender reassignment surgery
    55–6
real-life experience
    forensic settings   113–17
    gender role change   71–3
    occupation issues   71–3
    psychotic illness   103–4
    reversion to former gender role   124–8
    speech and language therapy   141
rectal complications, genital surgery
    214–15
references, occupation issues   78
referral criteria, phalloplasty   235
referrals   9–10
    speech and language therapy   140–1
Reifenstein's syndrome, hormone
    treatment   160
relationship issues   84–9, 251–5
    female transsexuals   18–21
    gynaeandrophile man   87
    missing mores   252
    outcomes   84–9
    pre-operative relationship   88
    sexual relations, female transsexuals
        20–1
    'stage of life' difficulties   253
    unaltered   253–4
relationship motivated reversion to former
    gender role   257–8
religious matters   277–84
    Buddhist view   280–2
    Catholic view   278–9
    Church of England view   278
    Evangelical Alliance's view   279–80
    Hindu view   282–3
    Islamic view   282
    Jehovah's Witness view   278
    Jewish view   277–8
religiously motivated presentation, lesbians
    58
religiously motivated reversion to former
    gender role   257
resonance, speech and language therapy
    148
reversion to former gender role   257–8
    assessment/diagnosis, inadequate   258
    to female role   127–8
    to male role   125–7
    real-life experience   124–8
    relationship context   125
    relationship motivated   257–8
    religiously motivated   257

role change, gender see gender role
    change
rubber fetish   60

sadomasochism   60–1
safety monitoring, hormone treatment
    177–8
schizoid personality
    gender identity disorder   66
    gender role change   89
    unaltered   89
schizophrenia
    emergent   48–9
    prevalence   65
scrotum, neo-   239–40
second opinions   3–5
serological investigations, diagnosis   16
sex worker, psychotherapy   96
sexual deviance   60–2
    autogynaephilia   35–7, 55
    hairstyling   61
    rubber fetish   60
    sadomasochism   60–1
    shifting pattern   61–2
sexual function, post operative care
    218–19
sexual relations, female transsexuals
    20–1
shifting pattern, sexual deviance   61–2
side-effects, hormone treatment   177,
    183–4
skin grafts, post operative care   243
sleep apnoea, hormone treatment   185
SLTs see speech and language therapists
social skills, speech and language therapy
    144–50
social state examination, diagnosis   12
socio-linguistic issues, speech and language
    therapy   149–50
somatic changes, hormone treatment
    182
Spanish man   57
speech and language therapists
    (SLTs)   139–56
    increasing requirement   139–40
    role   139–56
speech and language therapy   139–56
    communication skills   144–50
    counselling   150–1
    discharge criteria   153
    He Says, She Says   145
    initial assessment   141–3
    intonation   147–8
    length of intervention   152–3

speech and language therapy (*continued*)
  non-verbal communication   145, 149
  physical presentation   144
  pitch   146–7, 151–2
  real-life experience   141
  referrals   140–1
  resonance   148
  social skills   144–50
  socio-linguistic issues   149–50
  surgical voice modification   151–2,
    194–7
  treatment   143–51
  treatment aim   140
  voice education   144
speech impediments   110
steroid hormones, CAH   162–4
stockbroker, dementia   52
strictures, phalloplasty   243–4
supportive psychotherapy   97
surgery *see* gender reassignment surgery;
    genital surgery
surgical voice modification
  feminisation   194–7
  speech and language therapy   151–2

'third sex'   42–3
thromboembolic disease, hormone
    treatment   175, 179
thromboses, arterial/venous, phalloplasty
    244
thyroid chondroplasty, voice feminisation
    surgery   196–7
toilet question
  legal issues   265
  occupation issues   77–8
transsexualism/transvestism, differential
    diagnosis   17–18

transvestism   31–4
  dual-role   32–4
  fetishistic   23–5, 31–2
  military settings   31
transvestism/transsexualism, differential
    diagnosis   17–18

urethroplasty   238, 239

vaginectomy, phalloplasty   242
vaginoplasty   212–13
  patient advice   221–4
venous thrombosis, phalloplasty   244
verifying medical history, diagnosis   14–15
victimisation, gross   115
victims of crime   115
views
  gender identity disorder   1, 289–90
  mental illness   289–90
  religious   277–84
visual handicap   109–10
vocal cord attachment, voice feminisation
    surgery   194–5
vocal cord-shortening procedures, voice
    feminisation surgery   196
voice changes, hormone treatment   182–3
voice feminisation   191–7
  surgery   151–2, 194–7
voice production   193–4
voice therapy *see* speech and language
    therapy
vulvoplasty, patient advice   221–4

waiting times, gender reassignment surgery
    71–3
war settings *see* military service
welfare benefits, legal issues   263
work issues *see* occupation issues

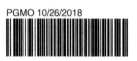